MW01517821

Jack Wilde is an artist, a scientist, a veterinarian, a traveller and a family man. After a humble upbringing in the North of England he chose an academic career and became a Veterinary Surgeon serving in the Colonial Service in Africa. A challenging wartime voyage to an unknown destination led to professional work which was concerned with managing tropical diseases of cattle in Africa and he had many significant scientific achievements, researching in the bush, building vaccine production units and researching on complex intracellular organisms. This all took place in the colourful African landscape that inspired his artistic talents. For many decades his painting, especially those of tropical Africa, became well known and many now hang in houses around the world.

He and his wife, Kathy, of over fifty years brought up two sons in Africa who shared the rich experiences of their parents. He has had a varied experience of the world and has documented his experiences from the early days to his retirement in the UK. This is an engaging snapshot of life in the British Colonial Service in the 20th Century.

SCIENCE
AND SAFARI

Jack Wilde

Science
And Safari

*To Denis
& Barbie

with best
wishes

Jack Wilde*

Vanguard Press

VANGUARD PAPERBACK

© Copyright 2005
Jack Wilde

A CIP catalogue record for this title is
available from the British Library

ISBN 1 84386 153 4

*Vanguard Press is an imprint of
Pegasus Elliot MacKenzie Publishers Ltd.*
www.pegasuspublishers.com

First Published in 2005

**Vanguard Press
Sheraton House Castle Park
Cambridge England**

Printed & Bound in Great Britain

Dedication

To the memory of my dear wife Kathy.

Contents

Foreword
By Dr W Plowright, CMG, DVSc, FRCVS, FRS.

Jack Wilde is one of those remarkably gifted individuals who, during a large part of their working lives, brought resourceful competence and a paternal tolerance to the Colonial Veterinary Service (later, part of Her Majesty's Overseas Civil Service).

His later contributions to the establishment of units for the study of major protozoal diseases of animals, first with the Wellcome Foundation in Kenya and, later at the Centre for Tropical Veterinary Medicine in Edinburgh University, were a reflection of the great esteem in which he was widely held after his first 'retirement'. He is now one of the small band of survivors from an imperial era, now long gone and regretted by few of later generations.

Much of Jack's story is a feat of memory and detailed family history, in which his dearly beloved wife, Kathy, played such a supporting role, an anchor through the many vicissitudes of his service overseas and in Britain, not to mention his long retirement in the West Country.

I remember Kathy from my days at Vom in North Nigeria in the early 1950s as a welcoming hostess who even undertook to make the curtains for my bachelor's house! My wife and I will always remember how the Wilde's acted '*in loco parentis*' and put their charming residence at Kabete at our disposal for our wedding reception.

Jack has provided some penetrating but usually kindly

insights into the character and behaviour of his colleagues, friends and other acquaintances, both in Africa and afterwards. Who amongst us has not sometimes fallen fowl of authorities; considered other to have been plagiaristic or worse; judged alien peoples in a less kindly light or regretted the passing of empire and subsequent deterioration in ex-colonies?

Through it all Jack has remained addicted to his painting, which has provided him with purpose, pleasure and I'm sure solace through many decades. We treasure a painting of his Kabete period that was a generous gift and is now a constant reminder of an old colleague and friend of fifty years.

Swahili Lullaby

Mtoto alilia nini?
Huyo Bwana Huyo,
Mtoto alilia nini?
Huyo Bwana Huyo,
Kuimba na kutikia,
Firimba ngoma kompania,
Sisi sote tumemshangulia.

This is a Swahili lullaby which I was taught by Bawani, a member of the Zanzibari Royal Family. I think he was a nephew of the Sultan. We were shipmates in the SS Madura in 1941

As is the case in many traditional songs and poems, literal translation is almost impossible. The nearest that I can get to a meaningful translation is as follows;

For what is the child crying?
There he is master, there he is,
For what is the child crying?
There he is master, there he is,
To sing and chime in,
With flute and drum everyone,
We all together have succeeded or have pacified him.

PREFACE

A friend suggested to me that I should write an autobiography, as my life seemed to have been varied and interesting. This rather surprised me as my own impression was very different and as I look back from my dotage I feel a degree of disappointment with what I have achieved. There have been so many points in my life when, given the opportunity, I would have taken a different course.

Throughout life, one is faced with choices; to take this road or that; to go straight ahead or to diverge to right or left. Life's progress can be likened to the growth of a tree. The bole of the tree comes from its roots and the branches take off in various directions, the twigs similarly producing dichotomies at intervals until the mature tree occupies a large amount of space. Some of the peripheral buds are on one side, where they can greet the morning sun, others will be diametrically opposite so that they are warmed by the sun in its daily decline. But there the metaphor ends and can only be regarded as a very inadequate model.

In our human lives, the decisions made at the various dichotomies facing us have, or more truly can have, a moulding effect on the human subject concerned. Thus one has to trace one's life back as it happened and be content with its beginning, over which we can have had no influence, and, more importantly, to accept its reality of ups and downs, failures and successes, disappointments and triumphs, if one is fortunate enough to be accorded any such reward.

CHAPTER 1

Early Days

My knowledge of my antecedents is scrappy. I came into this world very much as an afterthought having been preceded by a brother who died soon after birth and two sisters, the elder being thirteen years and the younger ten years older than me. I think that these two sisters had a lot to do with my upbringing as my mother and father were working hard to make a corner shop in Blackpool successful enough to give their family a reasonable start in life. I understand that soon after my birth I suffered an attack of what was possibly meningitis but, amazingly, I recovered without any obviously serious after effects. However, as I grew older, my sight proved to be defective and long-sight had to be corrected by the use of spectacles. With hindsight I have felt that the defect was possibly a result of my earlier illness. My earliest memory is of being taken at the age of about two years to a children's playground by my younger sister Lily. I was unfortunately taken short and can remember running along a street in an attempt to reach home before a calamity occurred. I didn't avoid the calamity.

When I was a little older, perhaps about three years of age, supplies were delivered to our shop by horse and cart and a photograph was taken of me, my hair curly and very fair, sitting on the back of one of the horses. This was at the time of the First World War and I have vague memories of my father in khaki uniform. As far as I know, he did not go to the front but was a member of a unit called the Volunteers, rather like, I suppose, Dad's army of the Second World War. I also vaguely remember seeing a Zeppelin at that time. I do remember Armistice Day in

1918 when I was five years old and I can still visualise the bunting hanging across the streets. About this time we had moved to Burnley, a Lancashire cotton-spinning town. I was later to understand that the move had been made necessary by an illness suffered by my father, brought on by the stresses and strains of the business. The doctor had told him he would have to sell his business and find a job that took him out into the open air. He, therefore, took a job, which was then styled 'Commercial Traveller', nowadays the name 'Rep' would apply, with a well-known biscuit manufacturing company, William Crawford and my father was based in Burnley.

We lived in what I remember as a large house on a corner overlooking some allotments with a little shopping centre nearby. The shop which made the greatest impact on me was a bakery run by a Mrs Duxberry, who made lovely custard pies and delicious Cornish pasties. I started my primary school education in Burnley but my only memory of that school is of the first day of my attendance when I was taken to the school by my mother. I do retain a few vivid memories of Burnley. One was of visits to the barber's shop where large brushes were actuated by a rotating shaft. The brushes were applied to the customer's head at the end of the barbering process and one's scalp was subjected to a vigorous brushing. Another was of large lorries carrying bales of cotton from which some small cigar shaped wads of cotton fell onto the road. We children used to pick them up and light the ends and then swing them round in the air until they were nearly burned through. I also remember my father indulging his hobby of oil painting, though he didn't seem to have much time to give to this hobby. I still have one of his pictures in my possession. We had some friends called Maybury and once when I picked up a very painful infection of one of my fingers he took me to the doctor, presumably when my father was away on business. The doctor called the affliction 'blood poisoning'. He took a sharp scalpel and made a continuous incision from the knuckle of my finger to the tip, through the nail and down to the palm of my hand. This, he said, was to 'let out the poison'. I well remember having to hold my hand over a bowl into which the blood flowed copiously. Mr Maybury, in appreciation of my fortitude, gave me a toy wheelbarrow of which I was inordinately proud.

When I was about eight years old, my father was transferred by his firm to Sheffield. Here we acquired a house in Glencoe Road where we had a long back garden with, at its end, a large and gnarled tree beyond which was a field and a wood, separated from the garden by a wall. This wall and the old tree provided the props for advancing my climbing skills and those of my friends. In an old barn where we used to play, one of our favourite games was to climb up onto the roof beams and to dive into the hay below. One of our group conceived the idea of diving and somersaulting into the hay. He did it quite expertly but when I tried I didn't go far enough over and landed on my neck. At first I thought I had broken it and was so afraid that I never told my parents of the incident. I have often wondered if that had anything to do with a fibrocytis in my neck, from which I have suffered intermittently in my later years.

Our house was in what I suppose was a terrace but where each pair had a passage separating the two houses but where the first storey was contiguous with that of its neighbour. There was a second storey forming a rather capacious attic under a single roof, which ran the whole length of the terrace. Opposite was a wall surrounding parkland, which was the site of a large house. Our next door neighbours were Joe and Hilda Lindsay. Joe was a piano tuner but he adopted the style of professor of music. He used to sit at his open window on warm summer days ostensibly playing piano works very competently. In reality, the piano was a pianola and he was peddling his way through the difficult works, controlling the volume and tempo by means of two small levers in front of the keyboard. The Lindsays had two sons, the elder, Hildred, the second Alwyn, and a slightly younger daughter, Olive. They were my playmates in those days although my mother did not really approve of them. My bedroom was one of the attics, which had a dormer window in the front. The two boys next door had the corresponding attic in their house and we used to make the old string and treacle tin telephones and pretend to send messages to each other. One day, I decided to cross the intervening piece of roof from my window to theirs and climbed out of my dormer onto the slates. It just happened that

21

my Dad was coming up the road and saw me. I was about to let go of my window frame when he shouted and told me to get back into my room and stay there until he arrived. When he arrived he was carrying a razor strop and he gave me a good belting on the bum. That was the only time I was ever beaten and I realised then that it was understandable. I learned the lesson. Had he not seen me in time it is possible that my career might have come to an early end and I would not have been writing this. I suppose that I was about ten at the time.

During our period in Sheffield, a young girl, about my age came to live with us. Her name was Billie. There was something about her relationship with our family, which was never fully explained to me. I was given to understand that she was my cousin but I think she was probably adopted by my Dad's sister, Mary who was married to a lawyer in Winchester. Mary was a Christian Scientist who suffered, what I later realised, was very crippling arthritis which made it impossible for her to look after Billie who, it was hinted, was no better than she should be. She was a very active, boisterous child and she introduced me to the differences between little boys and little girls. In this, she was ably assisted by Olive. I'm afraid I must have been very ill informed at that time. It was a school friend of primary days who dispelled my original ignorance on the matter of procreation by explaining to me that babies were born through a split in the woman's belly starting at the belly button.

My informant in this matter of procreation was Maurice Board, whose father ran a pub in Charles Street near the centre of the city. Maurice and I became good friends when we were in primary school and we moved into secondary school at the same time. Maurice had no intention of going further than matriculation in school. He was a brainy boy and he told me that as soon as he passed the matriculation exams, he would leave school and enter his elder brother's profession. This brother had a very lucrative practice in accountancy in Sheffield and Maurice intended to be part of that business. He told me that he would be articled to his brother and become a Chartered Accountant. He had every intention of being worth £60,000 before he was thirty. This, to me, was an astronomical sum which I regarded as an exaggeration. He left school after his fourth year and we lost touch with each other. It was only in recent years when I had retired and moved to Dorset that I heard of Maurice again. Roland Saunderson, from Sheffield, came to live in the neighbouring village of Yetminster and I met him in connection with the establishment of a benefice magazine. I asked him if he had ever come across Maurice Board. To my surprise, he knew him well. Maurice had been instrumental in the winding up of some companies in which Roland had some financial interests. He gave me Maurice's address and I arranged to go and see him when next Kathy, my wife, and I made the journey to Yorkshire.

We found him living with his wife Barbara in an attractive house in the village of Dore, quite near to where my home had been in Totley. Maurice's Rolls Royce was in the drive. He expressed delight at seeing us and we reciprocated. It transpired that he had achieved his aim of qualifying as a Chartered Accountant at a younger age than anyone before him and when we visited nobody else had yet achieved the same distinction. He had developed a great interest in classical music and had adapted a large room in his house as a music room with under bench cupboards all around the walls. In these he stored his records and his collection was such that he said that he could reproduce the music from any programme which was presented in the concert halls or on the TV and radio. I was most impressed. Maurice had, by now, retired but retained his connection with his company by doing consultancy jobs provided, he said, they were big enough and financially worth while. Maurice also was, for many years, a director of Sheffield United Football Club. Sadly, he died two years after we had re-established contact with each other.

Another close friend of mine lived next door but one from us. He was Bobby MacKay, whose father was the manager of a business in Sheffield. Bobby used to have rather sophisticated presents for his birthdays and Christmas like the kit he had one year for making torch batteries. We had great ideas about manufacturing batteries but the scheme didn't work out. We spent most of our spare time wrestling, rolling about the floor firmly embraced. Bobby had a particularly effective neck lock. When not confined to the house by the weather, we and our

23

other friends spent a lot of time digging trenches and fighting battles with air guns and catapults. I remember on one occasion, I let fly with my catapult, the missile being an airgun pellet. The idea that my shot would go anywhere near the 'enemy' camp didn't enter my mind as our shooting was far from accurate. I didn't even aim but to our collective horror the pellet penetrated the scalp of one of our friends. Closer inspection showed that the missile had made a small hole in the skin and was lying against the skull. I retrieved it with the aid of my penknife. There was no blood and we all decided that we had better not tell anyone about the accident. Fortunately the little wound healed very quickly and our wounded friend suffered no pain and basked in a little bit of heroic glory. These cowboy and Indian campaigns and battles were interspersed with making campfires and trying to cook chips in an old frying pan.

In Sheffield, I attended the Manor Primary School whence, after taking the 'eleven plus' I went to the Sheffield Central School for Boys that provided me with a very happy secondary education and some very good friends. It is a tribute to that school that all members of my group obtained scholarships to Cambridge, Oxford, Leeds, Sheffield or London. In my fourth year class at the Central School, I was studying for the Matriculation Examination, when Jimmy Brown, Chemistry Master, asked me what I intended to do after matriculation. I said that I wasn't sure but that my brother-in-law had suggested that I should apply for a post in his company, Alliance Assurance, in which he felt sure I would be able to be employed. I wasn't enthusiastic about an office job and said so to Jimmy. He suggested that I should consider going into the sixth form with the object of taking the Higher School Certificate in Biology. I had attended some after school lectures organised by Jimmy Brown who had initiated a science club which I had joined. The lectures were given by Jimmy but from time to time he persuaded a pupil to present a short dissertation or demonstration. I was fascinated by this and asked my parents if I could continue at school for a further two years. They readily acceded to the suggestion in spite of the fact that it meant another two years during which I would be dependent on them. I went into the sixth form after matriculating. In this form we were tutored by Jimmy in Chemistry and Biology. Jimmy took us out at weekends into the Derbyshire countryside and captivated us with his encyclopaedic knowledge of animals and plants and our environment. He was a natural teacher.

In the sixth form of the previous year, Jimmy had entered some students for university scholarships and all of them were successful. One of the scholarships was an open one, of the Royal Scholarships in engineering, chemistry, physics, biology and geology. Of these, only two were offered in biology and, if my memory serves me correctly, only two in geology. In that year two of the students were entered for the biology awards and one for the geology. All three were successful. In my year, Jimmy entered three of us for the biology awards and one for the geology. There was, of course, a very keen sense of competition. Two scholarships and at least three of us and goodness knows how many more from other schools and polytechnics and even the first year of universities. My fellow pupils and I were not very sanguine about success. We had to spend two years in the sixth form during which time Jimmy coached us assiduously.

When the time came for the examinations, our feelings were intense. One of us in the biology set, at least, would be disappointed. Indeed, we felt that it would be a great triumph if we secured one of the scholarships. At the very best, it appeared that one of us, at least, would fail and would have to try for a scholarship of a lower order.

The examinations were finished and the term ended. The first weeks of the summer holiday were a time of nervousness for me and I suspect that my schoolmates were similarly affected. One morning I cycled to the home of my friend Graham Keyworth as we kept in touch and went on rides together in the holidays. That morning, the post arrived when I was with Graham. One of the letters announced that Graham had been selected for a Royal Scholarship in Biology. No sooner had he read this news than the phone rang and it was our other co-examinee. Monty had also been offered a similar scholarship. My feelings might well be imagined and I cycled home in a spirit of great despondency. I arrived home to find that the mail had been delivered and wonder of wonders, I also had been awarded a Royal Scholarship. We learned afterwards that the standard of the entries had been so high that the examining board had decided to provide three scholarships in biology – all going to Jimmy's pupils. To crown it all, we learned that our friend who had opted for geology had won the geology award. This success was almost entirely the result of Jimmy's superb tuition and his dedication to his calling as a teacher. I feel that I owe him a great debt of gratitude. Our group, of course, became scattered after we left school and we entered our several universities, but all were more than averagely successful in their respective fields. However, the prize for eminence has to go to Fred Dainton who became a brilliant scientist of great importance to the government in the Second World War and was later elevated to the peerage as the Lord Dainton of Hallam. Sadly Freddie died in 1998. He and his wife, Barbara came to visit us in Leigh and we corresponded on several subjects. I was able to provide him with some photographs of our schooldays which he used in his autobiography, 'Doubts and Certainties' published by the Sheffield Academic Press.

In my schooldays of course, my sisters had grown up and like Richmal Crompton's William I had to deal with the situations brought about by the frequent visits of young men who had interests in nubile and not unattractive young ladies. Win was a very competent pianist with a remarkable ability to sight-read and turn any piano music into lovely sound. I well remember listening to her playing Beethoven and Chopin on summer evenings when I was in bed. She worked in the office of the well-known music shop of Wilson Peck in Sheffield and when prospective purchasers of a piano turned up, she was often asked by the management to demonstrate the quality of the instruments on display. Lily was quite reasonable on the piano but leaned more towards singing. She had a good soprano voice that she used to good effect in amateur concerts. The first time I ever heard a radio broadcast was when we had crystal sets and I heard a concert given by the local 'Opera Opptimists'. The entertainment was broadcast by the then Sheffield 2FL Radio, and Lily was the soubrette. Elder sisters did, of course, have their uses and I did benefit by the odd half crown to go to the pictures and leave the young lovers in peace.

One of the young suitors was a bank clerk whose home was

in Melborne in Derbyshire. He used to go home at the weekends on his motorbike and he offered to take me with him on the pillion one weekend. I thought this was a great idea and so off we went one Friday evening. The young man's father was the Station Master at Melborne and so I had the great pleasure of riding on the footplate and even, one heavenly day, of spending the whole day on a shunting engine being allowed by the engine driver to drive the old shunter and move some trucks around the yard. It is easy to imagine with what great pleasure I described my activities to my pals when I went back to school.

Another, rather more mature man who met Win in the course of her work, was a Canadian who was a member of Sir Thomas Beecham's entourage on an opera season in England. He became a frequent visitor to our house and I was held spell bound by his descriptions of his exploits as a professional ice-hockey player in Canada. His lurid account of matches in which players resorted to all sorts of vicious attacks on opposing players went down very well when I relayed them to my pals at school. Another advantage of having older sisters was when I was getting to my higher teens, I could go with them on holidays in the Co-operative Holiday Association and the Holiday Fellowship. I enjoyed some very happy times mountain climbing and trekking in interesting places, and met people who broadened my outlook. The man who eventually married my sister Lily, was the son of a rope manufacturer who had a ropewalk in Sheffield. When the Buffalo Bill circus came to the city the services of a rope maker were in demand and my future brother-in-law's father got to know Buffalo Bill very well. He gave me an ivory handled Colt revolver, which he had received from the famous cowboy. The barrel was blocked up so that it could not be fired but it was a very prized possession of mine.

One day when my mother had gone out with my father, I arrived home from school to find that I could not open the front door with my key, so I went round to the back door and found that this door was jammed by a drawer of a fixed cupboard just inside the doorway. I managed to insert my arm in the gap and eventually, with much effort and banging, I managed to open the door and enter the house. The place was in a state of disruption. Drawers had been pulled out and emptied onto the floor and books were strewn about. It was the same in all the downstairs rooms. I picked a stout iron poker out of one of the fireplaces and made for the stairs which I climbed silently. My bedroom door, facing the stairs was open and I could see that the built in wardrobe door was also open and I could see a pair of feet in the space under the door. I did a swift rush at the door pushing it to with all the force I could muster. It clattered to. No one was there nor were they anywhere else upstairs. The feet I had seen were a pair of my own shoes. I went down the stairs and found the front door closed but not locked and so the birds must have flown while I was clattering away at the back door. My parents arrived home very shortly afterwards and we examined the damage. The police were called and arrived soon after and started investigations. We heard nothing for several days and so my father called in at the police station. He began to complain and the sergeant told him that he must mind his words. Some of the stolen items had been found in a nearby front garden and among them was a colt revolver. Did my father have a licence for a handgun? No. Well he had better keep his trap shut or they would charge him with unlawful possession of an unlicensed firearm. That was the end of that.

Our school had a great reputation for the production of Shakespeare's plays. This was due to the fact that a great Thespian, Benny Marshman, produced one of the plays every year. He was a marvellous man, large and portly and a mine of knowledge on every detail of the Bard's work. In my first year the play was the twenty-first produced by Benny with not one repeat. Work on the annual play started in the autumn term when those of us volunteering for the job spent hours every afternoon and evening after school converting the large assembly hall into a stage and auditorium. I was enthusiastic in this work as were all of us volunteers, including Freddy, helping with stage construction, properties and scenery. I was involved in seven of the productions, my greatest contributions being made behind the scenes but in several of the plays I took small parts, the most prestigious of which was that of Dogberry in, 'Much Ado About Nothing'. All the female parts were played by boys and some lovely female characters they made. The annual play was a great occasion and invariably the six performances were played to packed houses. It was during my time at the school that a book was published about the Sheffield Central School's run of plays entitled, 'All right on the Night', in the publishing of which Freddy Dainton played an important part.

At school I didn't excel at sports. I played football and cricket for the house but I was restricted by the fact that I had to wear spectacles for long-sight. I did fairly well in athletics and swimming. In my last year at school I won the mile race and I still have the cutting from the Sheffield Telegraph with a press photo of me breasting the tape. The report in the paper said, 'Wilde ran a well judged race to win the mile'. No time was given but I imagine it was not particularly brilliant. I did, for a short time, play for an old boys' rugby team, but again I was not very good mainly because of my hypermetropia. .

While I was still at school my family moved to a new house in Dore and Totley on the Derbyshire side of Sheffield. It was delightful to be able to walk out of the house, through the woods and onto the moors. When at home during university vacations, some of our group used to forgather at our house and either walk or cycle through the pleasant county of Derbyshire. We went rock climbing and cave exploring and indeed discovered and reconnoitred a cave of which we had not heard before. We originally found this cave as a hole in the moors near Mam Tor. It caught our attention because we were following a stream which suddenly disappeared. We scrabbled about in the surrounding scrub and discovered that the stream ran into the ground through a hole in the rocks. We followed the stream into the hole and found that we were in a narrow water worn cleft in the limestone. On that particular occasion we were not equipped for underground exploration and so we marked the spot and determined to make another visit in order to explore the situation more fully. The day arrived when we had gathered our very primitive and inadequate 'caving gear', and started our expedition. None of us was experienced in underground exploration but we had a good idea of how to set about it. For illumination we had acquired a couple of acetylene headlamps and a few battery torches. We were clothed in jerseys, old trousers and knitted woollen bonnets. On our feet we wore stout walking boots. We knew that it might be possible to get lost underground and so we took the precaution of taking with us a large ball of white string.

Our route was a streambed running along the bottom of an obviously water-worn cave. The walls were beautifully smooth and tortuous, sometimes the cave was deep and very narrow, at others wider and the ceiling was lower. It seemed marvellous to us that this stream must have been running along its self-made channel for thousands of years. I don't know how far we penetrated or how deep down we had gone but from memory I imagine we had progressed some two hundred yards into the earth and possibly thirty or forty feet deep, but we came to a point where the tunnel opened into a cavern about ten to fifteen feet wide. The water here ceased to be an obvious stream and formed a pool about five feet deep. We considered the situation. It seemed possible that the tunnel or a cavern might continue on the other side of what could be a rock wall. We had a coil of rope with us and so I volunteered to go under the water and try to find an opening in the roof. I took all my clothes off except for my boots. The rope was tied round my middle. My companions said that if I gave no sign of returning within a minute or so they would pull me out. I submerged myself and with a torch in my hand, which amazingly produced a beam of light under water, I proceeded cautiously, with my lungs full of air, under the roof which seemed to be fairly horizontal. I felt the roof above my head with my hands and tried to see to the sides through the now murky water. I suppose I must have gone forward about ten or fifteen feet without finding any outlet and so crawled back into the cave. When I came out of the water I was frozen and had no towel or other means of drying myself and so had to put my clothes on again. It took a long time for me to warm up and I was very glad to get out into the outside air which was, at least, a few degrees warmer than that inside the cave. However, this episode gave us a taste for underground exploration and we did quite a lot of crawling about in caves in various types of situation before I left Derbyshire for my University life in London. I do remember one episode when we were in a cavern with several interconnecting passages. We were crawling along one of the passages when our dim lights picked out a horizontal line ahead. When we got nearer we found that it was our trusty string. We had come round in a circle and thanks to the string we found our way out safely. Being away in London and subsequently taking up my career abroad, I lost touch with most of my caving friends. Many years later I heard that our discovery of the entrance to a cave on the moor, which had become known as Giant's Hole, was followed by more expert exploration of the site. This, I understand, led to the discovery of another very large cavern which I believe, is now open to the public as an attraction comparable with the Peak Cavern in Castleton.

Of our caving group, Graham Keyworth and Clifford Bingham, contributed in the academic world to research in botany and rural economic education. Tom Wilson graduated in geology at the Royal School of Mines and went to South America to work in oil exploration. George Wright studied medicine at Sheffield University and was an accomplished performer on several wind instruments, especially the clarinet and saxophone. He became a much loved General Practitioner in Falmouth where he also took Holy Orders in the Church of England. He died in the nineties and was mourned widely in the town where he was a part time priest. Clifford and Graham have also died but I have completely lost touch with Tom.

My scholarship was a Royal Scholarship to Imperial College where, in the Royal College of Science, (RCS), I studied for a degree in Zoology. I shared digs in Fulham with Graham Keyworth. Our landlady, Mrs Edwards was a great woman in more senses than one and we were really well-fed and had some hilarious experiences as she was a great practical joker. Everything, including the practical jokes, cost us twenty-five shillings a week. Of course, we students were three to a bedroom. Mrs Edwards was a widow and had to take in lodgers in order to make a living. In those days there were not many people who had pensions. Every bedroom in the house was occupied by students or young people in local employment. Mrs Edwards even went so far as to provide a bed for a young woman who was making a very modest living in a shop. She had to share the main bedroom with our landlady and was supposed to help Mrs Edwards from time to time with a hand in the housework. She didn't seem to be over energetic in this direction, however, she did sometimes help with the bedrooms and so was involved in one of Mrs Edwards's practical jokes. One day the pair of them made apple pie beds in our bedroom and even went so far as to loosen the mattresses from the bedheads with the idea that the beds might collapse when we climbed into them. By good fortune, the beds did not collapse even when one of the chaps sat on his bed and tried to pare a corn on his foot with my cutthroat razor. We discovered the plot before any harm was done but had to undo and remake the beds before we could settle for the night. We said nothing next morning but in the lab at college I prepared a batch of nitrogen tri-iodide. This is a very unstable compound which, when dry, explodes at the lightest touch. While wet it is quite stable and so I took the substance back to our digs in a test-tube of water. When the ladies were out, we spread this material in various places in their bedroom. We put it on the chamber pots and on Mrs Edwards's tooth mug and on any places that might be contacted while they were undressing and preparing for bed. When the ladies retired that night, we crept down the passage to listen at their bedroom door. We had to stifle our mirth when the fusilade commenced. Nitrogen tri-iodide, when it does explode, does not cause any serious damage but, unfortunately, it does spread iodine about. I, therefore, hoist with my own petard, had to obtain a supply of sodium hyposulphite and spent several hours removing iodine stains from all over the bedroom.

We didn't have a lot to spend in those days but we managed to have a good time and to take part in college affairs. I was a member of the RCS Dramatic Society playing several roles in our productions. In sport I opted for cross-country running and ran for the college for four years finishing up as captain of the club. We had a very useful arrangement with the Chelsea Football Club which permitted us to train on one day a week, running round the cinder track which surrounded the football pitch at Stamford Bridge. This was a great privilege as we also had the services of Charley Harris, the Chelsea masseur who gave us valuable coaching and also massaged us after the training sessions. He gave me some instruction in athletic massaging and this proved very useful as in my last year with the club I massaged the team at our weekly matches against the other London clubs with whom we had fixtures.

I joined the University of London Officers Training Corps (OTC) that was attached to the 47th Second London Regiment of Light Infantry. The camps and various activities provided me with some happy days and many good friends. We were actively involved in several University and national occasions. When His Majesty King George V laid the foundation stone of the new University of London Building we formed the guard of honour, proudly marching behind the band of the Scots Guards having been vigorously trained by our Sergeant Instructors who were seconded to us by the Grenadier Guards. At this time in my youth, I suffered a series of boils in my ears. The pain was intense and I don't know why I was so dreadfully afflicted unless it was because when I went swimming in the public baths I enjoyed diving and swimming underwater. Possibly, I picked up an infection that was exacerbated by submitting myself to increased pressure. In those days there were no antibiotics or specific chemotherapeutics. I suffered this affliction for several months and I was in the middle of a most painful earache when we were on the guard of honour to His Majesty. It was an unusually hot day and my suffering was intense but I would not have missed the experience and honour.

We were also on duty for the Royal Silver Jubilee and on a sadder occasion at the funeral of His Majesty, about a year later, when my unit was lining the route outside Green Park. The crowd had been pushed down behind us so that there was a good deal of pressure on our backs. The police appeared to be pushing the crowd along the park railings, much to the annoyance of those who had established their advantageous position much earlier. I still have a vivid memory, while we were 'resting on arms reversed', of one old lady hanging onto the back of my belt and saying, "Don't let them push me away, soldier, I've been here for hours." One of our summer camps left an indelible memory on me and on, I suspect, all the other members of our contingent, when we endured a more sordid episode. We were camped on the cliffs near Beachy Head and a branch of the NAAFI provided our messing. One day, the menu for the evening meal contained the item, 'savoury mince'. This was very savoury. After the meal, in the delightful evening sun, most of the unit walked into Eastbourne. Violent diarrhoea struck. Almost everyone from the camp was affected. We made our way back to the camp as best we could despite the journey being punctuated by frequent violent calls of nature, all modesty or decorum being completely ignored. The attack persisted through the night with a constant stream of sufferers rushing from the tents to the latrines. The medical parade in the morning showed an unprecedented attendance. The Medical Sergeant passed down the line each person being addressed with the same question "What symptoms?" the reply from all except two individuals was "Diarrhoea." The two exceptions were suffering from constipation. Every man on that parade including the two with constipation received the same medication, 'Number Nine!' While this parade was in process, the NAAFI manager appeared outside the cookhouse in his pinstriped trousers and black morning coat. The parade with one accord broke up and overpowered him and then his pinstriped trousers could be seen being hoisted to the top of the flagstaff. The facts eventually emerged that the savoury mince had been made from a batch of meat that had definitely 'gone off', the spices being intended to disguise the rotten taste of the item. The manager wisely didn't press charges about his 'debagging'. I was a member of the Corps for my four years in Imperial College and enjoyed the training, obtained certificates A and B issued for infantry instruction and also qualified, first class for rifle shooting at Princes Risborough firing range. Our rifle in those days was the Lee-Enfield 303, soon to be replaced in the British Army. In drill, of course, we formed fours not threes.

The main zoology course in the Royal College of Science was slanted towards entomology. Three of us in my year wished to graduate in pure Zoology and so in our fourth and final year we were allocated a small separate laboratory where we were left to our own devices to carry out research projects. Our lab was in the Huxley Building next to the Royal College of Art in Exhibition Road. The main laboratory was next to ours and there the routine laboratory teaching was carried on. This Huxley Laboratory was the one in which H.G.Wells had studied and the one in which he set his short story entitled 'The Slip Under the Microscope'. In my time the Professor of Zoology was James MacBride who has been described as the 'last of the Lamarckians'. He was a martinet and frightened us all with his aggressive manner. MacBride was not a very organised lecturer and it was lucky for us that he left the major part of the teaching to his younger colleagues. When he was on the rostrum he doddled about with a long pointer in his right hand, the thicker end of which was repeatedly banged on the floor of the rostrum while the narrow end waved erratically in the air from time to time striking the lamp shade above his head. We students all watched this wavering end of the pointer with fascinated anticipation of seeing the electric light bulb being smashed. However, in our time, this hoped for eventuality never occurred.

Once in a while Professor MacBride came to inspect us when we were working in the laboratory. When this happened the atmosphere was electric and every student was quaking in his shoes. The bench in this lab was very long and accommodated about fifteen students. One day when the 'Old man' came in on one of his inspections we were dissecting earthworms and had to remove the ovaries, which lie in the thirteenth segment. The professor started at the bottom end of the lab and his rasping voice was heard, 'Show me an ovary'. The poor unfortunate did his best but it was not good enough. 'That's not an ovary you idiot! It's just a bit of muck', howled MacBride. This sort of treatment was repeated as each successive student was subjected to the inquisition. I was about tenth in the line. Sweat poured off me as I feverishly prodded about in the entrails of the worm. By something like a miracle I found the ovary impaled on the point of my dissecting needle. I carefully washed it off into a watch glass and prepared it for placing on the microscope slide. A sudden explosion from the MacBride buccal orifice startled me into dropping the watch glass and I watched with horror and apprehension as its alcoholic contents began to flow over the side of the bench. With consummate skill I managed to spear the ovary on the end of my needle and get it onto the slide, rapidly covering it with a coverslip. Meanwhile, the old curmudgeon was drawing ever nearer. I adjusted the focus of the microscope and in my nervous state over compensated and the cover slip, fortunately still intact, stuck to the microscope nosepiece. I grabbed it with forceps and replaced it on the slide hoping against hope that the ovary was still adhering to it. My neighbour was receiving the last of his ear bashing as I took a pace backward to allow the professor to get to my microscope. He grabbed the course adjustment with a fist rather as though he was grasping a hammer. I muttered with some alarm, "That's the course adjustment, Sir!"

"I know, I know, you stupid boy, do you think I don't know how to use a microscope?" He peered intensely down the tube and then declared that was the best specimen he had seen this morning. I breathed again and the great man passed on to terrify the next victim.

My two zoology colleagues were Nevil Chapman and Alan Ford. They were both quite brilliant students. Alan had a photographic memory which was a great help, especially in the learning of all the details of type species. Nevil had a very sharp intellect which enabled him to sort out and retain the important characteristics of any part of the syllabus and learn accordingly. Like me, they were both active members of the dramatic society and Alan showed a flare for producing. He really was more interested in drama than in zoology. I felt somewhat inadequate in comparison with these two companions and I suppose as a consequence, probably worked harder and more assiduously. As we approached the final examinations we all began to become more and more apprehensive about our chances of getting a good degree. I felt that Alan would get a first and that, possibly, Nevil would get either a first or a second. I hoped that, at least I might manage to pass. We all had to submit a thesis on our research project. My project was on the feeding mechanisms of *Pecten maximus*, the scallop, and I had received scallops from the vicinity of the Eddystone lighthouse for use in my research which involved the microscopic observation of the streams of suspended particles drawn into the inside structures of the animal. I had always had the ability to draw so that my thesis contained a lot of very detailed and explanatory diagrams which were presented in a fairly professional manner. I have always had a strong belief that it was this work of mine that contributed largely to my success in the examination. The results were, remarkable and, in my opinion, quite unexpected, Chapman 2nd Class, Ford 2nd Class and Wilde 1st Class.

My landlady benefited from my choice of thesis subject in that she was very partial to scallops and had all mine after I had finished with them. She cooked them in butter between two saucers, so she said. I have never taken to shellfish though this might be regarded as odd in someone whose special subject in zoology was the Mollusca. During one vacation I spent some time with the oyster fishing boats in the Blackwater. Hand dredging for the oysters was exceedingly hard work and played havoc with one's hands but all the ways of wresting a living from the sea are not only very hard but also fraught with considerable danger and real hardship. During another vacation I signed on as a deck hand in an Aberdeen trawler. I arrived in Aberdeen by train very early one cold August morning and made my way to the fishing docks. I was looking for a trawler called the George Stroud, one of the fleet belonging to the Stroud Fishing Company, but I first had breakfast, a rather fatty and greasy mix of bacon and eggs, in a very basic eating house over the fish market. I found the George Stroud tied up to bollards in the harbour. There was a lot of activity on the foredeck with mechanics repairing the large winch in front of the wheelhouse. Tools lay scattered about with apparent reckless abandon and people came along and flung boxes and other bundles aboard. I dumped my rucksack on a pile of nets and jumped down onto the deck. No one took any notice of me. After an hour or so some men, who later proved to be crewmembers, drifted along and carefully lowered themselves aboard. I found out later that they were all suffering from an excess of alcohol, their imbibing of which had taken up the forty-eight hours between trips. Eventually, the mechanics and their tools and accessories disappeared and I made myself known to those still aboard who were to be my shipmates. A gentleman in a bowler hat, a cardigan and yellow winkle-picker shoes arrived and stood on the edge of the wharf.

"Aren't you coming on?" shouted one of the hands.

"Not until the boat's alongside," he replied. The vessel was about eleven inches from the edge of the wharf. This was the skipper. The boat slowly drifted nearer to the sea wall and the skipper stepped delicately aboard. He disappeared below and the next time I saw him he was attired in dirty trousers, seaboots and a thick grey sweater. On his head was an old flat cap and we were now ready to go to sea.

We moved out and turned north. I now discovered that three of the cases, which had been put aboard earlier contained spirits, to whit, thirty-six bottles of whisky delivered from bond. I'm pretty sure that the first bottle was broached before we were out of the three-mile limit. However, apart from one man in the wheelhouse, presumably steering the ship, and the two firemen in the engine room, the rest of us, eight in number, were congregated in the trapeze shaped after cabin situated immediately over the propellers. In the centre of this cabin was a correspondingly trapeze shaped table fixed to the deck. This was fitted with what are called fiddles, very necessary to prevent dishes and mugs from being shot about when the ship responded to the roll and pitch of even a fairly calm sea. The seats around this table were fixed and behind them were three bunks, one on each side and the rear one athwartship. As a working "guest" I had been allocated one of these bunks which were regarded as the 'officers' sleeping quarters. Forward of this space were two minute cabins, one on the port side for the skipper and the other on the starboard side for the 'Chief' engineer. These were provided with the luxury of doors. A stove on which a very large kettle boiled day and night took up the bulkhead between the two doors. Into this were thrown, from time to time, large handfuls of tea. Milk and sugar were similarly added and only when there was no room left for fluid in the kettle were the used tealeaves thrown out. The routine followed as we started steaming, as opposed to fishing, commencing with the opening of the first bottle of whisky.

There was only one glass on the ship and this was a four-ounce medicine glass, which had lost its base and consequently could not be stood up. The skipper filled the glass and drained it and then filled it again and passed it to the Chief. He drained it and handed it back for a refill after which each man had his four ounces of the golden liquor when the whole process was repeated. I declined my share from the start. The atmosphere in the cabin was becoming thick with cigarette smoke and whisky fumes and we had now got into a smart swell. I made my excuses and moved aloft onto the deck and promptly emptied my bacon and egg breakfast into the North Sea. I wrapped myself up in the warmest clothes that I could muster and lay down in the lifeboat, which appeared to be permanently screwed down to the deck. I stayed put there for most of the day only moving hurriedly to the side of the ship at intervals necessitated by my revolting stomach. The libations continued in the cabin below and I could hear the increased noise as the drinkers became more and more oiled. The Chief Engineer, normally referred to as 'Chiefy', must have remembered me and felt that I needed something as he came up on deck and gave me what turned out the be a mug of his homemade rhubarb wine. I felt at that point that I would like to die but I was once more constrained to crawl to the ship's side to get rid of the home-brew. I must have dozed but as evening drew on I began to feel a little more alive and I staggered up into the wheelhouse where the first fisherman, Jock, he would be designated the bosun on an English ship, was in charge of the navigation at that time. I still felt queasy but the atmosphere was fresh in the wheelhouse and to be much preferred to that in the after cabin.

En route to the fishing grounds, the trawler is said to be steaming as opposed to trawling which is the actual process of fishing. During steaming the course and its various changes are set by the skipper and it is the duty of the helmsman to keep the ship pointing in the right heading. We were making for the rich fishing grounds around the Faroe Islands. Our steaming speed was about twelve to sixteen knots depending on tides, wind and weather. Our journey from Aberdeen to the place where we started fishing was about six hundred miles. During this steaming period I began to feel better and was rapidly finding my sea legs. As I didn't want to sleep in the after cabin, I was allocated a bunk in the fo'c'sle. It was in the forepeak, immediately against the iron side of the ship, just under the aperture through which the anchor chain passed, the hawsehole. The bunk was provided with some slightly damp blankets and had a stout board at the side to prevent the occupant from being thrown onto the deck. The noise of the water hitting the bows was terrific, it sounded just as though tons of stone and rubble were being thrown at the ship. The other occupants of the fo'c'sle were the two firemen and a deck hand called Nathan. The latter, curiously, described himself as a teetotaller and was doing his first trip since coming out of prison where he had served a spell for burglary. When I first poked my nose into this area of the accommodation the two firemen were rolling about the deck in their own vomit. At that time I was of the opinion that Nathan and I were the only sober members of the ship's company. I returned to the wheelhouse.

As evening drew in and the world became dark, Jock was still on watch as we steamed towards the Pentland Firth. He was certainly 'feeling no pain' having had a good share of the whisky. He rather woosily pointed out the headlands and lights. 'Duncansby heed – Pentland Skerries – Dunnet Heed' and so on. At one point we seemed to be steering directly towards a bright flashing light. We drew nearer and nearer and I began to be seriously worried, especially as Jock was certainly not sober.

I pointed to the light and with some diffidence said, "We're a bit near to that light aren't we?"

"Och aye" he replied, "we've got to steer as near to the rocks as we can to catch the tide. If we can do that all right we can be through the Firth in forty-five minutes, otherwise we could take four hours." We certainly were very near the light. I still have a vivid memory of looking down on the waves crashing over the rocks at the foot of the lighthouse. This was the Pentland Skerries Light, I seem to remember Jock referring to it as the 'North Rock'. After another hour or two in the wheelhouse, I decided to try my bunk in the fo'c'sle. I suppose I did get a little sleep but as dawn was breaking I pulled on my boots and went back to the wheelhouse to find that we had turned north, leaving the Dunnet Head light astern.

Jock seemed to be almost sober now, which was more than could be said about most of the rest of the crew. As I looked back out of the wheelhouse, the skipper staggered out of the galley door, across the deck and vomited over the side. Harry, the cook had been incapacitated by his alcoholic haze so that no food, as yet, had been cooked. Mac, the second fisherman, had taken over from Jock and he also was feeling rather frail. The sea was becoming a little rough and Harry, the cook, staggered out of the galley and clambered precariously up the companionway to the bridge carrying a large mug. I opened the wheelhouse door and he came in and presented the mug to Mac. I discovered that the mug was half full of steaming hot water with a toothbrush standing in it and in the bottom reclined Mac's dentures. Harry fished out of his pocket a tin of Gibb's Dentifrice which he also handed to Mac. The second fisherman declared, "Ah'm awfu' partic'lar aboot me teeth. I allus like to clean em once or twice a trip." It was at this point that I displayed my youthful naiveté.

"Oh yes," I said, "I'm very particular about mine but I have forgotten my toothbrush." I realised my mistake immediately but it was too late.

"Och," said Mac, "use mine," and he handed me the mug and its contents. In my delicate position, I felt that I might offend if I didn't accept the generous offer.

"Thanks a lot," I said and took the mug and the toothpaste and opening the window, I rubbed the brush vigorously on the pink slab of Gibb's, stirred the toothbrush in the hot water, spat out onto the deck and turned round to hand the mug, toothbrush and paste to Mac. He handed the wheel over to me with the instruction to 'Keep her steady on nor' b' west a half west' and proceeded to clean the green off his dentures.

At this stage I found that being active helped to dispel the remains of my seasickness and I was very willing to be shown how to steer the ship. The basic technique was to keep the binnacle needle steady on the heading given. At first it was not easy as, if the ship diverged from the correct heading, it was difficult for a novice to avoid over compensation. This could produce a sort of left/right wave motion appearing in the wake of the vessel. However, I soon became reasonably proficient as a helmsman and after a few days was left to take spells of watch when we appeared to be alone in a wide expanse of sea. At one point a large whale surfaced near the ship and travelled alongside for some ten minutes diving and surfacing and blowing. Eventually it turned away and left us.

Harry was soon back to his routine job and we had our first hot meal. I had developed an appetite and was only too ready to sit at the table in the after cabin next to Chiefy and enjoy the results of Harry's cooking. He certainly was good at his job and had a reputation for his hot rolls, 'morny rowies' in the vernacular. These were produced every morning for the first meal after dawn. How he did it I do not know. His galley, just off the deck at the head of the companionway down to the cabin, was minute and was equipped with the minimum of the essentials of cooking. I had now become accustomed to getting into my bunk and getting an hour or two of sleep when the opportunity presented. Towards evening we sighted the Faroes on our starboard bow. The skipper did much of his navigation by dead reckoning which means setting the course by visual observation of the land because angles and distances can be calculated by noting gaps between mountains and valleys and distinctive configurations of the coastline. The business of fishing now commenced.

The George Stroud carried two trawl nets, one on the starboard side and the other on the port. Normally the starboard net was used, the port acting as a spare to be shot when the damage to the starboard net was so bad as to demand lengthy repairs. On this trip there seemed to be a lot of damage to the nets and hours were taken up with net repairing. This was a very skilled operation at which most of the crew were experts. I was given the job of filling the needles that are quite large, specially shaped pieces of wood on which the coarse twine has to be wound. The trawl net used in the George Stroud, as in most of the British trawling fleet, was of the 'otter board' type. The mouth of the net on each side was attached to a large wooden door, heavily cladded with lead on its lower edge. As the net was towed, these doors were forced apart and so kept the net mouth open and on the bottom of the seabed. It is snagging on rocks and wrecks that wears through the rope and netting causing the damage which is such a time consuming problem. Each door was attached to a long heavy steel warp which passed forward over a pulley hanging from two strong bowed steel structures at the ship's side, one fore and one aft, called gallows. From these the warps were directed to the drum of the steam winch, which was firmly bolted to the deck in front of the wheelhouse. When the net was shot it was, naturally carried away abeam, as the ship was stationary, a comparative term only, and the steel warps were unwound. The ship was then put underway and the tackle was drawn aft until the warps were alongside the ship. It was then the hazardous job of the first fisherman to lean far over the stern and fix them into a large shackle from which they diverged backwards and downwards to the doors. As the vessel gathered speed forwards, the doors were pulled apart so opening the net into which the fish were swept. The net narrowed to a bag at its distal end called the cod end. This was closed at its extreme end by a specially tied and readily releasable knot. A trawl usually lasted about three hours and then the skipper would give the signal for the ship to 'heave to' and the winch started to haul in the net. The sound of the winch starting up was the signal for all hands to leave their bunks and turn out on deck. As the winch drew in the warps, the tension on these increased until the first fisherman had to carry out the even more hazardous operation of releasing the shackle block. He did this by leaning over the stern and knocking out the shackle pin with a hammer. The outer warp would flash through the sea like lightening. I was given to understand that this has often been fatal for the operator. I was told of mates who had had their bodies cut in half by warps either as a result of the above operation or when a warp had actually snapped in two under the great strain of the trawl. As the net came up to the side of the ship, the doors were swung on board and a rope which passed over a pulley fixed high on the foremast or gilson was lashed round the neck of the cod end and the mass of fish, if the trawl had been successful, was pulled high over the deck by the winch. It was then the job of someone, to go under the cod end and release the cod end knot. A shower of flapping fish would then cascade over the unfortunate crewmember and every one had to set about gutting and cleaning the fish. The foredeck was divided by boards into pounds and the fish were thrown into these according to species and size. If the net had not suffered serious damage, it was immediately reshot. If it was slightly damaged then it was repaired as soon as possible and shot again. If it was very badly damaged, the port net was shot and all hands carried on with the work of cleaning up and storing the fish on ice.

The George Stroud, for its time, was quite an up to date trawler, it had an echometer and a ship to ship and ship to shore radio. It was also equipped with a steam boiler for extracting the cod liver oil. This was an unsavoury operation in which steam was forced at high pressure through the accumulated mass of livers. After the fish had been stowed and the mess cleaned up, there remained the job of net mending and ice breaking in the ice hold. It was only after these chores had been completed that the crew could expect to get some food and, if lucky, an hour or so of sleep. As a rule there would be four or five trawls in twenty-four hours. In that period, there would be five hot meals, mostly fried fish and potatoes followed by plain boiled duff pudding. Sunday was notable because the meal nearest to midday provided meat and the duff contained currants. On the trip I am describing, the meat was turtle. This had come up in the net on the previous voyage and had been kept on ice. Hot, stewed, sweet tea was available at all hours. The lid of the teapot was the usual vessel for the drink and any left in that was poured back into the pot. Trawlers are built to roll and the George Stroud was no exception. It rolled and pitched like a very lively corkscrew. While we were fishing we had almost constant rough seas. It was the time of the equinoctial gales and the decks were mostly awash. Some of the waves must have been thirty or forty feet high and it was common to get the sea breaking as high as the wheelhouse. The strong roll of a trawler is very beneficial during the hand hauling in of the net as when the trawler rolls side under the net floats up and all hands grab it and push it down towards the deck. Then all stand on it so that as the reverse roll takes place the movement of the ship pulls the net in. This is repeated several times until the cod end arrives at the ship's side and the rope can be made fast. During this operation the sea often came over our heads.

There were times when I wondered just why I had been foolish enough to sign on. It certainly wasn't for the money. I didn't get any pay, the rate for a deckhand was 9s.6p per day, and I had also to pay for my food. A plethora of fried fish and chips wasn't doing any good for my digestion. I suggested to Harry one day that we might have a change and have steamed or boiled fish. We had one meal of boiled cod and it wasn't popular, nothing like my mother used to cook.

I got on very well with the skipper and crew. I had had the

forethought to take on board, large supplies of Black Cat cigarettes, which I dispensed freely. I also had a go at everything except net making, of course. I gutted and packed and broke ice and helped to haul in at every trawl. I spent a lot of time when I could have been sleeping, on watch during the trawls and became quite reliable at the wheel. Conversation was not of an intellectual kind and the subjects rarely rose much above the belt. The language was not only broad Scots but also was liberally sprinkled with unmentionable expletives. One was wet permanently and got used to sleeping in moist clothes. Hands were constantly wet and sore and streaked with blood, fish scales and tar. Washing was an unknown phenomenon. I was told that the Chief Engineer was a chronic syphilitic, the Second Engineer had a woman in most of the Scottish fishing ports and I have mentioned Nathan who had just done a stretch. All members of the crew said they would like to get out of the trawling job. One told me that his son had a great job delivering milk, he wished he could get a cushy job like that. Apparently, what happened to these intentions when their boat arrived back in port was that after unloading they went to the nearest pub and got completely sloshed, finding themselves forty-eight hours later in an alcoholic haze, back on the trawler and waiting for the skipper to broach the out of bond liquor.

There are many things that remain in my memory about the Scottish trawlers and trawler men. One is the consummate skill shown in finding the best fishing grounds and their navigation in those grounds. Rarely is a chart used. The skipper looks at the sky and the sea and then announces the course, speed and time, after which he disappears into his cabin, presumably to sleep, and apparently completely confident of his bearings. If a trawl has produced a good yield he might put out a dan (or buoy) and steer away from it. After three hundred yards, one of these slender markers was invisible to me, but not to the skipper and crew. They would steer away from it for three hours, turn round and come back directly to it. Moreover, if when the dan was put out no other ships whatsoever were visible one could be sure that before your ship had had time to get back to pick up the buoy there would be three, four or five other trawlers steaming in the area. For this reason skippers were loathe to put out a dan if they had a good catch because it attracted competitors. The decision of the skipper as to when to stow the nets and make for the home port was governed by several considerations, not the least of which was news from the port with reference to market prices. Their share of the profits of the trip increased the wages of all the crew. If the skipper were not the owner, he received the largest share. The officers, that is the First and Second fishermen and the Chief and Second engineers got a lower share and the deckhands and firemen got a flat rate depending on the proceeds of the fish sale. Thus when prices were high it became a sort of poker game and then came the hectic run for home. On our voyage we didn't have a very big catch but we left the grounds after about sixteen days of trawling. All the crew were pleased when the skipper poked his head through the window and gave the signal to stow the tackle. After we had passed through the Firth I was accorded the privilege of steering the ship most of the way from off Rattray Head to Aberdeen. The weather had become quite warm and the sea was calm so when I had come off my watch I hauled up a bucket of sea water and stripped off my clothes for the first time since boarding the ship and had an all over wash, but, of course, with no soap. This caused huge amusement for the crew who gathered on deck to enjoy this phenomenal performance.

When we arrived in Aberdeen harbour I gathered my rather smelly and damp belongings into my kit-bag and after a sad farewell to my shipmates who, incidentally, tried to persuade me to go back for the next trip, I made my way to the Stroud office and paid my dues for the food I had eaten.

It's queer what odd things one can do in unusual situations. I went to the station to catch a train to Sheffield and went into a restaurant for a meal as I had an hour or so to spare and what did I order? Grilled cod and chips! The waiter told me it would take about a quarter of an hour to get it cooked and so I went to the washroom and looked in the mirror. I was filthy. The black on my neck had to be rubbed off in rolls with my fingers.

There is rather a sad tailpiece to this story. The George Stroud, after being unloaded at the end of our voyage, had to move to the coaling station at Torry to load up with coal for the next trip. On the way there she suffered an accident and sank.

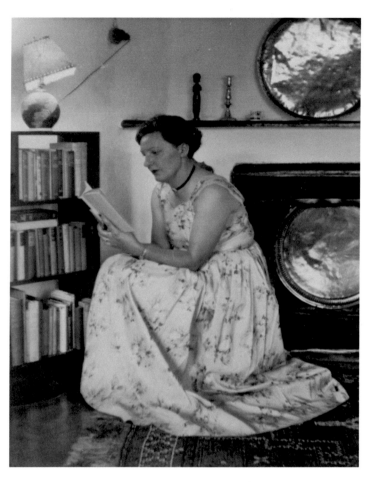

Kathy at home in Mpwapwa.

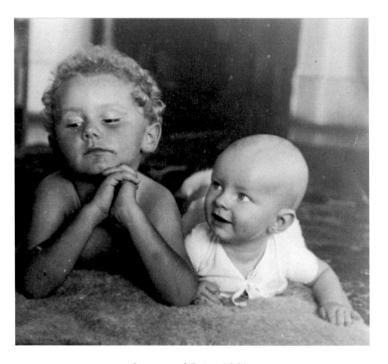

James and Peter 1951

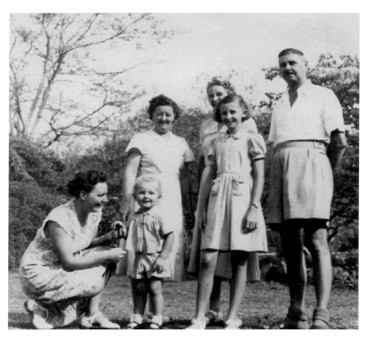

Kathy and James with Win, Ann and Laurie Griffiths.

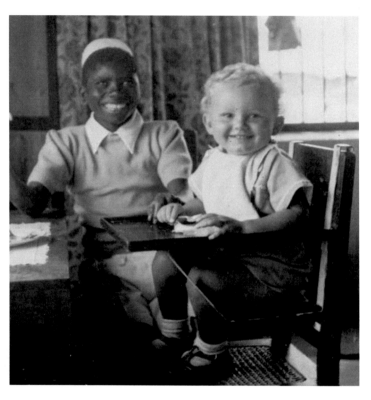

James with the nanny.

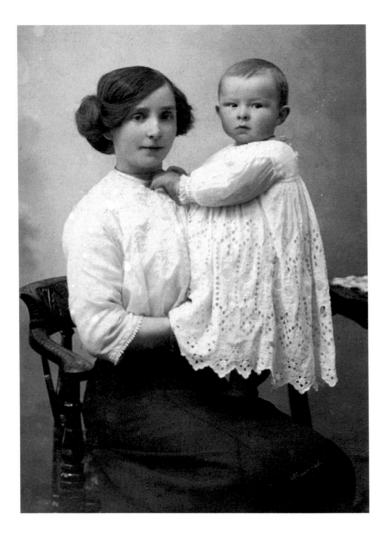

Jack, a few months old with Nanjie Comber

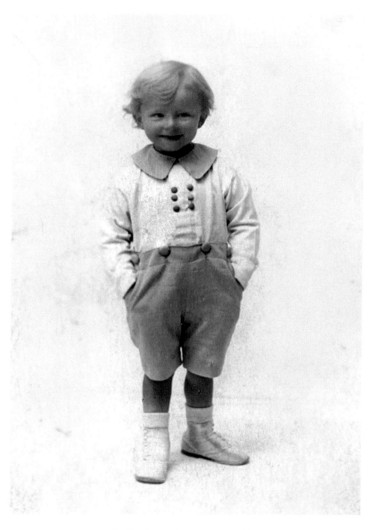

Jack about three years old.

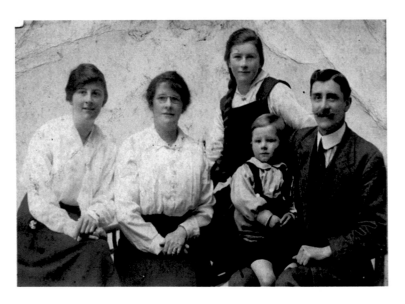

Win, Mum, Lily, Jack and Dad

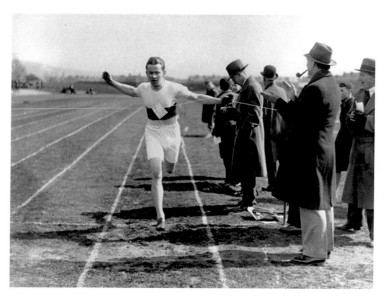

Last year at school – winning the school mile.

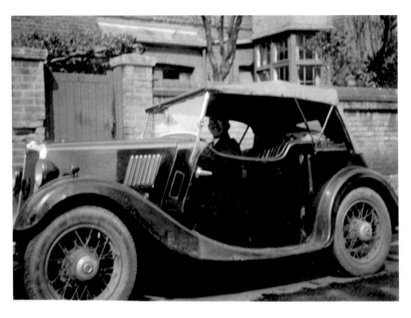

First car – a Morris Minor

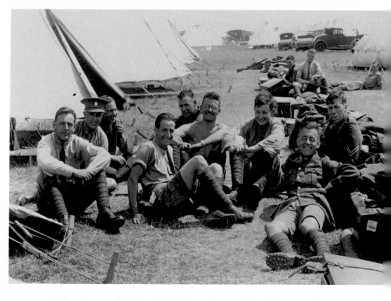

Relaxing at Officer Training Camp, Beachy Head

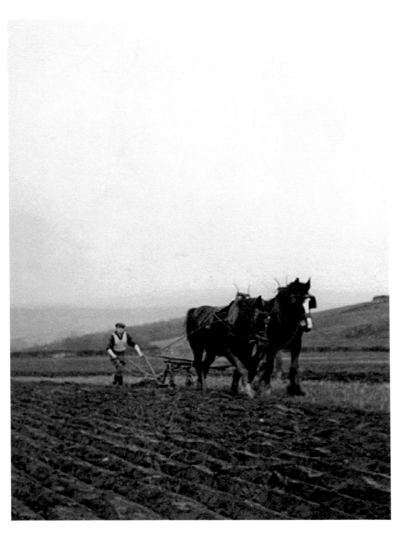
Jack ploughing in Derbyshire. There can't be many people now alive who have ploughed behind a pair of horses.

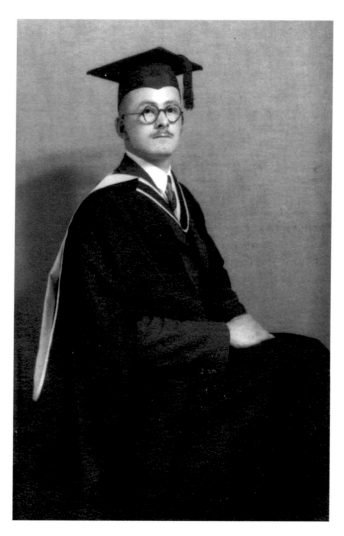

Graduation from Imperial College.

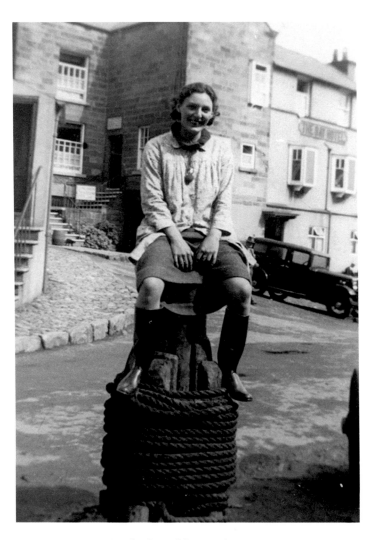

Kathy in Robin Hood's Bay.

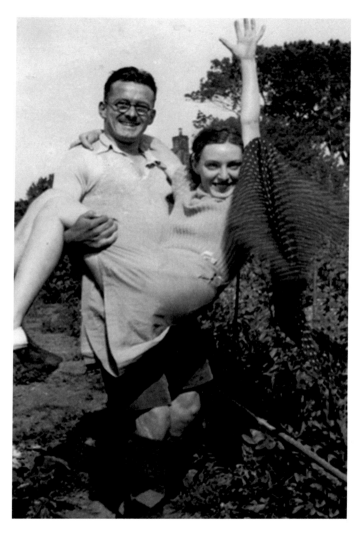

Happy Days in Fylingthorpe.

CHAPTER 2

Veterinary Training

Our graduation was in 1936 and we received our degrees in the Royal Albert Hall. The economy at that time was far from robust and I had to look around for a job in marine zoology in which I had decided to make my career. There was just nothing doing in that line and so I decided to stay on for a while in London where I would be more in touch with the academic job market. I had in mind the idea of finding a job as a chauffeur, which would enable me to live in or around London and so be available for any interviews which might arise. I discussed the situation with my Assistant Professor, Hewer, who told me about some scholarships in veterinary medicine, which were being offered by the Colonial Office. He asked me if I might be interested in doing the veterinary course. I said I certainly would be interested as I had spent quite a lot of my vacations working on farms but that the chances of going into veterinary medicine with its long course and the expense had never been presented to me as a possibility. Hewer said that this might be the very means of opening the veterinary field to me if I could face another four or five years as a student. I said I would be prepared to accept the idea. I, therefore, made enquiries and obtained the necessary forms of application and accordingly was invited to an interview.

I had little concept of the administrative situation with regard to colonies, dominions and dependencies but made my way to an office in Whitehall where I was ushered into an austere room with a large central table along three sides of which were disposed five important looking gentlemen. The fourth side

was furnished with an empty chair to which I was directed with the invitation to be seated. Opposite me, at the other end of the table, was seated the chairman who I later discovered was The Lord Irby. He asked me several questions about such things as whether I read books and if so what kind of books, what authors, what subjects and other aspects of my literary leanings. I was then quizzed on the subject of my interest in the colonies, and was required to recount why I wanted to work in the colonies. I pointed out that having completed my degree in zoology I wanted a job and I was prepared to start another course in Veterinary Medicine and Surgery if this was going to lead to a satisfactory and fulfilling career.

My inquisitors didn't appear to be thrilled with my interview and showed a certain degree of somnolence, probably due to having been persuaded to attend this interview by the offer of a good lunch. The chairman seemed to be winding up and asked me how I felt that I had got on in my final examinations. By a coincidence, I had received the news only that morning that I had obtained a First Class Honours degree. The members of the interviewing committee suddenly seemed to waken up and five pens were picked up and applied to the papers in front of them. They wished me well and I departed. Some days later I received a letter from the Colonial Office informing me that I had not been selected for a Veterinary Scholarship. This was very disheartening, but I decided to stay in London for a time and search around for some sort of job. Someone brought to my attention an advert for a job in the Burma Frontier Service. I had no idea what this service was and all I could find out about it was that it was a sort of military cum administrative service, apparently in the north of Burma. I decided to apply and I was offered an appointment. However, as I was about to accept the offer, another letter arrived from the Colonial Office saying that my application for a scholarship to the Royal Veterinary College had been reviewed. Details about the scholarship were given. If my memory serves me correctly, the scholarship would provide me with all college fees, £10 for books and the princely sum of £250 per annum to cover living expenses. I also had to provide someone to act as surety for what was quite a large sum of money against my either failing my professional exams or

failing to take up any post offered on my qualifying or failing to complete three years service in the post. My brother-in-law, Dr Laurence Griffith, who was an eminent sylviculturist in the Indian Civil Service agreed to act as my surety. I was most grateful to him and, of course, accepted the offer.

Accordingly, I entered the Royal Veterinary College in September 1936. In those days the only way of becoming a qualified veterinary surgeon in Britain was by completing the courses at one of the veterinary colleges and passing the examinations of the Royal College of Veterinary Surgeons. The whole course was one of five years and professional examinations were taken each year. The final examinations in medicine and surgery were taken at the end of the fifth year of study. Failure at the end of any one-year meant referral in the subject concerned and this could be repeated after six months further study. Failure in any subject twice meant expulsion from the college and the sinking of any hope of qualifying. In the light of my having a degree in Zoology I was exempted from the first year course and started my training in the second year. It was to be another twelve years before the veterinary colleges were incorporated into their corresponding universities. Then, the qualification, the Membership of the Royal College of Veterinary Surgeons, was replaced by a degree of the university and the diploma of membership, MRCVS, was automatically conferred. The Royal College of Veterinary Surgeons retained the function of visiting the various colleges to ensure that the standards of the MRCVS were maintained. I found myself among students approximately five years my junior in age as they had entered the college straight from school having obtained the necessary standards in 'A' levels. The standard of attainment in these 'A' Levels was and, I think, still is the highest required for any faculty in any British University. This is partly because there are only six Veterinary Colleges in the British Isles and the Republic of Ireland.

I found the courses in the veterinary college very different from those in the faculty in which I had studied previously. This was because the actual amount of factual knowledge that had to be memorised was vastly in excess of that in other faculties, except, of course in Medicine. The mass of material to be

absorbed was, as one might expect, very much increased by the necessity to study the anatomy, physiology, husbandry and diseases of all the major domestic animals, as diverse as the horse and the chicken. Lectures were, therefore, packed with detail and most students who had not had the benefit of a university education made a valiant attempt to get the lectures transferred to their note books verbatim. It certainly was a gruelling course. A further requirement of the qualification is that students must spend six months in a veterinary practice. This was usually fitted into vacations and one of the difficulties was finding practitioners prepared to take one on and give one real clinical experience. I was not seriously handicapped by missing the first year tuition as I had, in my vacations from Imperial College, spent quite a lot of time on a mixed farm in Derbyshire. I lived in at the farm on occasions and worked as a farm labourer. While doing this, I gained experience in handling heavy horses and was even instructed in the process of ploughing with their aid.

Very soon after starting in the RVC. I met another mature student who was also a Colonial Scholar, Fred Bell, a graduate in agriculture of Armstrong College, Newcastle. Fred and I became firm friends and remained so until long after we both retired. Fred was Emeritus Professor of Physiology of our old college and University. He died, sadly, of Alzheimer's disease in 1999. One of our first considerations was to find somewhere to live. While it was possible for me to return to Mrs Edwards', Fulham was rather a long way from Camden Town where the Royal Veterinary College was situated. The cost of transport by the Underground was also a matter of importance; however, I managed to get Mrs Edwards to take the two of us until we could find more conveniently situated digs, so we searched around for suitable accommodation nearer to the College. We tried a succession of rooms in and around the Camden Town, Highgate and Hampstead Heath areas. Most of them were unsatisfactory in various ways, but at last we settled for some digs in Dartmouth Park Avenue. The house was run by a retired Naval Officer who regaled us with graphic accounts of his heroic exploits in the First World War. We referred to him as the 'Commander'. His wife was a great admirer of Dr Marie Stopes.

She apparently regarded us as young men liable to fall by the wayside with unsuitable female acquaintances. She brought up to our room masses of books by Dr Stopes and pointed out to us the passages describing the various methods of contraception.

Another inmate of this lodging was a chap who worked in some rather obscure department of the civil service or an obscure organisation affiliated to it. He was a strange person and gave us advice on any matter which happened to turn up in conversation. He made his own marmalade and so we referred to him as Marmalade Joe. Our digs were cold and we were generally cold in them. Marmalade Joe, while also suffering from the frigidity of our rooms, had what he presented as a sovereign remedy for our reaction to the low temperatures which we had to suffer. His method was to strip off on arrival in his room in the evening and give himself a vigorous towelling. This method did not, to put it mildly, appeal to us and we resorted to wearing our dressing gowns and crouching over our very inadequate single bar electric fire. We bought a bottle of Big Tree Burgundy and a packet of panatela cheroots and persuaded ourselves that we were living the life of indigent but sophisticated students. Included in our lodgings were breakfast and an evening meal, which the Commander dignified with the title 'dinner'. One day we had a rabbit stew in the evening and we, ill advisedly as it proved, complimented the Commander on the tastiness of the dish. Thereafter we had rabbit stew about four times a week, rabbit being the cheapest meat available at that time. After a few weeks of this dish we found another lodging and bade the Commander and his wife a sad farewell. Our new landlady was a Mrs Lomond who had a house near the Parliament Hill Fields. Mrs Lomond was more the Mrs Edwards type and made us feel at home so that we became more like members of the family.

At that time there were about a dozen students in the college who were left over from the days when the veterinary course was one of four years and there was a much more relaxed curriculum with no provision for the expulsion of failers. Some of these students were the offspring of wealthy parents who could afford to pay the fees for tuition and all the other financial demands of student life as long as their sons, they were all sons,

were apparently occupied in some college or other and would eventually become capable enough to take over the family estates or businesses. The majority of them had cars, usually expensive ones. I remember one of them turning up at the college in a very large Rolls Bentley which took up much of the limited parking space available for staff and students. Their lifestyle was expensive and their attitude to lectures and practical work was casual in the extreme. They spent much of their time in the student's common room playing poker and devised various plans for arranging to have their names recorded in the attendance registers. Some of the more indigent students were attracted to this style of life but having been registered in the five year system could not afford to fail and so, as the time of the examinations approached there was a hectic and agonised resort to swatting with feverish approaches to the more industrious of their colleagues for the loan of notes and help with revision. Sadly, several of them fell by the wayside and had to repeat six months later at special Christmas exams. A few managed to scrape through at the second attempt but others disappeared from our ken forever.

The old four-year remnant was the cause of some noteworthy disturbances. On one occasion there was a near riot, which started in the 'ride', a covered area of soft bark and soil on which horses were exercised or tested for their action or for signs of lameness. The incident was triggered off by the stripping of one disliked student. This unfortunate individual was stripped stark naked and painted with an assortment of stains from the pathology lab, particular attention being paid to his genitals. I wasn't present at the time but I was informed that several of the female students were and that they took a lively interest in the activities. However, the fracas spread out of the ride and into the college buildings where one professor was damaged by a metal locker, dropped onto him from the stairs above. More students became involved and the performance went on well into the night. The following morning the casualties were assessed and I was given a graphic account of one of the wealthy students sitting in the office of Jimmy McCunn, the professor of anatomy, having a large scalp wound stitched up. The victim refused to go to the hospital and would

only rely on copious libations of whisky as an anaesthetic during the operation. The professor, Jimmy McCunn was not only a vet but also was medically qualified.

Formerly, almost all-veterinary students were males. It was not considered that the profession was a suitable one for the fairer sex. By the time I became a student, more females were being accepted into the veterinary colleges and in my year they made up about twenty-five per cent of the student intake. Most of them were good students and pleasant enough company. They broadly fell into two classes, the larger of which comprised those who were very assiduous in their studies, never missing a lecture, practical class or demonstration. They considered themselves the equals of any male students and made it quite obvious that they did not want any of the gentlemanly courtesies which most of us males, in those days, considered the rights of ladies, such as the raising of a hat or the deferring to their sex in the matter of seats in a crowded public vehicle. However, they were always at the front when it came to demonstrations or assisting at operations, when they would elbow their way to the front pushing other students, male or female, to one side. The remaining female students were those who exercised their charms on fellow students and even on lecturers and professors and who were very ready to accept assistance when the subject became a little difficult for them. Some of these made themselves very attractive to their fellow students. On the whole, most of the male students accepted the females comfortably and the atmosphere was harmonious and industrious. Most of the females in our year succeeded academically and made noteworthy members of their chosen profession. I'm ashamed to say that Fred and I played a rather dirty trick on a couple of the brightest members of the class who were females, Anne Russell and Stella Salmon.

The incident took place in the dissection room and we were at the stage of doing the anatomy of the dog. We students worked in pairs on the small animals and Anne and Stella occupied the slab next to us. When we came to open the cadaver abdomen, it was obvious that our dog, a male, had died with a full bladder. On pressing the full bladder I found that the penis delivered a stream of formalised urine in a vertical fountain.

Such a state called for proper investigation and so we emitted interested sounds such as ooh! and aah! and we peered intensely into the abdominal cavity. The reaction was as we had anticipated; the two girls rushed over and got their heads down over the abdomen at which point I pressed the bladder. It seemed funny at the time but as I indicated above, we were rather ashamed of our joke. The girls took it very well and they had a laugh themselves. Anne was a rather mysterious character. I think she was of German extraction and had been employed in some way or another by the British secret service. She was a good squash player and she and I had several games together at a local squash club, she almost always beat me. I have to say that our friendship was never more than completely platonic.

The abdication of Edward and the succession to the throne of George VI still provided a major subject of discussion among my new student friends in the RVC as, of course, the process was not complete until the end of my first term. Arguments continued heatedly in the students' common room. Soon, however, the intensity of the demands of this very exacting course of study pushed public affairs as subjects of discussion, very much into the background.

In the first year of our time at the RVC work of reconstruction to convert the old college into a modern building was nearing completion. We had to use temporary accommodation for some of our activities but were able to move into the new building in 1937. In November 1937, the new college was opened by His Majesty King George VI accompanied by Queen Elizabeth, later the Queen Mother. We were privileged to be guests at the ceremony and I will always remember the Queen waiting for the King who was in the gentlemen's cloakroom putting on his overcoat. She was standing next to me in the foyer and made pleasant conversation with those of us standing nearby. I was most impressed by the seeming normality of a wife waiting for her husband as in a theatre foyer after a performance.

We had, in our year, a Burmese student, Maung Hla Kyaw (pronounced Mowng Hla Jaw). He was young and inexperienced and so Fred and I took him under our wings and helped him over the strangeness of life in London for a newly arrived youth from

57

Burma. We got him a place in our digs and he soon found his feet. In the vacations we took him on holiday and introduced him to friends and veterinary surgeons who could help him out with seeing practice. He learned quickly and very soon was off on his own. One of his first adventures was a visit to Paris. On his return he regaled us with vivid descriptions of activities in certain sex dives, the likes of which I have never experienced to this day. He decided to move off on his own and found his own digs, which was a relief to us. He found a practice where he could go for his *extramural* experience in Yorkshire and there he married his landlady's daughter who was, presumably, carried away by this apparently exotic foreigner. After he had graduated he returned to Burma. I don't think he took his English wife with him but I suppose Burma swallowed him in the turmoil of the war and he never communicated with us again.

Our class contemporaries were, as one might expect, a mixed bunch. As I have said most of them had come to the college straight from school and quite a number were financed by affluent parents and consequently their studies were not as motivated towards academic success as were Fred's and mine. We found ourselves relating to junior lecturers more easily than the majority did. There was one member of the staff, Professor Amoroso, who, when he realised we were already graduates, would tack himself onto us when we decided to go to Kings Cross for a lunch or a beer at the pub. He never happened to have any cash on him and so 'borrowed' from us and conveniently forgot his debts. Amoroso was a West Indian, qualified in medicine and was quite brilliant as a scientist. The main subject of his research and what I suspect kept him in his job in the RVC was the embryology of various mammalian species. His methods of researching were manifestly lacking in organisation and, as I found out later in my career, he was a most unreliable academic.

One member of our class, Derek Greaves, became a close friend of Fred and me. His father was a very successful market gardener in north Lincolnshire. Derek was possessed of a brilliant brain and in terminal and annual class exams was always first in all subjects, carrying off almost all the gold medals and yet he never seemed to do much studying until the

week before the exams. Fred spent quite a lot of term time playing poker with those who were similarly inclined and being more mature than most of the other players did fairly well in the financial sense. He worked sporadically throughout the term and then towards the end of term relied heavily on my notes and underlines in the text books. Derek was an inveterate gambler. He would gamble on anything but his great delight, while we others were swatting, was to get to White City and gamble on the dogs. There was a little of the *loco parentis* in me for Derek and so he tried to hide from me his visits to the dog track. He joined us in our digs and watched my movements carefully so that he could slip out to the local betting shop without my knowing. We caught him one evening at the Archway Tavern playing darts with a rather mixed bunch of unsavoury individuals. He was feeling no pain as he had thrown three darts into the triple tops and all his cronies had celebrated with him in his success. At the end of term, Derek usually found himself in debt and with no cash and so he would pawn his rather expensive microscope rather than let it lie idle while he was away at home, a circumstance that he concealed from his father in the cause of family peace. On return from vacation with his normal monthly allowance he had to borrow from someone the necessary sum to redeem his microscope. I fortunately was able to help him out with a loan.

Some of our classmates led a rather sophisticated type of life. Three or four of the males joined up with three or four of the females and rented a large old house in which they ran their own domestic arrangements and cohabited in a rather relaxed and haphazard way. As far as we could gather there was no rigid linkage but a free-for-all based on convenience and interests of the moment. Their mode of life was regarded by the rest of us with varying degrees of envy. Towards the end of our college life, at the beginning of our fifth and final year, seven of us veterinary students found ourselves in digs in a house near the Archway Road run by a lady called, believe it or not, Mrs Boggis. One of our number was a most gentlemanly chap called Charles. He was what ordinary people in those days called a highbrow. He was very interested in ballet and opera and on some occasions I accompanied him to the ballet or theatre but

none of the others had much interest in such art forms. Foden often seemed to go off in the evenings and he was somewhat uncommunicative about his destinations. Sometimes we would hear him come in late at night, usually accompanied and we used to say 'Lucky for some, there's old Charles with one of his dollybirds'.

Sometime later, he and I were in the tube on our way to the ballet and Charles nudged me and, indicating a man in the seat opposite, whispered, "He's one of us. We can always tell." I, in my naivety, didn't understand and then suddenly the penny dropped and I realised he was talking about homosexuality. After that he told me all about his condition and that when we were at the ballet he was watching the crotches of the male dancers while he supposed I was interested in the anatomy of the ballerinas. He told me that he went for weekly visits to a consultant in Harley Street, the fees being paid by his mother who was under the impression that he was suffering from a nervous disease. When he went on his evenings out he was consorting with waiters and men at the docks and this also applied to the visitors whom he brought into his room.

Les Harries, from Wales, was another of our number in the Boggis digs. He was extremely temperamental and could be sent into a paroxysm of apprehension by a quiet remark and of course was ragged repeatedly without his realising it. He was always the last up in the morning but without any ablutions or shaving he would crash down the stairs into the dining room where the rest of us were halfway through breakfast. In his dressing gown he would flop into his chair and by the time we had finished our breakfast he would be in an easy chair reading the newspaper having gollupped his bacon, eggs, toast and coffee in five minutes flat. One day Les told us he had a girlfriend and he would like us to meet her. Mrs Boggis very kindly suggested that the lady should come and have her evening meal with us one day. She went to the length of making some very good cream confections for the sweet. The great day dawned and the young lady arrived. She was a lovely girl. We all thought her too good for Les. The first course was excellent and Mrs Boggis came in and asked if anyone would like a second helping. Several of the others said they would and so Mrs Boggis

gathered up the plates and went back into the kitchen returning in due course with the plates replenished.

Les immediately wolfed into the food before one of us, I can't remember who it was, looked at Les's plate and said, "Wasn't that your plate Charles?"

"Yes I think it was. I recognise that piece of bone on the side." Les stopped eating at once and slowly put his knife and fork on the plate and pushed it away.

When the cream confections arrived they were greeted with great anticipation and were undoubtedly appreciated. The snag was that the person sitting next to the young lady made a derogatory remark about Les and the lovely girl immediately sprang to his defence by planting a cream bun well and truly into his nostrils. Within seconds a bun fight ensued and buns were all over the room including the walls. As might be expected, Mrs Boggis was not amused and sanctions were imposed and reparations made but we all agreed that we had had a good party.

In my second year at the RVC my dad helped me to buy a small car. It was an old Morris Minor tourer which I bought with guidance from the garage proprietor who looked after my father's car. It cost about £150. I supported this expensive deal with the idea that I could use the car for my journeys to London and back home and also that it would facilitate my seeing practice as I could use my own car and live at home, travelling by its means to the Norfolk Street practice in Sheffield. The idea proved to be sound as the principal of the practice contributed financially to my expenses and gave me the opportunity to go on my own to see farmers and other clients in the area. My father had taught me to drive and I had held a driving licence since my seventeenth birthday.

In the summer of 1939 I was spending my vacation, as usual, in the Sheffield veterinary practice. I had passed my fourth year exams and was now prepared to do my final year. This was the position when World War II broke out in September. RVC students were informed by the College that the buildings at Camden Town would be closed down. Arrangements were being made for the final year students to continue their studies in temporary facilities in Streatley on Thames, however, necessary arrangements could not be in place

until January 1940 and students were advised to continue seeing practice until the end of the year.

The principal of the Norfolk Street practice, David Caldwell, was very happy to keep me on and paid me a small wage, reimbursing me for the use of my car. I was thus employed as a trainee assistant and acquired some very useful experience. Fred Bell, having been referred in one subject took the opportunity to repeat the last term of the fourth year course at the Edinburgh Royal Dick Veterinary School and passed and so could start up with us at Streatley. The normal three terms of the final year were crammed into the six months to June when we took our finals. It was a very hard and onerous academic six months.

In addition to our studies almost the entire male membership of the year joined the Upper Thames Patrol of the newly formed Local Defence Volunteers which later became generally known as 'Dad's Army'. We had to do night patrols and get our studies done between very much abbreviated periods of sleep. One of the class, Brian Leach, refused to join. He said that this was not his war as he was Irish and in any case he wanted all the time he could get for swatting. Like Fred and me he was a Colonial Scholar being supported by the British Government.

The summer of 1940 was a good one so that much of our night patrol duty was done in the dry. We were warned to keep a keen lookout for Germans who, it was said, might be parachuted into the south of England disguised as nuns. I think that it was at that point that we were issued with five rounds of live ammunition. To my discredit I must say that one night I fell asleep and was later wakened by my partner on the patrol and found myself nestled in a pile of stone chippings. Amazingly, in spite of the demanding nature of our days in Streatley, we had quite a lot of fun and high spirited rough and tumble.

Despite entering into the 'Dad's Army' effort with energy and strong will, we felt that we should be getting into the armed forces. I wrote to Lord Irby explaining my feelings and putting forward my qualifications gained in the OTC. I stressed my A and B certificates and my first class marksmanship success, which latter I think was probably obtained more by good luck than skill. I asked to be relieved of my bond in order that I could

enlist in the infantry. The reply was polite and appreciative but I was informed that my veterinary training made my completion of qualification and posting to the Colonial Service of much greater importance than my training as an infantryman. I accepted this and buckled down to the necessity of passing my final exams. Later, when I was in my post in Tanganyika, I did take up the matter again with the Colonial Office in London and also with the Chief Secretary in Dar es Salaam. Again I was told that my job in Tanganyika and the work of getting food to our troops in North Africa overrode my attempts to get into the fighting services. My effort also caused a little friction with my Director.

During this final year Fred and I and some of our friends were living in Streatley House that had been converted into classrooms and labs with dormitories on the third storey. Professor Wright, universally known as 'John George' who was head of surgery, was designated 'Warden' for the duration. As a fire safety measure, some contraptions for lowering the upstairs inmates to the ground had been installed. These were fixed near to the windows and so naturally we felt the need to try them out In order to make the descent one had to hitch oneself into a sling and slide off the windowsill. The weight of the body pulled the rope down through a geared device, which enabled the escapee to sink slowly to the ground. Meanwhile the sling at the other end of the rope came up ready for the next person to make the descent. It was decided that Derek Greaves should be the first to try the device and so he got into the sling and sat on the windowsill. "You'll be all right," we said, "we will hold on here if it goes down too quickly." Accordingly he slid off the windowsill and started down. He showed a tendency to twist round and swing into the wall: by the time he was halfway down he was twisting rather rapidly. We stopped the rope from going through the gear and Derek swung round smartly and put his foot straight through the windowpane, which was alongside. This proved to be the window of John George's study. We were all called to the professorial study and asked for an explanation. We were suitably contrite and explained that we were only trying the safety mechanism to make sure that we would be able to use it in an emergency. John George, normally a rather severe

pedant, said that he accepted our explanation and we were not even made to pay for a new windowpane.

A colourful contemporary Colonial Scholar was Bill Luke. He was a great character and an entertaining companion. He was given to a little excess of alcohol intake from time to time and when in his cups was very amusing. He formed an attachment with Alison Esdaile, one of our classmates. She was a bundle of fun and naughtiness and could be outrageously entertaining at a party. She passed her final exams at the first shot but Bill was referred in one subject owing more to his inclination for fun rather than to any lack of intellectual ability. When we qualified in June 1940, Fred and I were among those living in Streatley House. The house was near to the Swan Inn. Bill joined up with Alison in a job, running the Swan until he was successful in his exams at Christmas 1940. I well remember on the day when Fred and I and our successful colleagues were informed that we had qualified, there was a great euphoria and celebration. Bill's referral did not deter him from joining in the rejoicing. I can see him now in one of the dormitories where we were gathered together. He was stark naked except for a straw boater on his head, proposing a toast to his friends who had passed. The door opened and in strode Professor John George Wright. Without batting an eyelid, the professor addressed Bill in his usual precise terms on some subject of a completely impersonal matter, which he wished to discuss with Bill. Some time later, when Bill and Alison, now honourably married, were in Kenya, we arrived in the same country having just left Nigeria. We became good friends. The pair by this time had become very domesticated with a growing family. We learned that it was in one of the dormitories in Streatley House that Sue, their first child, had been conceived.

Another friend, who was a bit of a harum scarum character, was John Scott. He was involved in an incident that we found amusing. He was picked up by the police in the West End one evening when he had drunk rather too much and was causing a nuisance. When he arrived at the desk in a well-known police station the desk sergeant asked him for his name, which he gave. When he was asked for his address he replied. "Maidstone Jail." As one might expect this sort of nonsense did not meet with

approval. However, the misunderstanding was cleared up when John explained that his father was the governor of Maidstone Jail and that indeed was his home. He was let off with a caution. When he qualified, John Scott joined the Royal Army Veterinary Corps. He was eventually posted to Burma and served on the infamous Burma Road campaign. We lost touch with John as well as with Derek Greaves who also joined up as soon as he had qualified. I met John many years later in Ethiopia where he was working in a United Nations research laboratory helping in the campaign against foot and mouth disease in cattle. It was from him that I had the last news of Derek. He also had been posted to the same theatre of war. He, in his usual way decided to do 'something different', I am sure that it must have been just for risk and the excitement. He wangled a trip in one of the RAF planes, which were flying across the frightening Patkai Mountain range. These flights were initiated by Squadrons 31 and 194 transporting materials from Northeast India to China, the 'Hump Crossing'. The flight on which Derek hitched a lift never came back. Major John Scott OBE had no more details. Unfortunately he is no longer with us. Derek's last gamble meant the loss of someone who would have made a real contribution to veterinary science. A sad and unnecessary adventure.

The time for the final examinations came and the usual stress and apprehension attacked us all. No matter how hard one has worked and how assiduous one has been, the anxiety of final exams is an awful episode in life. The writtens are completed; the chances of mistakes are turned over and over in one's mind, failure is imminent. I think that this state of mind is present in all serious students, whatever they might say subsequently. I am sure that the anxiety and stress is worse for medical and veterinary students than for those in any other faculties. I feel that this is due to the very mass and variety of facts that must be committed to memory in these subjects. When it came to my *viva* in veterinary medicine I nearly flopped. My external examiner was a Major in the RAVC and he was a bastard in addition to being a very bad examiner. The first question that he put to me was, "What makes a cow vomit?" In our course we had been told that the cow does not vomit, it merely ruminates. This formed the basis of my answer to the question. "Well," said

the major. "I tell you that a cow can vomit, so what causes vomiting in a cow?" I thrashed about in my brain for some possible cause of vomiting in the cow including the possibility of an excess of unripe apples in an orchard. This was all to no effect. My state of mind at this point can be easily visualised.

My professor of medicine, affectionately called 'Uncle George' who was internal examiner said, "Don't you think, Major Wortley, that it would be a good idea if you tried to find out what Wilde knows rather than flog a dead horse that he doesn't know?" It transpired that a letter had appeared in the Veterinary Record a few weeks earlier from a practitioner who had treated a cow vomiting due to bracken poisoning. This was so unusual as to stimulate the vet concerned to write to the Record about it. It could have caused my downfall in the hands of such an incompetent examiner. Many years later when I was examining students for higher post graduate degrees and diplomas I made sure at the beginning of the *viva* that I put the candidate at ease and usually after, a preliminary chat, went into the subject in question gently and smoothly.

Immediately before the final examinations, Brian Leach, to whom I have referred before, received a letter from the Colonial Office informing him that if he passed his finals satisfactorily he would be posted to Nyasaland at once. Fred Bell, who it will be remembered, had to resit one of his fourth year subjects, also received from the Colonial Office, intimation that he would be posted to Uganda, subject to his qualifying in the forthcoming exams. I naturally expected similar intimation, though none arrived for me. Naturally I was somewhat annoyed. Here were an Irish republican and a student who had failed one of his examinations given the fillip of knowing that they had a job to go to while I who had passed all the stages in the curriculum mostly with high positions in the class and with some medal awards apparently was not to receive an immediate posting. I was, naturally, very upset but thought it better to take no action about the situation and concentrated on getting qualified. When the results came out and all three of us had passed satisfactorily, I made an appointment with Lord Irby, the appropriate authority, and visited him as I passed through London on my journey home. I put my views to him and he was apparently very

understanding. He explained that a post in research was expected to become vacant in the near future and that the Colonial Office had earmarked me for the job. I remember vividly that he said to me that of the three Colonial Scholars, who had just qualified, I was the one they expected to make a career of the Service and make a mark in tropical diseases. He advised me to go home and keep my hand in by taking a temporary job in practice. I would shortly be appointed and would have to hold myself ready to go out to Africa to a research job. I was, of course, mollified and departed for King's Cross station to take the first train home. Irby's forecast, whether he meant it seriously or not, was proved correct as Fred did only the required one tour in Uganda and I believe that I was the only Colonial Scholar to serve to retirement.

In the last year, much of the teaching had been devoted to surgery. I had used my artistic ability to record most of the operations in a special notebook. Each operation was illustrated in colour showing all the stages from first incision to the last suture. One of our classmates, Albert True, who had failed his surgery and had to repeat in the following December, asked me if I would lend him my surgery notes. In the euphoria I agreed to lend him my book of illustrations. Sadly, that was the last I ever saw of it. Many were the times in my career when I regretted the loss of my surgery notebook.

My old friends in the Sheffield practice were pleased to take me on in a temporary capacity until such time as I received my sailing orders. I was therefore, accorded the remuneration of one guinea per day and an allowance for petrol. This was not bad for a starter in those days and as my home was on the Derbyshire outskirts of Sheffield, I was able to live at home and manage on the pay, which I received. The Principal of the practice had been a very experienced vet but had died of heart failure in my arms on the floor of his office during one of my 'seeing practice' spells when I was a student. The future of the practice had been very unpredictable but the assistant, David Caldwell, who had only qualified a few years before I did was enabled to take over the practice and he employed another young vet, David Thomson. This David was a very Scottish Scot. He felt it necessary to instruct me in all the features of Scotland and the Scots that

made the Scottish nation and Scottish achievements the finest in the world and certainly superior to those of the miserable English. I took this with a grain of salt and managed to retain my equanimity and, indeed we became firm friends.

Of course, the war was now on in no uncertain terms and the German bombing had begun. My father had erected an Anderson shelter in the garden and when the raids started on the cities other than London, my mother and father, and my sister Win and her daughter Ann, who were on leave from India when the war broke out, were all ready to use the shelter when necessary. I well remember the night when the bombers made Sheffield their target. This was not only a case of the sirens going off but was the real thing. In our shelter we listened to the sound of the bombing coming ever nearer. At one point we realised that something had been left in the sitting room that we required, I forget what it was, but I decided to go into the house and retrieve it. I was in the sitting room when there was an almighty crash. I distinctly remember the large heavy sofa literally jumping off the floor. I thought the bomb must have fallen in our garden and hastened out to see if the rest of the family had been damaged. It transpired that this bomb had fallen just under a mile away on the road to the city. In the morning I tried to get in to our surgery that was in the centre of Sheffield. It was impossible to drive any further than Beauchief and so from there I made my way on foot having to climb over rubble and avoid bomb craters. It was a scene of devastation. Apparently, sticks of bombs had been dropped along the main road from the centre of the city to the south, the pilots having overrun their obvious targets that were the great steel works on the north east of the city. Our surgery was unscathed and so we set to work as well as we could with the transport available. As veterinary surgeons we were authorised to perform special services in connection with livestock. I still have my certificate of authority signed by the Chief Constable. The clearing up of the extensive damage to Sheffield took quite a long time and this made our job of getting out to the farms and other places where we had veterinary work to do, difficult and time consuming. It was most impressive, however, how repairs and renovations were rapidly carried out and how we and everyone else managed to improvise and

surmount the obstacles posed to our routine life.

During my spell of a few months in the Sheffield practice there were some interesting and bizarre occasions. One of my jobs was the inspection of the large numbers of pit-ponies used in the coalmines. For this purpose I had to go down into the mines to the underground stables in order to examine all the animals in the pits. The inspection had to be made at the weekend before the last shift had come up on Saturday morning. The stables were invariably in the oldest part of the pit and were reached by walking, theoretically, along the main roads. In several of the pits, the stables could be reached by taking short cuts through old workings. The Veterinary Inspector was very much in the hands of the chief horsekeeper on these occasions and so, most often, the short cut was taken. This often entailed crawling under low and frighteningly ominously old and creaking wooden supports. The ponies were always in very good condition, sleek, well-fed and groomed, with shiny coats. The miners who handled them were very proud of their charges and took a pride in their fitness and well being. I went down several pits and became used to the process of being dropped at great speed down the shafts. Only once did I have a really disagreeable job to do. That was with a pony that had fallen into a grease box and broken its leg. I had to destroy the poor creature.

I was introduced to the pit-pony inspection duty by David Thomson who had been doing it before I qualified. He took me to do the inspection at Tinsley Main pit one Saturday morning. We came up with the last shift for the weekend. David felt that we should take the horsekeeper, as a friendly gesture, for a drink, and so we repaired to the Fisherman's Arms. David, who was wiser in these circumstances than I, ordered the first round of drinks.

"Three pints of bitter."

"No no! Bill" interjected our horsekeeper (we'll call him George for the purpose of this anecdote.) "Three specials," he said. Accordingly, three pints of black liquor were served to us, I must say it was a very smooth drink. George demolished his pint in very short time, telling us that he usually had eight of these libations of a Saturday before he went home for his dinner. I felt

that it was up to me to buy a round and so I ordered three specials. It was heavy going for me but I struggled on and tried to diminish the black liquor in my glass. David, who was driving, as unobtrusively as possible, tipped most of his pint into my glass. George called up another three pints in spite of all my efforts to restrain him. I could stand up in the pub but when we stepped out into the fresh air, my legs gave way. The result was that I became completely drunk for the first and last time in my life. David got me into the back of the car where I remained asleep for about six hours.

Another job, which fell to me, was to act as track surgeon to one of the greyhound racetracks. This I found rather boring as I had to examine all the dogs in their racing kennels in the late afternoon of the race meeting and then had to examine each dog when it came out for the parade before each race. It was also imperative that I was present until the last race was run. I then had the business of getting away in my car among the crowds of race patrons, often only to find, when I arrived back at the surgery that there was a message for me to visit a farm miles out of town for a clinical job, possibly a calving, a milk fever or a horse with colic.

During this period of my assistantship I experienced one of the situations which come into the life of people who find themselves carrying what seems to be an inordinately heavy responsibility. It happened in this way. In our practice we held contracts with the two registered greyhound tracks in Sheffield. The bigger of the two was Owlerton Greyhound Racing Track, which was looked after by the principal, David Caldwell. I was assigned to the Darnall track. This was under the chairmanship of an ex-naval Commander, who had a reputation for brooking no opposition. The track, training and racing kennels were ruled by the Commander with a rod of iron. Everything had to be right or he would want to know why the hell it wasn't. All the trainers and kennel lads held the Commander in great awe. The big day of the year for the Darnall Track was Boxing Day when every greyhound on the books had to be available for a once a year occasion. Instead of having the normal Saturday evening card of six races, the great Boxing Day meeting started at 2p.m. and consisted of (if my memory serves me rightly) eighteen races.

That meant that there had to be in the region of a hundred dogs fit to run. The racing kennels were full to capacity and the race cards for the occasion were printed, the turnstiles were manned and the car parks were cleared as large crowds of excited dog racing fans were expected. It was the biggest money spinner of the year for the Darnall track.

At 6a.m. on Boxing Day I was awakened from my post Christmas slumbers by a telephone call from the racing kennels. Nearly half the dogs in the kennels were scouring that meant that they were in the throes of a severe attack of diarrhoea. The significance of this news was indeed dire in more senses than one. I shook off the somnolence of the night after Christmas, dragged on some clothes, jumped into my small car and drove to the practice surgery. My mind was a turmoil of thoughts on what could be done for diarrhoea in the canine subject. The obvious treatments could, with luck, have the dog on its feet and beginning to look normal in a couple of days but we didn't have two days nor did we have enough of the normal medicaments to dose fifty odd squittering greyhounds. I opened up the surgery and sought and found a large carton of powdered china clay, used for making up bottles of diarrhoea mixture. I acquired, I don't remember how or where, a bottle of brandy and raced away to the kennels. The whole kennel staff was anxiously awaiting my arrival. I set up a treatment table and got the staff to find for me a large washing bowl into which I transferred copious amounts of the chalky powder, stirred to a cream with water. I mixed into it a liberal dose of brandy and dished out a mug or two of the golden liquid to the distraught staff and then had the boys bring the affected dogs to me. I gave each one a rapid examination and then spooned into it a large dose of the mixture. This treatment having been completed on all the affected dogs I left with the instruction that all the animals must be kept under observation especially as regards any bowel evacuations which occurred, until I returned three hours later.

When I did get back after my breakfast, there was a distinct improvement in most of the dogs. I examined each one and watched them carefully as they were walked up and down for me. It must be easy to imagine what a turmoil was going on in my mind. Here was I, a very recently qualified vet, with the

critical decision of immense importance in my hands. Were the dogs going to be fit enough to race in about five hours time or were they not? The entire weight of the Boxing Day meeting was fairly and squarely on my shoulders. If I said "No" then the whole meeting with all its implications, would be cancelled. I examined all the dogs again, clinically. I went into the office. The Commander had already been informed by telephone. I rang his number and told him the position saying that I would stay and observe the animals closely for an hour and then let him have my decision. That was an anxious hour. The scouring had stopped and the dogs were looking brighter and, indeed appeared to be quite normal. All the staff, of course, were anxiously watching with me. The chief trainer said to me, "If the meeting is on, some of these dogs will be shitting china plates on the parade." This was a reference to the custom at greyhound races of parading the participants in each race, immediately before the race, in front of the stands. Several of the dog race cognoscente based their choice of a possible winner on whether or not the animal emptied its bowel or bladder during the pre-race parade. The critical moment came and I decided to let the dogs run. The meeting was a great success as a sport and financially. In expansive mood at the end of the evening the Commander sought me out and asked me, somewhat *soto voce* if I had given the dogs anything to pep them up as quite a lot of them had turned in unexpectedly good times.

During my fairly brief sojourn in the Sheffield practice I became somewhat of an expert in performing an operation for 'jumped toe' in racing greyhounds. This entailed the removal of one of the dislocated bones in the digits while retaining the pad so that the animal could return to racing without losing any of his speed. There was, undoubtedly some skulduggery among the unlicensed dog racing community and even in my short time in practice I was approached by one of these people with an offer for me to do something to slow a dog down. He didn't try it on a second time. Some of these people, I understand, adopted the idea of putting a tight rubber band round two of the toes to effect a slowing in a race.

In those days a lot of use was made of heavy horse breeds both on the farm and in the city where horse drays were a

common means of transport. Our practice was contracted to a lot of these heavy horse users including the railway, the breweries and the steel and engineering works. We had an extensive farm and small animal practice, which covered large areas of south Yorkshire and north and east Derbyshire. We had clients as far north as Wakefield and south into the Sherwood area and sometimes had to go into Lincolnshire, so the practice gave us a great variety of work.

Visits to remote farms could be a source of real difficulty especially at night and in snowy weather. The difficulties were exacerbated by the war as direction signs were none existent and at night we had to drive by the faint illumination afforded by shielded lights. I remember one day being called out to a farm in south Yorkshire to examine a young heifer with a haemorrhage. Believe it or not, the owners of the farm were two brothers called Hezekiah and Ebor Crapper. It was a very foggy day and so Hezekiah, who was my caller, gave me explicit instructions as to how to find the farm and said he would be at the lane end sitting on a sack of potatoes. Sure enough, when I found the farm there was Hezekiah in the fog, sitting on his sack of potatoes. We went down to the cattle shed where my prospective patient was tied up in a stall. I realised that a rectal examination was necessary and so asked Hezekiah to bring a bucket of hot water with soap and a towel whilst I divested myself of my upper garments. The farmer brought the necessaries and while I proceeded with the intrusion of my arm into the rectum Hezekiah marched up and down the shed behind me singing out in a loud voice, "When the lord came over the Jordan..." He paused to inform me that he and his brother were strong Wesleyans and sang every Sunday in the chapel choir. As the strains of the hymn resounded through the shed the heifer decided to let out at me with one of her hind hooves, catching me in a vulnerable place. I let out a rather un-Wesleyan expletive. At this, the farmer stopped in the middle of his rendition and said, "Young man, never worry about your bad language, me and my brother are aces at it ourselves." The heifer made a good recovery and no doubt I was regarded as a reasonable young vet.

The short period during which I was in veterinary practice

was very interesting and instructive. Apart from the fact that we were at war and I was champing at the bit about getting to my future work in the Colonial Service, I really enjoyed the work and established very happy relations with my fellow vets and many of the clients. I particularly enjoyed the heavy horse and farm animal side of the practice and, as far as I was involved with heavy horses, I was fortunate, as these loveable animals were soon to disappear from the general farm and transport scene.

In late November I received a letter from the Colonial Office to inform me that I was to be appointed as a Veterinary Research Officer to the Government of Tanganyika. I was instructed to hold myself in readiness to embark at short notice for the journey to East Africa. My excitement was intense and I poured over maps of Africa and discovered where this exotic country was. A telegram arrived in early December giving me a date of sailing from Glasgow. I received advice as to what things I should take with me and these included clothing and household effects such as crockery, bed linen, mosquito nets and mosquito boots and there were many more pieces of advice most of which were found, subsequently, to be useless. My sister, Win who, as I mentioned before, was home on leave from India, insisted on taking me to Liverpool where there was a tropical outfitters establishment. So, off we went to Messrs Lawn and Alder in Liverpool, staying overnight at the Adelphi Hotel. My sister, having lived in India for some years, advised on the items to be purchased. Two of these items she rated as of utmost importance, namely a pair of mosquito boots and a solar topee. Accordingly I purchased a very fine pair of boots made of soft Morocco leather. The hat which she chose was what, in the Indian Service was called a 'pig-sticker'. This was a handsome pith helmet with a quilted cover and Win assured me that it was the approved headgear of all European Officers in India. When I appeared in this magnificent hat after I arrived in Africa, it caused such mirth that I promptly gave it away to an Indian duka wallah in the village. As for the mosquito boots, I wore these on a few occasions but they caused such an amount of incredulous interest among my fellow officers that I put them away and, indeed I still have them practically as new as they were on the

day when I purchased them.

There then followed a string of telegrams from the Colonial Office alternately giving instructions for embarking and cancelling these instructions. This happened several times and I began to think that I would never get away. At last I received instructions to present myself and my baggage at a dock in Liverpool. As this had not been rescinded the day before the date given in the telegram I realised that this was it. I had been given no details as to the ship in which I was to sail and so in the darkness of a cold January morning, my father took me to our local station together with my trunk and cases and I started on my journey to Liverpool and beyond. It was an emotional parting. My mother, particularly, was very upset. Here was her only son bound for far away and unknown parts over a sea, which, at the best of times, had its dangers but which in wartime, was virtually lethal. I have to admit that I was a bit choked myself but once on the journey my mood turned to an anticipatory excitement.

I had to cross from one station in Manchester to another and then found myself in Lime Street, Liverpool. There was a scene of great activity. Many people seemed to be bound for Africa and a group of porters grabbed my trunk and cases with the question, "Madura, Sir?" It appeared that our ship must be called the 'Madura'. Everything at that time was so secret that I had been given not a hint of the name of the ship in which I was to travel but apparently everyone in Liverpool knew. The SS Madura was a liner of the British India Line (the BI). I hoped that providence would deliver my goods on board but I didn't know that they were safely there until several hours later when I was aboard myself. And so I found myself in a queue in the Princes Dock, slowly moving forward to pass through the gates where we were wished God speed by a clerical gentleman who, I was given to understand, was the Dean of the Cathedral. He had a very sad countenance as though he was bidding farewell to the condemned.

There followed a journey by sea that was, I suppose, unique. The first night we were aboard the SS Madura, we were moved away from the dockside and anchored in the middle of the river Mersey. There was an air raid on Liverpool but we were

unscathed and, surrounded by a large convoy of ships, moved out to sea on the morning of Sunday 12th January 1941. We were with the convoy until the 18th after which we were on our own. I have described this voyage in some detail in my book, 'Wilde Tales from Africa'. Suffice it to say that the voyage was certainly extraordinary in comparison with a voyage from Britain to East Africa in times of peace. What should have taken about eighteen days took fifty days, thanks to the wartime problems. Many ships were being sunk at that time but we were lucky and got to our destination unscathed. Recently (Year 2003) I have been watching a series of episodes on the television, showing the devastating destruction wreaked on allied shipping by the Nazi U-boats in 1940. Hundreds of British and allied ships were sunk and convoys were decimated in the Atlantic. The scenes of horror with people attempting to swim in burning oil or freezing, heaving seas were heart rending. It is possible that SS Madura came through unscathed because of the very fact that she was abandoned by our convey as her speed was so slow. The U-boats apparently concentrated their attacks on the conveys. Seeing all this has made me aware of the awful fears and heartaches which must have been suffered by my mother and father. Radio silence, of course, was strictly imposed and so they could have assumed that our ship had been sunk along with the others. I believe that SS Madura was put on the lost list until her arrival in Freetown was signalled to Britain. It is most likely that my parents did not even know the name of the ship in which I sailed.

After leaving Freetown, our voyage was reasonably normal. Of course, blackout was observed and all able-bodied male passengers had to perform lookout duties day and night in spells of, I seem to remember, four hours. The sight of Capetown, brilliantly illuminated at night, was wonderful to us and we went ashore with a strange sense of normality. Thereafter, the voyage resumed its wartime routine and faced the hazards of enemy action. The most dangerous part was the passage through the Beira Straights. We were given to understand that there was a well organised Nazi spy system operating in this area. Allied shipping suffered losses in the Mosambique Channel but we managed to make the passage without being attacked. We did not go into Dar es Salaam which was my official destination but

completed the voyage in Mombasa where we arrived on the 3rd of March. After a night in the Avenue Hotel, I made my way to Tanganyika via rail to Moshi with a night in the hotel there and then by rail to Korogwe. From there to Morogoro on the Tanganyika Central line I travelled by lorry. After a short stay in another hotel, I caught the main line train from Dar es Salaam, arriving at my station, Mpwapwa, on Friday the 7th March 1941.

CHAPTER 3

Colonial Service in Tanganyika

When I arrived in Mpwapwa, I was greeted by Sammy Evans, Senior Veterinary Research Officer and head of the laboratory. However, the Director of Veterinary Services, Bertie Lowe, was away and Sammy was temporarily Acting Director in charge of Head Office. He took me round the laboratory and its immediate environs and introduced me to the African Veterinary Assistants working in the laboratory and the Goan Clerk, Mr J.C.Almeida who would be my clerical assistant. After this, Sammy pushed off to Head Office, which was about a quarter of a mile away but was linked to the laboratory by a rather primitive telephone line. If I needed any help I was to call him on the phone. "Did I need any help?" was the understatement of the year. Mr Almeida and two of the senior Africans spoke English but it was in a limited and rather quaint manner.

In East Africa officers of all departments accepted that the indigenous people with all their problems were the first responsibilities. This attitude was fostered to its greatest extent in Tanganyika, which was not a colony but was administered by the British under a mandate of the League of Nations. The necessity for officers in the various services to be proficient in the *lingua franca* Swahili was therefore more rigorously adhered to than in the other East African territories. We had to pass the lower standard Swahili examination before we could be confirmed in our appointments. As far as I was concerned with the work of the laboratory I managed to grasp the essentials and carry on the routine work. I had spent much of my time on the voyage out learning Swahili with the aid of an Education

Officer, Ouseley from Uganda, who was returning in the Madura. I soon became fluent in the language and was even asked to act as an examiner in the oral tests of entrants for the Lower Standard qualification.

Swahili in its pure form as opposed to the so called 'kitchen Swahili' spoken by the Kenya settlers and most of the Asian population is a delightful musical language. It has a complicated, regular grammar and many incursions from English, Arabic, German and other languages which had been made necessary by the introduction of western inventions. An example of this is the word for a motor car, which is 'motokaa'. To cope with these introductions in some instances intriguing devices were resorted to as in 'gari ya moshi' for a railway train. Gari is the Swahili for a cart, ya means of, and moshi means smoke. The railway, of course, was a most significant introduction from the west.

Mpwapwa, a small outstation in the Central Province of Tanganyika Territory (as it was then, since, following amalgamation with Zanzibar, known as Tanzania.) was the Headquarters of the Veterinary Department. The main veterinary part of the station was in an area called, locally, Kikombo which was about half a mile from the actual village with its 'dukas' – Swahili for shops. At the opposite side of the village were the boma or administrative offices and one of the large secondary schools of the country.

Kikombo was a cupshaped valley (Kikombe is the Swahili word for a cup), reaching into an escarpment of rocky profile which sheltered the Veterinary station from the north. A stream arose from the foot of the escarpment and provided the water supply of the three areas. In the highest part of the valley were the buildings of the laboratory. Below these were the houses for the officers and the general workshops and further down still was the Head Office of the Department. A rough red earth road left the valley here and ran down alongside the stream to the village and thence for twelve miles through ragged thorn bush to the central railway line with its small station at Gulwe.

The function of the Veterinary Department, as in most tropical countries, is the control of disease in domestic animals and the development of a healthy and productive population of the country's livestock. An efficient veterinary service, therefore,

depended on a staff of veterinarians supported by livestock officers, technicians and administrative officers and in the case of countries with large wild animal populations, wild life experts. Tanganyika was a country of about 360,000 square miles of land with a massive variety of animals, vegetation, and topographical features as well as a great number of tribes with their own particular languages and tribal customs. Some of these are pastoralists, a large proportion nomadic and others are arable farmers but most of them live on a subsistence level.

As I remember, we had in the department eighteen qualified veterinary surgeons. They were, therefore, very thinly spread over the country and we had to supplement them with our own trained African staff. These were drawn from the two best schools in the country and were trained at the laboratory as African Veterinary Assistants. The field veterinarians were deployed in the provinces and districts of the territory. The functions of the laboratory were; back-up of the field officers by confirmation of diagnoses of diseases met with and reported from the field, provision of materials and vaccines, information and staff assistance and training of Veterinary assistants. The laboratory was responsible for research into the diseases encountered in the field, especially in the development of vaccines and treatments and the testing of new vaccines and specific chemotherapeutics and the manufacture of appropriate vaccines.

In Mpwapwa, work was carried out on the improvement of indigenous stock and the experimental introduction of exotic breeds. Efforts were also made to improve the feeding and husbandry of the native stock. Very little was done by the indigenous pastoralists to preserve animal feed when it was plentiful so that it could be made available in times of drought or in the dry season. In Mpwapwa we were able to demonstrate how fodder could be conserved by such methods as haymaking or the preparation of silage. To these ends we developed farms in which improved methods of husbandry could be demonstrated with the object of encouraging African farmers to adopt these improved methods and so raise their standard of living and produce healthier and more productive stock. Experiments were carried out on newly introduced grasses particularly with a view

to finding drought resistant strains and creeping grasses which could help to bind the soil and so reduce the ravages of erosion.

The animal disease of prime importance was rinderpest (cattle plague). This is a virus disease, which kills about ninety per cent of fully susceptible cattle. It causes a severe fever with very extensive excoriation of the mucous membranes of the whole body, mostly outwardly noticeable by ulceration of the mouth and stinking diarrhoea. The disease is extremely contagious so that it spreads rapidly through herds with devastating results. It had to be tackled by strict control of cattle movements and this was particularly difficult among nomadic tribes such as the Masai. At that time a crude vaccine against rinderpest had been developed and one of my responsibilities was the production of this prophylactic. This involved the maintenance of susceptible cattle, which had to be infected with the virus, and then slaughtered when the virus in their tissues was at its peak level. The appropriate tissues were removed and treated to inactivate the virus after which they were emulsified, processed and bottled for transmission to the field as vaccine.

The Veterinary Officers in the field were responsible for the organisation of immunisation campaigns in their own districts and provinces. This, of course, involved a tremendous amount of planning and liaison with the authorities in neighbouring areas and even with neighbouring countries. It was an extraordinarily difficult business and entailed the formation of teams of workers including African Veterinary Assistants, Veterinary Guards and manual workers. During these campaigns, the field Veterinary Officer spent most of his time on safari, sleeping under canvas and maintaining contact with the cattle owners. Many of these were antipathetic to vaccines of any sort and would resort to all manner of devious means to avoid having their cattle vaccinated. He also had to make sure that the supplies of vaccine were adequate and in the right place at the right time. The *modus operandi* was to send out messages to the owners in the districts to be treated, with instructions as to when and where they were to assemble their cattle. This was followed by a team of workers who moved onto the site and planned the area in which the vaccinations would be carried out. Then the team would cut bush poles from the surrounding bush and construct holding pens and

81

crushes. These had to be strong and made according to a very strict plan. The crushes had to be such that cattle could be packed into them without any of the animals being able to turn round or move freely. Then along would come the Veterinary Officer and his team of inoculaters. Their owners, under the supervision of the Veterinary Guards, would herd the cattle into the crushes. Often it was possible for the inoculaters to run along the backs of the cattle injecting each animal with a dose from a multidose syringe. Meanwhile, other assistants would be filling syringes. The method must be accepted as crude but it worked to the extent that a good team could inoculate two thousand or three thousand cattle in a day, working from dawn to dusk. It says a lot about the fifteen or sixteen British veterinarians in the field in Tanganyika when at the peak of our campaigns against rinderpest, some two to three million head of cattle were vaccinated in a year.

The true *raison d'etre* of the Veterinary Departments in British administered Africa was the raising of the standard of living of the indigenous people of the various countries. Our main efforts were directed towards making life for the tribal farmers better and more productive. The same objectives, of course, applied to all departments of the Colonial Service. We in the Veterinary Department and those in the Agriculture Department were probably closer to the tribal people than were others because we dealt with the basic livelihoods of people who were almost completely dependent on their livestock and the products of their land. The members of the Administration were, of course, responsible for all matters such as the civil life of the territories under British control but their activities depended to a great extent on the help and advice given by the technical departments and the police. Medical help was provided for the indigenous people but the qualified doctors were very thinly spread over the huge tracts of country constituting the tribal areas. Hospitals and clinics were established and manned by European doctors, helped by locally trained African medical assistants. Some of these, who usually came from the higher classes in the schools, were trained as specialists in certain disciplines. I know of one such who was trained to operate on cataracts, very common throughout the country. He travelled

from village to village operating from a van, which acted as a mobile surgery. He did a remarkable job and in his time restored the sight of thousands of his fellow Africans. The service also employed a number of Indian medical graduates who were posted to many of the smaller townships as Sub Assistant Surgeons. Some of them, with experience, became very useful practitioners, filling the gaps that could not be filled by the fewer numbers of British trained doctors. We had a succession of these S.A.S.'s in Mpwapwa. Some were very good; some were not so good and made us wonder just what their qualifications were. I remember one of them whose great interest was in surgery and he tackled any condition, which gave the slightest scope for the use of the scalpel, with gusto. His favourite subject was elephantiasis. Any poor soul turning up at his clinic with enlarged testicles was received with open arms and the large organs, sometimes huge, were promptly photographed and their unfortunate owners were lead to the operating table. After recovery from the anaesthetic a second photograph was taken before the hapless individual died. The S.A.S.'s office walls were covered with the photographs of 'before' and 'after' as a testimony to the great and heroic surgical activities of our man from Poona or Bombay or Madras. I once sent an African labourer, who had suffered an accident in which a spike had penetrated his leg, to the S.A.S. for an anti-tetanus injection. Roy Egerton who, at that time was in charge of our laboratory workshops, took the injured man down to the clinic in the lab pick-up. The S.A.S. had to open a new phial of the tetanus anti-serum and having injected the dose into the injured man, he promptly turned onto poor Roy and without more ado plunged the needle into him and injected the remainder of the phial. "It is not good to waste such valuable serum," he declared.

One of the S.A.S.'s who was posted to Mpwapwa, and, incidentally, one of the best I ever came across, was an Indian doctor from North India. His name was Dikshit. He was a very good tennis player and so was invited to play on our one and only, rather rough court. We used to play after tea and before sundown, once or twice a week in the dry season. There were a few seats at the side of the court on which those who were waiting for their turn to play rested. On one occasion an

archdeacon visited us from one of the mission churches in the province and was brought up to the tennis court by his host. Dr Dikshit was sitting out on a seat. He was introduced to the Archdeacon. "This is Dr Dikshit, Archdeacon."

"How do you do, Dr Dixie?" Said the Archdeacon extending his hand.

"Dikshit please, " said the good doctor, leaving no doubt in the mind of the cleric.

Some two or three years after my arrival, Sammy Evans, having completed twenty years in the Service, retired and went to work in the newly formed East African Veterinary Research Organisation, in the up-to-date laboratories in Kenya. I was left in charge of the Mpwapwa Laboratory and shortly after that, Neil Reid was promoted to the post of Director of Veterinary Services. In 1946 I also was promoted to become Chief Veterinary Research Officer which post ranked with that of a Deputy Director. I was, of course, very gratified but with hindsight, I feel the promotion was probably premature. It is true that after five years of management of the laboratory, I had acquired a good working knowledge of the diseases of animals in the East African tropics. I had also become adept at using our scant resources to the best advantage but I regretted not having had the opportunity to work alongside a more experienced researcher in a more sophisticated laboratory with more modern equipment. However, for the best part of thirteen years, I worked in Tanganyika and in that time I travelled widely over most of the territory. I came to know many of the tribespeople, especially those of the tribe in whose country we were situated. This was called Ugogo, the people were the Wagogo and their language, of which I learned a smattering, was Chigogo.

I have written a small book describing some of the more humorous and bizarre experiences encountered in my years in Tanganyika[*]. Workwise, my experiences in that country if included here would become almost a catalogue of tropical diseases. Those that stand out most in my memory, are

[*] Wilde, Jack K. H., *Wilde Tales From Africa*, Castle Cary Press (Somerset, 1990)   ISBN: 0 9 05903 20X

rinderpest, of course, trypanosomiasis, East Coast fever, anthrax, babesiosis, and rabies. There were many others, including diseases of humans in which I was involved either as a sufferer or as one able to help others who were infected. This, naturally, included malaria which was very common among both African and European people. Those in which microscopic examination was of diagnostic significance, were often diagnosed in my laboratory. In addition, we had the duty of confirming suspected rabies both in man and animals.

From time to time, my work demanded quite a lot of travelling. Departmental transport comprised either lorries or what we called pick-ups which were like small lorries with a cab and an open rear part which was ideal for carrying camping gear and the technical necessities required for the work to be done, for example, a small refrigerator. The latter would be actuated by means of a paraffin burner. There would usually have to be a microscope unless we were to be centred at one of the district veterinary offices, which would already be provided with much of the equipment, which would be needed. Often I would have to go to one of the provincial centres where I might enjoy the luxury of a rest house or even better where I might be accommodated by the Provincial Veterinary Officer in his own house. I would usually be accompanied by him on safari to investigate the problem, which had called for my visit. These visits were often very pleasant interludes as all one's fellow officers were friends and we enjoyed exchanges of views and discussions on topics of mutual interest. In the Northern Province there were some expatriate farmers who raised cattle for meat and milk. Their farms were on the lower slopes of Mount Kilimanjaro and Mount Meru, both of which were volcanic. Meru rose steeply from foothills around Arusha, one of the larger townships of Tanganyika which also was the administrative centre of the Northern Province. It was regarded by most officials as a very desirable station to which to be posted, the climate being comparatively cool and almost temperate. Mount Kilimanjaro, some miles east of Arusha, is, of course, the highest mountain in all Africa and is permanently snow-covered at its summit. At that time there were several European dairy farmers in the Arusha and Moshi areas who held

title to their lands on the lower foothills of the mountains, Meru and Kilimanjaro. They regarded themselves as entitled to the services of the Veterinary Department, as indeed was their right. Some of them expected a certain priority in this respect, but on the whole they were an asset to their areas and were hard working and serious in the management of their lands. Most of them were descendants of the Afrikaner Voortrekkers who had pushed north from South Africa in the early part of the nineteenth century and still retained their Boer names. Complaints came to Veterinary Headquarters from these farmers from time to time and Bertie Lowe (DVS) sent me up into the Northern Province to look into some of their disease problems. The Provincial Veterinary Officer, stationed at Arusha was Gordon Pevie and it fell to him to organise my safaris in the area and he decided to accompany me to the various farms. Gordon was a typical Glaswegian Scot with an appropriate sense of humour and a distinct interest in the ladies. He and I were very different in character but we hit it off well and when we were together our different senses of humour sparked off each other and we usually had people laughing when we were at parties. Gordon's organisation of our tented safari was excellent. He knew all the good campsites and where we could get fresh supplies and he was on good terms with most of the farmers whose places we were to visit. Some of the farmers were a bit lax about their animal hygiene and left the routine work to their African farm hands, so that the root of many of their troubles lay in their lack of attention to the details of the cleanliness of their farm practice. Most of the problems were of a simple nature, the difficulty being in the diplomacy necessary in advising the owners how best to overcome their troubles. I remember my difficulties sometimes in maintaining my equanimity in explaining the importance of avoiding the cows, when going into the milking parlour, from having to stagger knee-deep in mud and manure with their udders covered in the slime. However, we got over most of the difficulties despite Gordon being rather short fused on occasions. We arrived one day at a farm where the farmer's wife was a half-cast South African. She was plump and comely and certainly attracted Gordon. A good lunch was laid out for us on the veranda and we were certainly well fed.

After we had finished the meal, the farmer said, "Now you young fellas, what about some stories?"

"How do you mean, stories?" I asked.

"Come on," he said, "you know what I mean."

I looked at Gordon and he looked at me and we both looked at the lady. Our host laughed. "Don't worry about her," he said, "she's very broad-minded. You tell them one of yours, Maisie." And she did and it left us with no illusions about her views. We were both good raconteurs and we had a large repertoire between us. Our host and hostess fell about laughing. They insisted that we should go for dinner at a Mrs Foster's place at Taveta in Kenya. Her husband was on safari but she would be delighted if we went over. So, we set off for Taveta, Gordon and I reclining on some sacks of grain in the back of a truck, our farmer and his liberally minded wife in the front. It proved to be an extraordinary evening. At no notice whatever, Mrs Foster produced an excellent meal and afterwards we were asked to perform. One of us started with a story and this sparked another one and so on. Mrs Foster had a lady friend from Dar es Salaam staying with her for a holiday from the Coast. This lady laughed so much and so heartily that she couldn't control her bladder and had to rush off to the bathroom. It was very early in the morning when we got back to our camp and fell into our beds exhausted.

Whilst most of the safaris were done by lorry or car, if visiting Dar es Salaam I would go by train and on some occasions by plane. When I had to visit Kenya I would usually drive to Dodoma and then up the great north road through Arusha and on to Nairobi. The road from Mpwapwa to Dodoma was little more than a track through the bush, which was, more often than not in the wet season, completely impassable. The so-called 'great north road' was also a dirt road. It was graded by the Public Works Department at the beginning of the dry season but in very wet weather it was, to say the least, very hazardous. On one occasion, when I was driving from Dodoma to Arusha, there were two inches of rain in the previous night and it took me about fifteen hours to do two hundred miles of the two hundred and thirty from Dodoma to Arusha. At this point, disaster struck.

In the wet season the dirt roads become two wheel tracks. The depth of the ruts, of course, depends on the amount of rain

and the nature of the particular part of the road on which you are travelling. Often the ruts are as deep as the distance between the tyre surface and the axle height of the biggest lorries that have passed that way. In heavy rain these ruts would be full of liquid mud. When approaching an upward incline, it was necessary to get your vehicle moving as fast as was reasonably possible in order to stem the rapid flow of liquid mud and stay in the track. The dreadful condition of the lorries in those days and the reckless abandon of the drivers made it customary for any lorry to carry a driver's mate who was referred to as the 'turney-boy'. If the vehicle came to a halt on an uphill stretch, the turney-boy had to leap out and plant a block of wood or a convenient large rock behind the rear wheel. When the driver got the lorry moving forward again, there was no time to retrieve the block or shift the rock, which was left in the rut cunningly concealed by the flowing mud. This was the practice that proved to be my downfall on this occasion. I was driving a Ford pick-up truck, a pretty powerful and sturdy vehicle, and was revving hard up the liquid mud track when I hit one of these turney-boy chocks and so the Ford truck leapt into the air and crashed down breaking a half shaft. The incident occurred at about three o'clock in the morning and I was lucky to get a lift in a lorry which, fortuitously was also travelling north through the night. The truck was picked up later in the day by someone from the Public Works Department (PWD) workshops in Arusha and repaired.

Private transport was a bit of a problem for young officers in the service in those days. In my fourth year in Tanganyika, however, I had saved enough money to start considering having a vehicle of my own. One of my veterinary colleagues, David White, who was very much an expert with engines, found what he thought would be a good buy for me. It was an ancient Ford 4 open tourer with a canvas top. With great temerity I paid what seemed to be the huge sum of £170 and became the proud owner of this sturdy motorcar. It proved to be a tough vehicle with a 'dickie seat', and an accelerator operated by the foot or by hand on the steering column. The suspension was on laminated springs, the front ones fore and aft and the rear ones transverse. The rough nature of the terrain over which we had to drive caused a considerable amount of breakage of springs and so I

always carried a spare spring and several pieces of the laminae in the dickie seat compartment so that if a breakage occurred on safari, some sort of repair could be effected on the road, sufficient, at least to get me to home base. The shock absorbers were of a rather crude mechanical type and were, in my experience, not very effective.

In spite of its age and shortcomings, my Ford 4 was a most robust and reliable vehicle. I used it mostly for moving about in the Central Province and didn't take it on long safaris but it was a great workhorse. I have, on occasion, used it to pull other vehicles out of difficult situations such as mud and even in shallow rivers. In the wet season the main hazard of driving on the dirt roads was provided by mud. With practice, one learned the principles of driving in mud. In some parts it was a matter of keeping the front wheels in the deep ruts in the middle of the road. This demanded an intense vigilance and skill as the slightest deviation could mean a slide into the edge of the track, which was usually a river of liquid mud. Once in that and one could be completely stuck. Revving was of little avail and was tantamount to digging into an ever-enlarging hole. To get out of this hole and back into the central ruts required ingenuity, great skill and a good deal of luck. Often it was necessary to resort to digging and dragging stones and brushwood and packing these under the driving wheels. The whole process, especially in the dark, could be a nightmare and, of course, it sometimes meant getting back into the car and waiting for the return of daylight.

In the dry season, after the main roads had been graded, it was possible to drive at unexpectedly high speeds but this caused the appearance of another unpleasant phenomenon. Corrugations. A vehicle travelling at speed would hit an irregularity in the road surface causing the wheels to rise slightly or to lose a degree of road grip. As it came down onto the road surface with increased spin it would cause wear on the surface which developed with the passage of more traffic into a series of corrugations across the carriage way. On some stretches of straight main road this became so bad that it was almost impossible to drive over the road at speeds lower than 45mph. At speeds between fifteen and forty-five mph it became almost impossible to steer the vehicle and so one had to increase speed

and so exacerbate the condition. From the driving seat the corrugations appeared to be about six inches apart but in reality the distance between the tops of the ridges was nearer to thirty-six inches.

When I eventually decided to buy a new car, I acquired one of the first Morris 6's to be imported into Tanganyika. It was very smooth and comfortable but was not as tough and invincible as the Ford 4. That, I sold for £100 to Kay Hickson-Wood. She was a remarkable woman who earned her living by travelling widely about the Central Province in some of the roughest and toughest parts of the country. She worked as supervisor of village dispensaries and small hospitals. The old car carried her and her cook with all her camping gear and medicines. I believe the car gave her years of reliable service. Imagine a modern car crashing around Africa for more than twenty-five years and, when I left Tanganyika, still going strong.

A common source of discussion and speculation in those days was the subject of how car suspension could be improved. Little did we anticipate the tremendous advances that were to be made in later years in the matter of motor vehicle suspension and shock absorption. I discovered a vast improvement when, in 1950, I purchased my Morris 6. The smoothness of the drive in this car was like magic and everybody had to have a ride in my new car to experience it. However, even in this car, I had a disaster and the suspension was tested to destruction on a journey up the great north road to Kenya. There was heavy rain and as I was approaching a small bridge I found the road covered with water. The joint between the road and the bridge had been washed away and so the front of the car dropped into a large pothole and the front suspension was ripped out of its mounting in the chassis, the wheels splayed apart and the engine sank onto the road. I was fortunate enough to get a message to Nairobi through the help of a lorry driver who came past. At about 2 a.m., a recovery vehicle picked me up and took me to Nairobi where the car was repaired.

On one safari, I travelled by train to Mwanza at the south end of Lake Victoria. There, I embarked in a Lake Steamer, calling at Bukoba and then steamed on to Kampala in Uganda and thence to Kisumu in Kenya. I then took the train to Nairobi

and had the experience of travelling on a truly remarkable piece of railway engineering. In parts, the track was carried on spider-like steel erections crossing and turning over deep valleys. It was an awesome experience. On that safari, I spent about a month working alongside some of the very experienced veterinary research workers in the Kenya Veterinary Department Laboratories at Kabete. It was a valuable experience for me and enabled me to improve the equipment and techniques to be used henceforth in my own laboratory at Mpwapwa.

One of the most exciting safaris I completed was one made by air in an old Anson plane used for special journeys by the Government. I have described this safari in some detail in my book, 'Wilde Tales from Africa'. It is enough to say here that it was a really hairy trip in which, at one point, in a violent thunderstorm, I found myself poking my head out on the right side of the cockpit to check that we were high enough to miss the trees while the pilot had his head out at the other side doing the same thing. I then had, under the pilot's instruction, to work the hydraulics that operated the undercarriage.

After I had been out in Tanganyika for four and a half years I was away in the Northern Province, when a message came to me through the Arusha office from headquarters. It was to the effect that if I could get to Dar es Salaam in four days, there was a berth on a ship to take me home on leave. In the war years home had been very far away. Even communication with those at home was tenuous and infrequent. We were able to send and receive air letter cards and even these often were lost in transit. I received one letter from a friend in England, which had taken many months to reach me. That it reached me at all was amazing as it had been opened by the Wermacht and resealed and then had been opened by the South African authorities before being forwarded to me in Tanganyika. The letter had been posted by Air Mail and must have been captured at some point with mail in a British carrier and then it must have been handed over to some allied or neutral organisation, which passed it on to the South Africans. It seems that even in wartime, mail can be transmitted to the addressee after it has been examined and found to be innocuous. However, be that as it may, when I was given this opportunity to go home on leave, I grabbed it with both hands

and made sure that I got to Dar es Salaam in time to catch the ship. The vessel was the MV Castalia which was on charter to the Union Castle Line and bound for London via the Suez Canal.

Once more I found myself in a blacked out ship on the high seas. The voyage was unremarkable except for two factors, which are indelibly stamped on my memory. The first of these was my meeting and making friends with a remarkable man who was a fellow passenger. His name was Dr Leader Stirling and he was a medical missionary who had been for many years working in the south of Tanganyika. He described himself first as a missionary and secondly a medical doctor. He had come out to Africa as an Anglican but had transferred his religious affiliations to the Benedictines. He was perhaps the most dedicated Christian I have ever met. He gave his services to the mission for virtually no pecuniary reward and was quite impoverished with very little in the way of spare clothing and just sufficient funds to act as pocket money. Under the black velvet skies above the Indian Ocean and with no ships' lights to dim the brilliance of the phosphorescence swirling around the ship's bows and sides, Leader and I and Ian, the ship's doctor, forgathered on deck in the evenings and had long discussions. The subject matter ranged from music, literature, philosophy to life in general. As Ian was a young Scottish graduate with strong leanings to the Kirk, it was only natural that religion featured prominently in our discussions. Leader Stirling was obviously a man of profound faith, such faith is always impressive in a man of science. I had struggled with the concept of faith since my formative years but always I had to accept that any faith I could muster was very fragile. One evening we were discussing the infinite and space and the extent of the universe as far as that was known. In the course of this discussion, Leader made a statement which made me feel something akin to a revelation but strangely, even though I have thought back to that evening, I can not remember what it was that struck a chord in my thinking. I regret this but I just can not get back to that feeling I had, sailing up the Indian Ocean.

The second factor involves a coincidence so remarkable that I must include an account of it in these memoirs. As I have mentioned, before the war, my elder sister, Win was on leave

from India with her husband, Dr Arthur Laurence Griffith. On the outbreak of war, Laurie was called back to India for special duties but he was informed that he would have to leave his wife in England, she would have to join him later at an unspecified time. Sea passages were strictly limited. My sister resigned herself to the situation and was told by the authorities that she would be notified when she would be allocated a passage back to India. It was not until 1945 that she received news that a berth was available for her in a ship of the Bibby Line and she made the necessary arrangements to take up the offer. It was only after she had sailed that I got a message to my parents that I was embarking on my way home on leave. We steamed through the Red Sea and into the Suez Canal. By this time, I had made friends with several of the passengers and got on particularly well with a Naval Officer, Lt Comdr. Fred Ferris. When we arrived in Port Said, there was some doubt as to whether or not we would be allowed to go ashore. Several rumours flashed around the ship and eventually we were told that we could go ashore but that we would have to be back aboard in two hours. Fred and I went ashore together and made for the famous Simon Artz store. Fred was anxious to buy some toys for his children at home and he made for the appropriate department. I wandered round looking at the things on sale. I was not far from the main entrance of the store when I noticed a European lady making for the main exit. Seen from the back, she had something familiar about her and so I hastened towards the door and was in time to intercept her as she was moving out into the street. It was my sister, Win. Her ship had arrived in Port Said from the Mediterranean and the passengers had been given three hours of shore leave that had overlapped with our two hours of similar leave. Neither of us had any idea that the other was travelling at that time. It was our first meeting for four and a half years. It was an almost unbelievable coincidence. Had I gone with Fred to the toy department, or if I had not been where I was when Win was leaving the store, I should never have known that we were in Port Said for the same two hours and I wouldn't have met my sister again for many years little knowing that we almost bumped into one another in Port Said.

The rest of our voyage home was uneventful and I was

welcomed back by my mother and father with open arms. Most of my old friends had dispersed to other parts and those whom I did meet had moved into other spheres. After the first bit of conversation, subjects of mutual interest were thinned out and not very sustainable and dwindled to such remarks as, "When are you going back?" There had been a group of us who consorted together, girls and boys, in the later teens, in which there had been a natural sort of falling into pairs. One or two of these pairs went so far as to cement the bonds with marriage. Others drifted apart and went their individual ways. Tom Wilson who did a degree in geology and mining in the Royal School of Mines married Muriel and went off to South America to take up a career in the search for fossil fuels. George Wright qualified in medicine in Sheffield and married Barbara, finally settling in practice as a very popular GP in Cornwall. He, rather surprisingly, later took holy orders in the Church of England and combined the work of saving bodies and souls.

In our teenage activities, which mostly took the form of hiking expeditions over the Derbyshire moors, I had been paired up with a pleasant blonde girl called Jenny Illingworth. Our friendship never extended into the realms of romance and was uninterestingly platonic. There must have been something in our relationship as during my first tour of service in Tanganyika, Jenny made contact with my mother, found out where I was and started writing to me. A correspondence was thus initiated and, through this, the idea of our getting married gradually inserted itself. Soon after my arrival home we met again and resumed our old friendship. We became engaged and began to talk about the wedding. Jenny had studied engineering and had a very good job with Rolls Royce in Derby. She must have been very good at her work, as she was involved in the design of new engines. I was becoming extremely doubtful about the idea of this marriage. I began to feel that there was no love in this match and was becoming very apprehensive about the proposed union and felt that we were going to make a monumental mistake. In the course of our discussions, the idea of the future possibility of having a family arose. Jenny startled me by saying she would never want to have a child. She told me that the landlady of the house where she had digs in Derby was pregnant and she thought it was 'a

94

disgusting state for a woman to get into'. As may be well understood, alarm bells were now ringing loudly in my head. When we got onto the subject of the wedding and the honeymoon, Jenny stated emphatically that she would have to be back on such and such a date. "Why?" I enquired.

"Because I have only a fortnight leave and must be back at work on..." and she stipulated a date. I rather thought that if we were to be married, we would go back together to Tanganyika and I put this, what I thought to be a fairly reasonable point of view, to her. At this point our engagement was broken off and we never met again. I wonder what happened to her. Perhaps she was as doubtful about the suitability of a marriage to me as I was of one to her and this was her method of ending the relationship. Be that as it may, it was the end of our relationship.

Towards the end of my leave I wanted to give my mother a holiday. She had always worked hard bringing up the family with love and self-sacrifice. We had a comfortable home but our life style had never been lavish. We had most of the things we wanted but regular holidays were not considered very important and certainly not essential. Dad was working and so I booked a holiday in a cottage belonging to the Cockerills, who lived in Thorpe by Robin Hood's Bay near Whitby. We had been there before and the daughter, Kathleen and I had had a teenage crush on each other. This had dissolved when I went to University in London. Apparently, when Kathleen heard that we were going to her parents' cottage for a holiday, she said that she would have nothing to do with us as I had previously broken her heart once and she didn't want any further truck with me.

The reason for my choice of Robin Hood's Bay for a holiday was that it was easy to go there, we knew it well and my mother had enjoyed her stay there before. My return to Mpwapwa was imminent as I was near to the end of my leave and I had a very strong desire to see Kathy again. She was obviously the antithesis of Jenny Illingworth and our earlier, youthful sweetheart episode was very nostalgic. My memories of her were happy ones. She was so uncomplicated in comparison with the female students of my university and RVC days. When we met on this holiday there was no strangeness, no embarrassment between us and we were soon quite sure we were

in love. I was very apprehensive about her acceptance of me as a husband and her agreement to take what must have been the immense step of changing her simple country life for a more complicated one in an African environment. My courting was successful, so much so that she took the prospective change in her life and situation in her stride and by the end of the first week of our holiday, we had decided to get married, much to the delight of our several parents. Dad drove down over the last weekend of our holiday and transported Mum and me back to our house in Totley. I was due to be given sailing instructions at short notice and so the wedding was arranged at the parish church about a hundred yards from our house. It was a simple affair, my best man being my dentist, a man of many more years than me, Ellis Snow. As my departure was so imminent, our honeymoon was very short and not far away. We took the train from Dore and Totley Station through the tunnel to Grindleford about six miles away and we stayed in a Hotel in the Village. Incidentally, while we were there, the King and Queen arrived for the opening of the new Ladybower reservoir. All the flags were out in Grindleford and I told Kathy that this was for us! We attended the opening ceremony and had a very good view of the King and Queen.

Shortly after our return from honeymoon, I received instructions to embark in a ship, which would be sailing from Hull in a few days. The vessel turned out to be an old coal burner named the SS Adviser. She had recently, been hurriedly modified to carry passengers. Things were pretty rough and basic. The cabins were four berth and there was no interior trim. We had to sleep against the steel sides of the ship. The feeding arrangements were rather crude. Passengers were seated on benches alongside trestle tables. The service was pretty rough. The cutlery was 'washed' by being stirred vigorously in buckets of water at the ends of the tables. Certain improvements were made as the voyage progressed and conditions became more tolerable. We had to take on coal, I think that was at Port Said, but wherever it was it was a dusty and unpleasant activity. Many of the passengers were going out to Africa for the first time and so the conditions were accepted, especially as the post-war mind set had not yet been reconditioned.

When I got back to Mpwapwa, my friends were all interested to know if I had married while on leave. They expected that my new wife would be the blonde they had heard about in my first tour. I had to explain that my wife was not Jenny but Kathleen who had dark brown hair. Some two months later I heard that Kathy would be sailing in a troop ship, the Neahellas, which was bound for Kenya to dock at Mombasa. I arranged some local leave and organised my trip to meet the ship. I didn't know then that the ship was a pretty rough one full of troops. I learned later that things on this ship were poor indeed. For example, the drinking water was supplied in drums about the deck with a cup attached for the purpose of bailing out the water for whatever the need for it was. It was a very shattering first experience of foreign travel for Kathy.

Kathy was a country village girl. She was born in the gamekeeper's lodge on Lord Normanby's estate in Mulgrave Woods, some ten miles or so north-east of Whitby where her father was the gamekeeper. As a girl she had not been much further afield than Bridlington and York and was very much of a home girl. After the war commenced she volunteered for training as a nurse and was dispatched to Bradford, Manningham Lane Hospital where she was pushed into the thick of it without very much in the way of instruction or advice. She was given a clinical thermometer and told to take a patient's temperature. She had no idea of how to do it and so wrote on the chart the figure that had been entered for the previous reading. She didn't do very well there and was so obviously home-sick that when she was sent to attend to a child who had been smashed up in an accident, she just could not bear it when the child was screaming and shouting 'Get off mi foot Grandad'. The authorities decided that she should go for training nearer home and they sent her to Whitby Cottage Hospital. There she did a little better although she was a bit queasy about trimming the nails of a male corpse and then having to collect the nail clippings from the cracks in the floor. The final stroke, which put paid to a promising career in the nursing profession, came when a young butcher's boy had an accident on his bicycle and he was brought into the hospital in clothing well bespattered with blood. His clothes were removed and handed to Kathy with the order to take them to the

wash room and get them washed. She proceeded with the duty gingerly dropping the blood soaked garments into the tub and suddenly contacted a mass of soft tissue which she thought must have come from the boy's person. It happened to be a piece of pig's liver which was destined to be delivered at the time he had his accident. Kathy decided to go home and the Senior Sister apparently agreed that this would be best for all concerned but said that she should do something for the war effort and so she went home and signed on as a conductress on the local buses.

It was; therefore, quite amazing that she agreed to marry me knowing that she would have to go away, not only to an unknown place but one far away in the huge, African continent. It was all the more remarkable that she accepted the situation when she found that she could not journey out to Africa with me but would have to wait for a sailing and then travel, unaccompanied, among strangers in a steamship, the like of which she had not even seen before. When the time came to sail, her brother, Robert took her to Glasgow, where she was to embark. The voyage in the Nea Helas must have been quite traumatic for her. Kathy had not the benefit of higher education which makes it all the more creditable that when we reached Mpwapwa she slotted into the life on a small up-country station very quickly and soon had her African staff eating out of her hands. They took to Kathy very quickly and she became very popular because of her sympathetic and down to earth attitude. Kathy has never been able to dissemble and wherever we have been she has always retained her plain speaking attitude, calling a spade a spade and standing no assumed airs and graces. I was very delighted to find that she took a real interest in the Africans around us and rapidly gained a working knowledge of Swahili.

There was no delay in Kathy's introduction to life in the African bush. She had been no more than fourteen days in Mpwapwa when a lion killed an ox actually in the confines of the laboratory buildings. On occasions such as this we had to sit up at night and wait for the marauder to come to devour the carcase and give us a chance to shoot him or her. I therefore arranged for our two Italian collaborators, Araldi and Venturelli, to sit up with me armed with rifles in the appropriate place the next night. Kathy declared that she was not going to stay on her

own in our house with me out among lions. So I agreed that she should come and hold the lamp and direct it onto the kill at the appropriate moment. The details of this event are contained in my book 'Wilde Tales from Africa'. She certainly had a real experience with lions.

Not long after her arrival, Kathy had a very interesting experience of safari. Most District Officers had their pet ideas about making a name for themselves in some branch of their duties to the local people. At the time of Kathy's arrival, our District Officer (DO) was Rob Bell and he had a desire to make new roads. One of the highest prominences in his district was a 7000 feet hill called Wota. Someone had started to make a road intended to make visitation of the tribe which was located on the heights of Wota reasonably possible without the necessity for a long and arduous foot safari. Rob decided to survey the road which had been started and decide what should be done to complete the task. He invited me to go with him and as he was taking his wife why not take Kathy as well? A weekend safari was arranged, This first experience of a really rough tented safari appealed to Kathy and so she wrote an account of the adventure to send home to her family. I had my Goan clerk, J.C. Almeida, make a few typescript copies and I am including Kathy's impressions of her first safari here.

"Safari up the Wota road'.

Wota is a mountain of about 7000 feet some thirty miles from Mpwapwa. Recently a new 'road' has been made up the mountain by the Provincial Administration. The District Commissioner, Mr Robert Bell, wanted to go up Wota on a tour of inspection as on his last visit the road had not yet been completed. He asked us if we would like to go with him and try to get to the top.

It was therefore decided to begin our safari at 7a.m. on Saturday, the main reason for an early start being that it would be cooler in the early morning. Five of us were going with four or five servants. There were Mr and Mrs Bell and their three year old son, Michael, Jack and myself. Our transport was an old Dodge lorry, not very comfortable, perhaps, but in this country

people do not seem to worry about a comfortable ride – comfort is a sideline, the point is – will the vehicle hold together and get us to our destination? Well we had a lot of snags before we finally did at about 11a.m. get away. To start with, our lorry was not ready for the road, the two back wheels were off and our Italian mechanics, who are very efficient, were adjusting the brake drums. Anyway, after that job was done, we had what we thought was a reliable lorry, but later in the day, we found that we had built castles in the air. We were piled high with safari kit, tents, tables, chairs, pots and pans and last but not least, lots of food and water. Away we went bumping and shaking over these terrible roads, the sun pouring down on us as it was by now the middle of the day. Happily we caught a little breeze on the top otherwise, I think we would have gone up in smoke. We had done about thirty miles when we heard very disheartening sounds coming from the engine, Rob Bell was driving and he steadied up when he heard the noises. Thinking that it might just be a bit of dirt in the petrol, we started off again but were only able to do another couple of miles and then... Well it was plain to see that none of our party was mechanically minded. They unscrewed nuts and bolts, blew down pipes, took things to pieces, lost little parts. In fact they proved themselves to be fairly hopeless with a Dodge engine. While these investigations were taking place in the bowels of the engine, the servants got busy, made a fire and prepared a meal by the roadside. It was rather a novelty to me as it was my first safari, but it gave me rather a bad impression through this unfortunate halt. Well after many more pokes, turns, blows and pushes, it was obvious that nothing more could be done. As one very important part must have been lying in the road irrevocably lost in African soil and could not be found. We were two miles from a tiny native village called Mima and the one and only thing to do was to walk there. The lorry was unloaded and with the aid of seventeen porters and our own servants we arrived at Mima, bag and baggage. It was now about 6p m., not much daylight left and so we picked our camping site and prepared to make ourselves comfortable for the night out in the African bush. It was a lovely evening, rather windy, but that helped to blaze up our huge camp fire. Only one tent was pitched, after all, it is nice to have a roof

available if only a canvas one, if it should become necessary. Our beds were made up, lovely clean sheets and pillows and it looked like being a cosy camp for us all. The servants made us a hot meal of curry and fruit which we ate at about 9.30p.m. I was very hungry but the others didn't complain of hunger.

We had sent a message back to Mpwapwa asking someone to come and help us and so we went to bed. What a night! As long as people were moving about, I didn't mind but when people started snoring I began to feel very nervous. My bed was alongside Jack's but he was tired and went to sleep very quickly. I felt completely alone and felt that some wild animal would be leaping onto my bed at any moment. Then I thought that snakes would be curling round my bed legs and would eventually wind themselves round my throat and such unpleasant things. I didn't want to disturb Jack and break into his sleeping but I couldn't help it. In the end, I got into his bed, a bit squashed I must admit, but I felt safe. Sleep was fitful and was soon dispelled as it started to rain. We suffered in silence for a while then got out of our bed and carried it into the tent. We all seemed to go to sleep. I was awake and up and about at 7.30 a.m. and we had breakfast. Molly had a little walk and Rob and Jack practised a few golf strokes and I read a little.

About 10 a.m. we heard an engine coming towards us. We all rushed about and were happy to see Venturelli and Araldi, our two Italian mechanics, one in a Ford V8 lorry and the other in the old Dodge which had let us all down on the previous day. Now we were able to continue our journey and do the most exciting part. We were attempting to climb the mountain along the new road which had not been used by any vehicle before. It nearly makes my head ache when I think about that climb. Venturelli was our best driver and so he took the wheel. The first six miles were very bad but we were expecting rough going and so we were able to face it feeling fairly comfortable. After that it was terrific. Imagine sitting or standing in the back of a lorry moving very slowly around hairpin bends, creeping up hillsides which were about one in six and looking over the side to see an almost sheer drop of three hundred feet and at the same time feeling the lorry wheels sinking into the loose surface, the rear wheels slowly sliding towards the edge. It was a very near thing

101

at times but we in the back wasted no time in jumping out. We had to jump for it on several occasions. Some of the Africans were almost panicky, one in particular called Paulo, appeared to be terrified. I am sure that if he had been a white man he would have been green. Anyway it took all the next day for him to get over it and he had a day off duty.

We proceeded like this for two and a half hours and only progressed fifteen miles in that time. We made it to five miles from the summit and then had to give up, It was impossible to go any further. After lots of hazardous and intricate manoeuvring, the lorry was turned round and we started down. After a little way we stopped in the shade of a big tree and had some food. The two Italians had left Mpwapwa early in the morning before breakfast as they thought we were not far away. The poor fellows were exhausted and famished. We soon dealt with them as we had any amount of food, tinned fish, lettuce, tomatoes, eggs, a cold roast joint of mutton ,(some called it lamb), bread and butter, cakes, tea and beer. That meal was soon over and we set off again. Down, down, down, bump, bang, hang on, jump, oh dear! It was a most hazardous ride, skilfully manipulated by the Italians. I don't know how we all looked when we arrived at the bottom but I can safely say that I was not the only one who felt greatly relieved to be all in one piece.

It was very hot as you can imagine in October in the tropics and several of us were looking like Red Indians through being in the sun and dust for so long. We arrived home at about 7.30p.m. and we were very thankful for a hot bath, a comfortable meal and bed.

That is Kathy's account of the Wota safari. We were very fond of Venturelli and Araldi and were sorry to lose them when they were later repatriated to Italy. I understand their hometown was Bologna.

These most useful engineers were sadly missed, especially when I had to find someone capable of supervising our mechanical works which were very varied. Someone had to keep our laboratory generator going and our transport had to be maintained. We sent out enquiries and by a stroke of luck, these came to the notice of a young British soldier who had chosen to

be demobbed in East Africa. He was a Lancashire lad called Roy Egerton who had met and married a woman in South Africa. He was a great find and Marie, his wife was also a real asset to our community. They rapidly settled into our official and social lives. Roy was an amusing and cheerful chap who took everything in his stride. He developed a language of his own in the workshop, incorporating his own style of Swahili. He became very popular among his workers who came to understand his quaint names for the tools used in the daily work. With some trepidation, I give here two of Roy's names for tools, which are retained in my memory. A screw driver in Swahili is a 'bis bis'. Roy's name for it was 'ukojo ukojo' derived from 'piss piss' as 'ukojo' means urine. A less convoluted one was 'marvi ya panya' used to denote a ratchet. 'Marvi' means faeces and 'ya panya' means 'of rat'. Of course the vernacular for faeces is implied.

Life in Mpwapwa, compared with that in the larger stations and towns was simple and unsophisticated. At that time we didn't have a club but made our own entertainment in our houses and on our one tennis court of which we were inordinately proud. A large part of our development was based on the clearing of rough scrub and bush, of which we had about two thousand acres, and producing pasture with grass strains appropriate to our climate. At the laboratory we had to breed small animals such as guinea pigs, goats and sheep. We also introduced European breeds of pigs and some exotic breeds of cattle. It was comparatively simple to modify a few acres of new pasture to make a rough nine-hole golf course. Greens, of course, were out of the question and so we made do with 'browns' with a surface of mixed sand, murram and pulverised termite mounds. These were rolled tolerably flat with a dressing of old sump oil. We had to grow succulent grass and green fodder alfalfa and a few vegetables for the small animals. To do this we dug out an area of earth lying at the top of a gently sloping hill to produce a water tank for the purpose of irrigation of the terraces of succulent green fodder. Into this area we had to introduce shade trees and so what better than citrus's, oranges and grapefruit, and then, of course, what could be more sensible than to make the water tank into a quite nice small swimming

pool All this work made life much more interesting and we found that many people on official safaris found it important to visit the Veterinary Department in Mpwapwa.

I had accumulated a large collection of classical music on records and had taken these out to Mpwapwa. Those of us who were keen on the musical classics used to forgather in my house to spend the odd evening having a meal and then settling down to listen to a 'concert'. Sometimes, one of the others who had also brought out his collection of records, would bring a selection to our *soiree*. On other occasions we would organise a party in one of our houses or a treasure hunt with clues scattered about the station. Some of our parties were hilarious but on the whole they were fairly harmless and helped to pass the evenings which, of course in our almost equatorial situation, became dark between the hours of 6 p.m. and 7 p.m. After my first tour, when I returned to Mpwapwa and was joined by Kathy, more new appointees arrived on the station with more wives and life settled down into a pleasant cycle of social activity out of working hours. In 1946 Kathy became pregnant. We had no medical antenatal attention such as is now accepted as essential for the birth of a baby. We had to deal with any alarms and abnormalities as best we could, sometimes, with rather inexpert advice from the S.A.S. In the village where the major population was composed of Asian duka wallahs and their families, there was a marked antipathy to the idea of treatment by an Indian doctor, especially if the patient was a female. I had the embarrassing experience sometimes of being consulted over problems of health by some of the Asian families. I had to exercise a good deal of diplomacy in handling these approaches and giving advice. On some occasions, where a blood smear was necessary as, for example, in cases of malaria, I was in a better position to make a diagnosis than was the S.A.S. and could help him out with advice. Indeed on odd occasions I was visited by the S.A.S. who asked me for a diagnosis of his own illness and advice as to the treatment.

Looking back on those days in Tanganyika and other parts of tropical Africa, I am amazed and thankful that we came through without serious damage to our health from contact with so many diseases. We suffered attacks of malaria and PUO's

(Pyrexia of Unknown Origin) and even amoebic dysentery. Though we were careful and very moderate in our lifestyle we, including our sons, could have been and probably were, exposed to many other tropical diseases. We could have suffered much more in view of our living in and moving through areas where we were undoubtedly at risk of infection. We had inadequate medical coverage but we came through.

In my early days in Tanganyika, I did suffer one most peculiar episode. It took the form of a sudden attack of an apparently allergic reaction. The symptoms were distressing and very painful. Swelling occurred over my entire body and when I say 'entire' I mean entire. My eyes were almost closed and my arms and legs were swollen and very painful. My legs were so tender that I could not bear to have them covered by a sheet and blanket. My servants fabricated a sort of basket to cover my legs and so keep the clothes off them. My penis was so swollen and distorted that when I crawled to the loo on my hands and knees and tried to urinate, the stream shot up over my shoulder. The S.A.S. was sent for and he declared that he had never seen such a severe condition and he was at a loss as to what to do. I was, by this time, not able to think straight but I had a period of clarity and suggested that he should get some adrenaline and inject it into me as quickly as possible. This he did and I am sure that the injection saved my life. Immediately there was an improvement and in a few days I was restored to normality, I never discovered what the allergen was. I had been doing some cement work to repair some broken brickwork on the fireplace in my house and I attributed the trouble to the cement. For a long time I was apprehensive about handling cement but I have done lots of concrete work since and have not suffered such dreadful symptoms again. The skin of my hand is allergic to several substances such as garden soil and such mineral oils as paraffin and engine lubricants and particularly tomato plants, but I don't think there is any link with the extremely violent reaction that I suffered so many years ago in Mpwapwa.

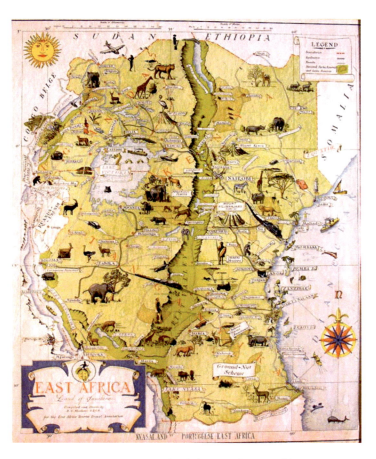

A contemporary colonial map of East Africa.

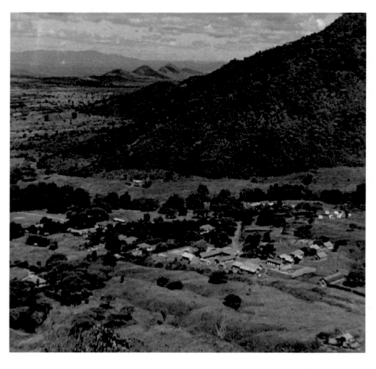

Mpwapwa veterinary station from the nearby hill.

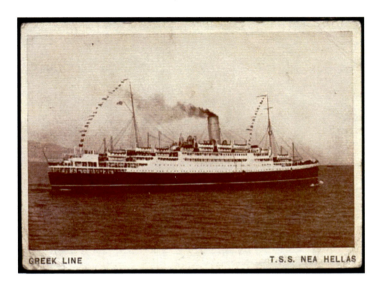

GREEK LINE

T.S.S. NEA HELLAS

T.S.S. Nea Hellas, the ship on which Kathy travelled to Africa.

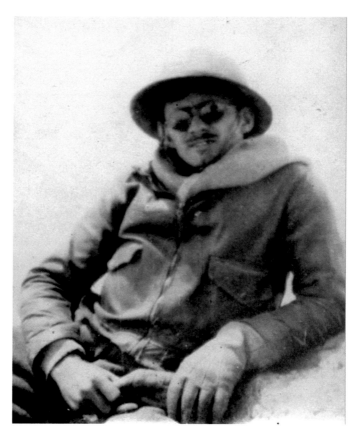

Jack on the summit of Kilimanjaro – the roof of Africa.

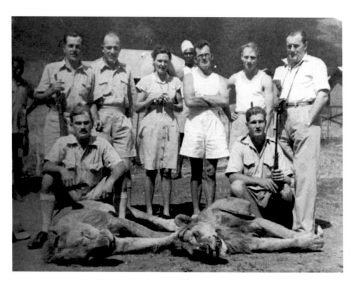

After a lion hunt
Back row: - Araldi, Venturelli, Kathy, Jack, Paul Fourie, Colin
Brown. Front row: - Alec Aycliffe and Pretorius.

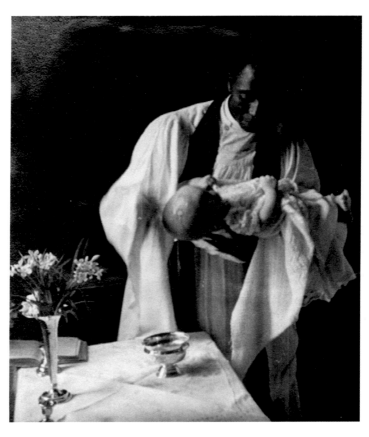

James' christening.

abroad who was addicted to bananas and ate them on stage and spoke his lines through mouthfuls of the fruit. Before the dress rehearsal, the property master informed me with great pride that he had bought three large hands of bananas and he had bought green ones so that they would not go off before we reached the last performance. I became heartily sick of eating my way through a mass of semi-ripe fruit until the final curtain. I have never been very keen on bananas since. The most notable contribution I made to the I.C. Dramatic Society was a tie which I designed for the members. It featured silver dramatic masks on a field of green. I still possess mine and I wonder if the tie is still used by members if, indeed, the society still exists.

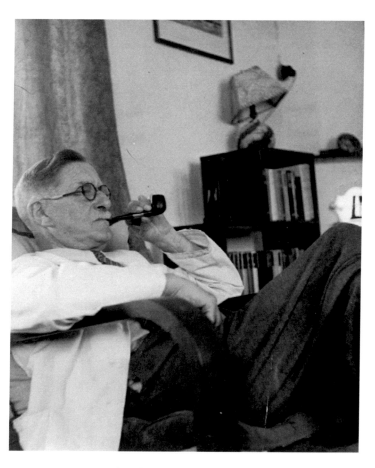

Jack's dad on his visit to Africa

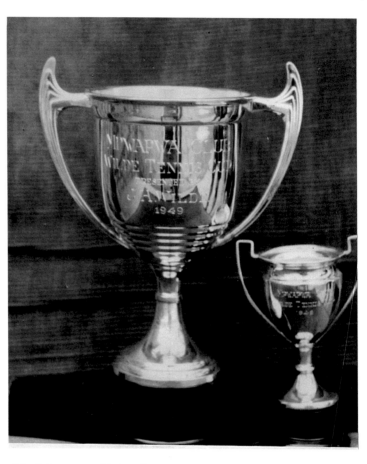

The Mpwapwa Club Wilde Tennis Cup, donated by Jack's dad.

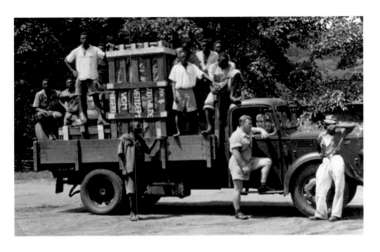

Departure from Tanganyika, the lorry loaded up and ready to go,
supervised by Roy Egerton.

CHAPTER 4

Young Family in Tanganyika

When Kathy was nearing the time for the birth of our first child in 1947, I took some local leave and we travelled to Dar es Salaam so that a hospital doctor could see her. We stayed with Tom and Fergie Walls who had become friends of ours. Tom was a PWD engineer and had been moved to Public Works Headquarters. He and Fergie had a pleasant bungalow at Oyster Bay and so we were able to stay in comparatively cool comfort. I had taken the Ford 4 down to Dar on the train so that we were mobile and could move around at the coast. It became apparent that Kathy was several days overdue. I took her on some rough rides in the hope that the delivery might be stimulated to begin. We went down to the sea and Kathy wallowed about in the Indian Ocean, appearing huge. I was not impressed by the hospital gynaecologist, a man called Hudd. Eventually he decided that the birth should be induced and on October the 19th at 11 30p.m. our son, weighing 9lbs 12.5oz was born. Had he been born thirty-one minutes later, he would have shared my mother's birthday. My Mum had sadly died in the spring of the same year without knowing that she was going to be a grandmother once again. My elder sister, Win already had a son, John and daughter, Ann and my second sister Lily, who had married Eric Brady, had a son, Tony.

When we got back to Mpwapwa, life went on as before but we were given a larger house with a large garden. We then had to employ more staff. Our menage now comprised Sudi, cook, Goliat, houseboy, a young cook's mate whose name I have now forgotten, Daniel, a young boy to look after the baby, Sunday, a rather indifferent gardener and a very tough labourer named Kaspal whose duty was to keep the kitchen supplied with fuel. The latter became well known for his ability to collect firewood. He was about five-foot tall and just about the same round the chest, a very strong and useful member of our household staff. He didn't believe in doing things by halves. When collecting firewood he usually picked one of the largest trees he could find and would come back to the house at a trot with a huge tree trunk balanced on his head. He was referred to as 'Muscles' Wilde. When I explained what this meant, he was delighted and proudly accepted it as his name.

When I first went to Mpwapwa, the nearest thing to a church that we had was a mission situated about half a mile outside the village. It was run by a Church Army officer who conducted services for the local people and any expatriates who cared to attend. From time to time we had a visit from a cleric from the main mission at Kongwa. The building itself consisted of a thatched roof supported by poles cut from the bush. The sides were open to the air and seating was on rough cut wooden benches. On weekdays, the cover did service as a school for children of the tribe. By the time James was born and we had to consider baptism, a new brick built church had been set up and we had visits from preachers in the surrounding areas and a local incumbent, who was one of the earliest Africans in the district to be ordained. His name was Padre Johanna. He spoke no English at the time. Incidentally, many years later, I met him in Kenya at an East African Synod, which he was attending, as a representative of Tanzania. Not only was he now speaking English fluently but he was also a bishop. However, when he baptised James the service was conducted in Swahili, which was a language in which I was fluent but which was not so well understood by some of our European friends. They drew my attention to this fact but I said that it wouldn't matter to James who had, as yet, no language apart from 'Mama. Goo goo etc'. So, the service and all the hymns were in Swahili, much to the delight of the local populace who crowded into the church.

When I had to go on safaris by road and it was reasonable for Kathy and the baby to accompany me, I would take a departmental pick-up so that the baby's cot could be carried in

107

the back with the servants and assistants while Kathy sat with me in the cab. When feeding time for young James came, he was taken from the cot and hitched up to Kathy in the cab and we proceeded on our journey. The longest such safari we did together was to Mbeya, some four hundred and fifty miles, all on dirt roads. Kathy had recently recovered from an attack of malaria but was fit and very anxious to go. Mbeya is a pleasant station situated near the southern border with what was then Northern Rhodesia; now, Zimbabwe. We stopped overnight at Dodoma and Iringa where I had some business to transact with my veterinary colleagues in charge of those stations. At Mbeya, was Mike Molloy, Provincial Veterinary Officer. He wanted me to join up with him in a safari to Sumbawanga near the south eastern shore of Lake Tanganyika. There was no direct road from Mbeya to Sumbawanga so that a route had to be taken over the border into Northern Rhodesia and thence on to Abercorn at the southern end of the lake and then back over the border and north to Sumbawanga. Unfortunately, in Mbeya, Kathy went down with malaria, most probably a relapse following her previous attack. That squashed the idea of her coming with us. Visiting Mbeya at that time was an old friend, John Hobday, who was Director of Veterinary Services in Northern Rhodesia. Kathy had to go into the small hospital in Mbeya in the charge of Dr Griffith-Jones, a Medical Officer whom I also knew. He had stayed with me in Mpwapwa in my first tour and I knew he would give Kathy and James all the attention he could.

We left Kathy's luggage with her in the hospital and Mike came with me in the pickup. Mike had a friend, Twiga Rogers, who was farming near to the road we were to follow and so he said we would be all right for a bed and food on the way. In the afternoon along the road, I noticed a small stone erection at the side of the road. It looked like a small memorial. "What's that?" I asked Mike.

In his Irish brogue he said, "Oh, that's where Stanley met Livingstone."

"It can't be, Stanley didn't meet Livingstone down here." I said. "They met at Ujiji near to Kigoma up the Lake." Mike thought he was right and I was wrong. At about 4p.m. we arrived at Sunzu, Mike's friend's farm, where there was a group of friends having tea in the garden. More chairs and cups and saucers were brought out and we were welcomed to tea. A guestroom was put at our disposal and so we washed and changed for dinner. I mentioned to our host the little memorial stone and asked him what it was.

"Oh that's to commemorate the capitulation of Von Lettow in the First World War.

"There you are, Mike," I said, "I told you it wasn't where Livingstone and Stanley met."

"Well," replied Mike. "You've got to say somtink."

The next day we went on through Abercorne and then back north towards Sumbawanga. We visited a farm about six miles from the township. This was owned by a German and his wife. The husband had been interned at the beginning of the war, the farm being left in the very able hands of his wife. She was a very attractive but tough looking woman who, Mike told me, was a very much sort after bedmate for some of the local officers who had been left without their wives in this very remote station. When we arrived at the farm we found Mrs Damm boiling a large cauldron over a fire in the paddock. Scattered around, were the dismembered remains of a couple of lions. The lady was boiling up the meat to feed her Rhodesian lion hounds, which were gathered, around the pot with their tongues hanging out. ready to consume the rather unsavoury stew. Mrs Damm was insistent that this diet made the dogs much more effective as lion hunters. One of her problems in this remote place was the killing of her livestock by these predators. We dealt with the problems, which had brought us on this safari and returned to Mbeya where I was pleased to find that Kathy had recovered from her attack of malaria and was ready to accompany me back to Mpwapwa.

While we were still in Mpwapwa in 1949 the Groundnut Scheme was introduced by John Strachey, the then Minister of Food in the British Labour government. The first we knew about the scheme was when three people representing the government came to see us in Mpwapwa. This, I believe, was the Wakefield Mission, comprised of Wakefield and two colleagues, Martin and Rosa. They had decided to set up the scheme in two areas, the first being at a place called Kongwa, about twenty-eight miles north of us in a very dry bush area. I think that they had been influenced in their choice of site by Tom Bain, one of the very few Europeans who had obtained permission to establish farms in the Central Province. Tom was a smart operator who, among other things, had set up a butchery at a place called Mlali, some twenty miles from Mpwapwa. He was a very keen South African business man and rapidly realised that a large scheme like that projected by Strachey would bring in a lot of potential for making money. The site at Kongwa was eventually chosen and work commenced. The idea was to clear thousands of acres of very tough bush and after much trial and error it was decided that the best method of doing this was to have very heavy bulldozers working in pairs with a heavy chain attached between them. By this method the bush was to be virtually dragged out by the roots. A huge consignment of heavy bulldozers, left lying about in the Far East after the war, began to arrive. Many of them did not work and as they could not be repaired they were just left where they were delivered. Many bulldozer drivers were recruited and brought to this remote bush area with their wives. Houses had to be built to accommodate the great influx of artisans and experts. A hospital had to be constructed and doctors had to be attracted to the job. One of the first of the medical team to arrive on the site was Dr Henderson-Begg. He was a pathologist and arrived with supplies of laboratory reagents and found that the hospital was far from completed and with no equipment. He came to me to see if I could save the situation, at least *pro tem*, by storing his materials in the laboratory refrigerators. This I managed to do.

The history of the setting up of the great groundnut scheme is a catalogue of disasters. Those responsible for the organisation of the scheme either did not consult the people in the services of the country or if they did, they ignored all the advice given. They very soon discovered that the small stream and waterhole which had just managed to sustain a small number of indigenous families was certainly not able to cope with a massive construction and development with a large and rapidly increasing population of expatriates, all used to having lashings of water at their disposal at the turn of a tap. Workshops were built, roads were bulldozed out, houses were built and masses of furnishings were imported and stacked in great piles in the cleared areas. And then, the rains came. Water was everywhere except in pipes and taps. The roads became canals, the workshops were deep in water and furniture and equipment were left standing in piles open to the ravages of the climate. The whole thing was a mess but eventually some order was restored and literally hundreds of African labourers were mustered. A few acres were planted with groundnuts but virtually no crop was achieved. The local tribes had never had much success with groundnuts and so did not normally plant them.

By now, there was a large population of Europeans of whom many were wives. Boreholes had been dug but the water, which was pumped out of them, proved to be a strong solution of Glauber's salts. This was no good for the washing of anything, especially ladies' hair. A source of good water was found at a distance of some ten miles. A road was constructed to this place and then a fleet of tankers was imported. These had to work day and night in order to maintain supplies for the growing population.

I could quote many examples of the sheer idiocy that reigned in this scheme, but as is now well known, the whole project collapsed with the loss of millions of pounds of British tax payers' money. Virtually no groundnut oil was produced in the scheme. My later experience emphasised the enormity of this waste. When, years later, I was transferred to Nigeria and visited Kano in the north, I was intrigued to see large pyramids of sacks, each one full of groundnuts. They were waiting to be freighted by rail to Lagos for transport by sea to Europe. They had been there for a long time as one could see on close inspection. The bags were rotting and the nuts were going to waste on the ground. I was told that the railway had insufficient freight stock to transport the loads. A few thousand pounds were needed so that new rolling stock could be ordered. The area was known as a good one for growing groundnuts. This rather inadequate description is, of course, the situation as I saw it in the Kongwa area. A much more reliable account of the groundnut scheme is to be found in an excellent book, 'The Groundnut Affair' by Alan Wood, (London, The Bodley Head, first published in 1950)

During this tour, work went ahead on various problems such as East Coast fever, trypanosomiasis and other diseases, which arose as either fresh problems, or as offshoots of other investigations and, of course, vaccine production had to proceed continuously. Constant work was being done on the development of more and better vaccines against rinderpest in my laboratory and in all the other veterinary laboratories in East Africa. It was the general view among those involved, that we would not be able to make real progress with all the other domestic animal diseases in the tropics while we were hag-ridden by rinderpest. A new type of vaccine against rinderpest had, by now become a practical proposition. This was a live but attenuated virus which had been adapted to goats and which was of reasonably reduced virulence to cattle. The early work on this vaccine had been done in India, primarily by J.T.Edwards. I think that the availability of this Goat Adapted Virus made possible, the turning point in our attack on this disease. The new vaccine was produced in the Veterinary Laboratories of the Kenya Veterinary Department situated at Kabete. For distribution, it was freeze dried and provided suitable refrigeration was available, it could be easily transported in the field making vaccine campaigns much more effective and expeditious.

During the war, certain overriding demands were made on the services in East Africa. We in the Veterinary Department of Tanganyika were well aware of the shortcomings of the husbandry of the indigenous livestock owners. The pastoral tribes regarded their animals more as a status symbol than as a source of meat. A man's status in the tribe was measured by the numbers of animals, which he owned, irrespective of the quality of the stock. The actual numbers of animals were much more important than their quality or their health status. The veterinary personnel had long been trying to alter this outlook and educate the stock owners to cull their third rate stock and so ensure more and better grazing for the more productive animals. In short, we wished to institute a system of selective breeding. Before the war the official government attitude had erred on the side of introducing methods of husbandry slowly and by gentle persuasion. The general idea was to interfere as little as possible with the ancient customs of the tribespeople. It was very difficult to make the people accept that it was much more satisfactory for them, their families and the environment to own smaller numbers of healthy, productive cattle than to be denuding their lands of vegetation by keeping alive scraggy beasts which were barely able to stand on four legs.

The conditions of global war affected the old views and we in the Veterinary Services were permitted to adopt a more pragmatic policy. We instituted a system of culling of stock and paying the owners a reasonable price for the animals culled. These animals were gathered into herds and moved along stock routes to centres where they could be slaughtered and tinned as corned beef for the allied forces fighting in North Africa. The whole operation involved the demarcation of stock routes furnished at appropriate intervals with veterinary treatment stations with dipping, veterinary inspection and treatment. The effort and expertise of the field officers engaged in the work were of a high standard and the results in providing food for our troops in the North African campaign, we were told, were of considerable help to the allies. At the laboratory we had to maintain supplies of the vaccines and medicaments for the field personnel carrying out the work.

Another aspect of policy, which was emphasised by the war, concerned South Africa. There was a considerable amount of sympathy for the Nazi cause among some of the Afrikaner people in what was then the Union of South Africa. It was important that the British Administration of East Africa handled affairs with the south extremely carefully. One of the provisos laid down was that rinderpest, then endemic in East Africa, should not be allowed to move south to the Rhodesias and further south where the disease had been eradicated by means of slaughter policies some time previously. We, in Tanganyika, were in the critical position in this matter. In a political agreement it was laid down that the Veterinary Department of Tanganyika would be responsible for seeing that no outbreaks of rinderpest occurred south of the Central Railway line from Dar es Salaam to Lake Victoria. If any outbreaks did occur south of this line, the Tanganyika Authorities had to inform the Government of South Africa immediately. It will be readily obvious that this put me and my laboratory, situated as we were, twelve miles north of the railway line, in a very critical position.

Any report of some suspicious disease in cattle in the south of the country demanded our immediate attention. I could be away on safari at a moments notice if there was any possibility of an atypical outbreak in this danger area. In the early days of the agreement, the Department established a camp in the south of the Territory where a small laboratory was set up and where rinderpest vaccine was prepared in large quantities and as much as possible of the cattle population south of the line was vaccinated. This happened shortly before I arrived in my post. It was carried out by a team of our Veterinary Officers organised by Gordon Pevie. The operation was a remarkable success but of course it was impossible to ensure that the virus was not present in the many plains, game animals acting as carriers of the disease. Accordingly, Neil Reid, a Senior Veterinary Officer, and later to become Director of Veterinary Services, devised a scheme which was almost incredible in concept. The idea was to build a stockade fence along the border of Tanganyika with Northern Rhodesia, to deter the movement of wild ungulates across the border. To anyone knowing the terrain it is an obviously impossible task. However, this did not deter Neil. He gathered a huge band of labourers and they started the job of cutting long poles from the surrounding bush and setting them upright to form a fence sufficiently sturdy and high to prevent antelopes and smaller animals from crossing the border. It proved impossible to complete the fencing of the whole border but the fence was erected to cover many miles of strategically important areas. One of the great problems was caused by elephants which irately demolished these intrusive obstacles to their free passage along routes which were their traditional 'rights of way' and did not recognise any sort of boundary, international or otherwise.

In Mpwapwa, one of the subjects of my research was trypanosomiasis in which the blood parasites are transmitted by various species of *Glossina* (Tsetse flies). This disease was a scourge of man and animals and although some new drugs had been found to be effective against the parasite in man (sleeping sickness) and cattle (nagana) there was a great need for more effective cures. A group of compounds called phenanthridines had shown promise but we were in need of more effective drugs, which would readily lend themselves to efficient and easy use for wide application throughout the vast areas of Africa where the disease was endemic.

It was, therefore, of great interest to me and my department when the pharmaceutical industries announced that a new trypanocide had been developed. I received a letter from the research branch of Boots saying that their chemists had done tests with three new compounds in the phenanthridine series, which appeared to show very marked activity against trypanosomes in mice. The letter was written by Dr Dai Hughes, who asked if I would be prepared to set up research into the trypanocidal effect of these compounds against *Trypanosoma congolense*, the most troublesome trypanosome of cattle in East Africa.

I replied that I would be prepared to do tests on cattle and a more detailed correspondence ensued. The Boots Research and Development Department was very agreeably surprised when I told them that I was prepared to involve at least a hundred cattle in the experiment. They had expected me to say that I might try it out on four or five animals. Consequently Dai Hughes and Gerry Wolfe, the chemist who had prepared the compounds, came out to Mpwapwa. I explained the methods I would use and the experiment was designed. Hughes and Wolfe were most interested to see how such an experiment could be set up and stayed with us until the first stages of the tests were under way. The compounds that had been developed by Gerry Wolfe were three quaternised derivatives of a substance called Dimidium, one of the phenanthridine series.

The experiment went very well, the work being done by me and my young veterinary colleague John Robson. The results showed that all three compounds were effective but one stood out from the rest. My report was in the form of a paper ready for publication and as I was due to go on leave I was invited to take the results home with me and to visit the Boots organisation in Nottingham.

My wife and I were given a very warm welcome by the company and were accommodated in the splendid Lenton House, formerly the home of Lord Trent better known as Jesse Boot. We were lavishly entertained under the personal direction of Sir Jack Drummond, a research director of the company. A special meeting was organised in the Head Office and I was asked to address the group of top executives and research personnel. I gave my interpretation of the results and confirmed that the trypanocidal properties were very marked and that the compounds appeared to be very safe to use. They were readily soluble in water and were stable in solution and so met the requirements of easy administration in the field. They asked me which I regarded as the best of the three compounds and I told them that in my opinion the best was the ethyl quaternised formula which was superior to the other two, methyl and propyl. On the strength of my recommendation it was agreed that the company would go into production of the ethyl compound and it was given the name 'Ethidium'. Our paper was published under the title 'The affect against *Tryanosoma congolense* in Zebu Cattle of three new Phenanthridine Compounds' by J.K.H.Wilde and John Robson.

A few years after this episode, Sir Jack Drummond, his wife and daughter were murdered while on a camping holiday in France. This crime was widely reported in the media and to us who had established a friendly relationship with Sir Jack, it was a particularly sad and shocking loss.

Another piece of research on the subject of trypanosomiasis, which we undertook at the Mpwapwa Laboratory, concerned the trypanosome of human sleeping sickness. This arose out of reports of outbreaks of the disease in a certain area of Tanganyika where it was not expected, as the tsetse transmitter was not known in the area. The question arose as to the possible transmission of the disease from cattle recently introduced into the district from a tsetse-infested area.

I was consulted by the administration who wondered if this transmission could occur but I could not find any appropriate reference to this in the literature. Cattle and other animals, particularly horses, could be infected by a species of trypanosome called *T.brucei,* which had been known since the splendid work of Bruce in the nineteenth century. *T.brucei,* which we often came across in our examinations of blood from domestic animals, was virtually indistinguishable from *T.rhodiense* under the microscope. It was decided, therefore, that we at Mpwapwa should do research in depth on this problem. I had, working with me in the lab, a very distinguished chemist, Dr Marcus French, and so we planned the work to include the chemical aspects of the infection as well as the clinical and pathological aspects. The work was exacting and time consuming especially as I was responsible for all the other activities of the laboratory at the same time. The research was completed and resulted in the publication of another paper, entitled, 'An experimental Study of *Trypanosoma rhodesiense* infection in Zebu cattle'. (Journal of Comparative Pathology, Vol. 55 pp206 – 228).

This research work, which was described by one medical expert in the field of tropical diseases as a 'classical piece of investigation', was rarely referred to in subsequent literature including text books on trypanosomiasis. I have found two references to the work in the book written by John Ford, and published by the Clarendon Press, Oxford 1971 entitled, 'The role of the Trypanosomiases in African Ecology'. In this book John Ford writes; 'The migrant cattle are not so much reservoirs of infection as carriers of infective strains along particular routes. The credit for demonstrating that this could happen with *T.brucei rhodesiense* belongs to Wilde and French (1945). They suggested that cattle could convey the parasites from endemic sleeping sickness areas to others where the disease was absent but the vector was present'. (p.450). Again on p.478 of the same publication, Ford writes 'No account was taken of the evidence of Wilde and French (1945) that cattle might act as reservoirs of *T.brucei rhodesiense* infection, while the confirmation of this in the Alego epidemic, by Onyango, van Hoeve and de Raadt (1966) had yet to be made'.

I have included details of the above research to exemplify what can occur in the research world where workers are not thorough in their searches of the literature. The 1945 paper produced by French and me had already presented evidence, which was resurrected by Onyango *et al* in 1966 as new. In addition, I was disappointed by the omission of any reference in the book produced by my good friend Col. Hugh Mulligan 'The African Trypanosomiases' (1970) to the first work on the drug Ethidium which I have described briefly above. This was undoubtedly due to the fact that the person responsible for the chapter on chemotherapy referred only to the papers written after the drug was named 'Ethidium' and his searches of the literature overlooked our work which was responsible for the establishment of this drug as a most successful means of saving the lives of what must be many thousands of animals suffering from trypanosomiasis over many years

By the time James attained the age of six months it was time for our home leave. Travel involving East Africa in those days demanded that the traveller had a valid Yellow Fever vaccination certificate. I already had such a certificate but, of course, James had not. I ascertained that one of the consultants at the Groundnut hospital had a supply of the vaccine and would do the necessary. So we went over to Kongwa where the consultant kindly gave the inoculation. However, he didn't have any of the official certificate forms so he made out a certificate of his own and signed and stamped it with the hospital stamp, giving all the details, including the vaccine batch number. Being aware of the convolutions of officialdom, especially in such places as Egypt, I was worried. We had to start our journey home by taking the train to Dar es Salaam. Whence we were to take an East African plane to Nairobi from where we were to fly by BOAC to London. When we arrived in Dar es Salaam I took the precaution of having James re-inoculated against yellow fever at the hospital where we were given an official certificate. From Nairobi we were flown in an old York plane that was rather rough, even having no inside trim. Before we took off, I made enquiries about the validity of James's vaccination, because I knew that we would touch down before the date when the Dar es Salaam inoculation could be accepted as being effective. The officials assured me that there would be no trouble, especially in the light of the Kongwa vaccination. I was still apprehensive and so, with our low flying over the desert, which was very bumpy, and with my worries, I was quite sick. We touched down at Khartoum where I again expressed to the authorities my nagging worry. Once again I was assured that there would be no trouble at Cairo where we were to make a stop. My apprehensions were entirely justified. The year was 1948, war with Israel was on and Britain was not the flavour of the month in Egypt.

The upshot was that we were subjected to rigorous examination in Egyptian customs control. Our baggage was taken off the plane and opened and thoroughly examined. Photographs, which I had taken in Tanganyika, were scattered about, ostensibly to see if we had spy pictures, which would be of use to the Israelis. After a long and trying interrogation and arguments, I was informed that I could carry on in the plane but that Kathy and James would have to be placed in quarantine. I refused to leave without them and so it was agreed that we should all be put into quarantine. The airway officials, meanwhile, had been doing their best to convince the Egyptian immigration officers that there was no real reason for our being held in quarantine but the locals were determined to make an anti-British example of us. The plane, which had been held up for all this time, much, I imagine to the irritation of the passengers, was released for take-off. Our baggage was locked in bond and held officially by BOAC and we with a minimum of personal hand luggage were bundled off, escorted by guards to the quarantine camp. This was a double row of brick huts surrounded by barbed wire entanglements manned by as rough a looking bunch of thugs as you could wish to see. We were assigned to a hut at the end of the row and over the fence was desert, I believe it was called Farouk Field. The heat was stifling. Our hut wall was one brick thick and the inside walls were too hot to touch. There was an entrance door and a window that was just a square hole in the wall fitted with a wooden shutter. There were two iron bedsteads each with a coarse blanket, a dirty cupboard and an opening into a small cubby hole with a squat toilet and a tap and a shower which was essentially a tin container with holes punched in its base. Our first priority was to keep James safe and cool. We had his carrycot, which we soaked with cold water and we kept him in that. There was a filthy so-called wash basin which Kathy cleaned, using sand from outside, scouring it with one of James's nappies.

We were told that we would have to stay in the quarantine camp until James's vaccination certificate became valid and that, according to my calculations, was four days. It was a very unpleasant time. We had no reading matter or news and we had no communications with the British Embassy or with the airline.

119

Every morning and afternoon a group of raggedly dressed individuals did a tour of the huts. One of the groups was supposed to be a doctor but he seemed to be a different individual on every visit. They were an unpleasant lot and we got the idea that they were looking for things which could make our lives more difficult. The wooden shutter to our 'window' was swung on two rings in the wall, which formed two hinges using two four-inch nails. The shutter was so hung that we could not keep it open. I therefore took the nail out of the lower hinge so that the shutter swung inwards against the wall and so remained open. When the next inspection took place the absence of the nail was immediately noted. There followed an animated and noisy altercation among the group. One of the members had a very limited vocabulary of English and with difficulty I was given to understand that we had stolen the nail, which was government property. I couldn't find it. I had put it on the brick ledge of the window but it wasn't there. I searched frantically and luckily I found it where it had fallen into the dust on the floor behind one of the beds. I had visions of being charged with theft and being clapped into jail, however, the nail was restored to its rightful place where it remained until the end of our stay.

Food was brought to us from a sort of mud hut café some way across the desert. It was unsavoury and not too hygienic looking material and so we did not eat it. We could buy bottled drinks but for sustenance we all three lived on baby food of which we had with us a large tin. We also purchased watermelons. I had a few pieces of paper and a pencil in my pocket and so spent some time sitting outside the hut trying to do some sketching. I had no india rubber and so cut off a piece of the sole of my shoe to act as an eraser. Other travellers were brought into the camp from time to time and sometimes we saw some inmates taken out and driven off in a taxi or airport bus and this brightened things up for us. One elderly English lady came over and spoke to us. She had been on her way to see her son in Northern Rhodesia but had been taken off the plane from London because her yellow fever certificate was signed by a doctor whose name was not on the list held by the Egyptian quarantine authorities. She couldn't eat the food presented to her and so we shared our baby food with her.

One rather funny thing occurred while we were in this camp. It must sound almost unbelievable but I can give the assurance that it was absolutely true. A very beautiful blonde English woman of about thirty years of age was delivered to the quarantine. It transpired that she was the wife of an Airwork pilot living in India where her husband was posted. Airwork planes had to be sent, periodically to the UK for their certificate of airworthiness. One of their planes was due for such a routine inspection and was being flown home to England by its pilot. The blonde had managed to get a trip home in this plane and apparently she was doing a line with the pilot. I think that the arrangement had been made hurriedly because she had not had a valid vaccination for cholera. For this reason she had been put into quarantine for one day and night, which was the regulation, so, her Airwork plane had to stay over the twenty-four hours and her pilot friend would call for her on the following day. Quite extraordinarily, she approached me as I was sitting outside our hut and without further ado she asked me if I would shave her legs. I was flabbergasted but my reputation for always being prepared to help anyone who asked for my help was at stake, and so I agreed to help this damsel in distress. I explained to her that I only used a cut throat razor but that did not seem to worry her, I must have inspired great confidence. She explained her situation and was anxious to appear at her best on the onward flight. Kathy came out of the hut to see our visitor and I explained the situation. She was not particularly gushing but we went inside and I got out my shaving kit. Kathy sat down with the obvious intention of supervising the operation. Our visitor, whose name, incidentally, we never knew, reclined on a blanket on one of the bedsteads and revealed her nether limbs. The revelation was complete from ankle to pubic region and I was requested to remove the hair from top to bottom. This I did, and considering the situation, I made a pretty good job of it with not a single cut. The young lady was highly gratified and the next morning waved goodbye to us as she was collected by her pilot boy friend. I hope he was fully appreciative of my efforts.

We had, by the way, ventured to open the cupboard in our hut to find in it some discarded female clothes. I suppose there was nothing remarkable about that but at the time we tended to regard these sad remnants as somewhat sinister. We were not sorry when the time came for us to depart. A BOAC coach came for us and took us back to Cairo airport where our luggage was restored to us and we boarded a DC3 plane and heaved a sigh of relief as we rose into the air and left Cairo airport behind. On the plane I appeared to have lost my hat, a green pork pie affair, which was, in those days the fashionable head gear for young gentlemen. The stewardess joined in the search for the missing garment but I said, not to worry, no doubt some porter or other in Cairo was now sporting it on his head to protect him from the remorseless Egyptian sun. However, when we were well over the Mediterranean, the door to the cockpit opened and the Captain came through gingerly dangling between his thumb and forefinger my lost hat, rather battered, dusty and the worse for wear. "Is this what all the fuss has been about?" he asked. I thanked him and told him that it was great to have such an old friend restored to one.

We stopped at Malta and stayed the night in the very posh Phoenicia Hotel. What a difference. One night in a dirty brick hut and the next night in a sumptuous hotel with a black marble bathroom *en suite*. The next day we flew to London and went up to Yorkshire by train.

Whilst I was in Yorkshire I decided to purchase a car in order that we would be mobile and free to explore the country visiting friends and relations. I decided on a Ford Popular, the cheapest new car that I could find. In order to avoid paying the purchase tax I bought it on the understanding that I would be exporting it to East Africa at the end of our leave. We went to my old home in Totley to see my father and to visit my old friends in the Sheffield practice. Our little car enabled us to make a holiday tour of parts of England, some of which I knew but many had not been visited by Kathy. We started off by driving over the Pennines to the Lake District and then south making a point of taking a look at some of the great cathedrals. We stayed at small hotels and motored along in a leisurely way, stopping where the mood dictated. Our list of cathedrals included Lichfield, Worcester, Gloucester, Exeter, Truro, Winchester, Ely and Lincoln. The only one among these, which was unsatisfactory, was Worcester. Here we were not allowed to enter the building. The doors were open and a lot of activity was evident. As we tried to walk in through the open door we were stopped by a verger – we presumed he was an official of some sort as he was wearing a black cassock. He informed us that they were preparing the cathedral for the Three Choirs Festival and members of the public were not allowed in. I said that we had come from Tanganyika and it would be nice if we could just go in through the door and no further. He was quite inflexible and would not let us step even six steps from the entrance. I felt very annoyed by this, as we thought, very unnecessary officiousness, and at the end of our tour wrote to the Bishop with our mildly expressed complaint, but received no reply. The upshot was that we have never entered Worcester Cathedral and I don't suppose we ever will. In Exeter we stayed in a small hotel in the close and having settled in our room and washed and changed, we walked over to the cathedral where the organist was practising. We sat in a pew in the transept and listened with great pleasure. Indeed we were privileged to enjoy an organ concert on our own. I will always remember the great base pipes which sat in the transept. Their notes were more of a sensation than a sound.

Kathy and I thought it would be a nice thing to do when we returned from leave to take Dad with us. He was somewhat lost since Mum had died in the previous year and he was being looked after by Mum's sister-in-law, my Aunt Lou whose husband had died many years before. When we suggested this to him he was delighted and so I made arrangements for him to travel with us and stay for whatever length of time would suit him. We were booked in the Union Castle ship, Durban Castle, scheduled to sail from Southampton. I also arranged for our car to be shipped from Southampton at the same time. We would drive down to the port from Yorkshire and stop off for a few days at Bury-St-Edmunds where my sister, Lil was living. My brother-in-law, Eric Brady had been promoted by his company, Alliance Assurance, to be Manager of their Bury St Edmunds branch. Lil was suffering from cancer of the spine and so it was a sad visit for us knowing that the chances of our seeing her again were slender indeed. Rob Lee, one of my colleagues in the Tanganyika Veterinary Service, had left the service as he was ill and had to go into hospital for an operation for TB of the lung.

He was spending some time with friends in practice near to Cambridge and so we were pleased to get him to visit us when we were in Bury St Edmunds. My Director in Tanganyika had suggested that on my return from leave we should sail via South Africa and that I should disembark at Durban and spend a month in Pretoria working at the Onderstepoort laboratories of the South African Veterinary Department. These laboratories were regarded as the foremost research laboratories in the field of tropical animal diseases. Some of the workers in Onderstepoort had names, which were associated with the most advanced work in tropical veterinary research.

Before we left home on our journey back to Africa, Dad had asked if there was anything he could bring with him that would be of use in Mpwapwa. A relative of his had a harmonium, which he could have for a very cheap price, would that be useful? The Mission in Mpwapwa had just built a new stone church and I thought that a harmonium would be a great gift for this. So, Dad had a joiner build a strong crate and pack the instrument for shipment with us in Southampton. The crate cost about three times the cost of the instrument and it looked as though it would stand up to the worst treatment that the shippers could throw at it. Of course, the break in our journey added to the complications of dealing with our luggage and the harmonium crate. As the various goods and supplies were being loaded onto the Durban Castle we watched anxiously as the items were hauled up in the great nets and we held our breath as the very characteristically shaped crate was swung aboard.

It happened that the Durban Castle was the ship in which Gay Gibson, a film star, met her death at the hands, it appeared, of one of the cabin stewards. It was alleged that she was murdered and her body was pushed through the porthole. I understand from information from one of the officers which I received after we had sailed, that several elderly ladies enquired if they could be assigned to the cabin which had been occupied on the fateful voyage which was the one immediately preceding our trip. The purser steadfastly refused to let anyone know which had been Gay Gibson's cabin, and in any case, all the cabin numbers had been changed. The voyage was the usual very comfortable and enjoyable journey. Only one incident of interest to us stands out in our memory and that was that James walked unaided for the first time on the table tennis table before we reached Durban.

We had to disembark at Durban for our stay in Pretoria and so all our baggage had to be offloaded and with the exception of the luggage that we needed for our stay, all our effects, including the harmonium, were placed in a bonded store. We settled into a small but comfortable hotel in Pretoria. Whatever one can say about Pretoria, this very modern city, built on the square block pattern, has the crowning glory of what must be the finest of all displays of Jacaranda blossom when the trees are in bloom. We were fortunate enough to witness this breathtaking haze of the unique Jacaranda blue. We have seen these trees in bloom in other parts of Africa, but nowhere have we seen it like it can be seen in Pretoria.

During our month's stay in Pretoria, I travelled by the official Onderstepoort Laboratories coach to the labs every working day. The Onderstepoort Laboratories were truly impressive, an outstanding centre of research with a world-wide reputation. The names of the scientists on the staff command the attention of all who have been involved in tropical veterinary research. Willi Neitz, with whom I was to spend most of my time, was a mine of information on the tick-borne diseases. He was very welcoming to me and introduced me to most of his colleagues who, on the whole, were polite but who could not help but indicate a degree of antipathy to a Britisher. I should say that about seventy or eighty percent of the staff were of Afrikaans stock with no particular time for someone from the UK. At about 10.30 each morning the senior staff assembled in a common room for coffee and general conversation and discussion. Willi Neitz took me along with him and introduced me to the various colleagues who happened to be in our vicinity. They would politely acknowledge my presence but would then continue their conversation in Africaans in spite of the fact that they all were fluent in English and indeed used English in all their publications. I regarded this as pointed rudeness and it left me with an unpleasant taste in my mouth. This anti-British attitude was very noticeable in other walks of life in the Transvaal as, for example, when one had to deal with people who were of what one might describe as lower middle class with poor education. A ticket clerk at the railway station once told me that there was no seat available on a certain train only to hand out tickets for the same train to Afrikaners in the same queue. Apart from this aspect, we enjoyed our stay in Pretoria, and on certain occasions when we were in the country we were most hospitably entertained at the homes and on the farms of Afrikaner farmers.

At the end of our stay, we were booked to embark in one of the smaller Union Castle merchant ships, which had accommodation for twelve passengers. Our vessel was The Good Hope Castle. Again we had to watch with bated breath the crated organ being hauled aboard and being lowered into the hold. Our voyage lasted about a week and terminated at Zanzibar as the Good Hope was not calling at Dar es Salaam. At Zanzibar the baggage had, once more, to be swung out of the ship onto the harbour side. My sister and her husband, Laurie were living in Zanzibar at that time as Laurie was doing a job for the Sultan involving a survey of the coastal mangrove swamps and so we were able to stay with them for the few days before we once more embarked on a freighter for the one day crossing to Dar Es Salaam. When I look back to this voyage from the UK to Tanganyika I marvel that it went with so little trouble. I would hate to think of doing it again. It was very complicated and yet it was the voyage on which we chose to take such an article of luggage as a crate containing a harmonium. However, for the last time, we watched the instrument being hoisted out to be lowered onto the dock in Dar es Salaam.

When it came to getting through customs we came up against the beaurocratic delights of Asian Customs Officials. "What is that?" enquired the important looking uniformed Mr Patel.

I said, "It is a harmonium."

"What is this arminium?" I explained that it was a second-hand instrument, worked by foot pedals and sounding something like an organ. I told the official that it was used in churches for the singing of hymns.

"That is not organ, it is piano and so is subject to import duty. You must open it up for my inspection," said Customs

126

Officer Patel. I tried to explain how difficult and expensive it would be to dismantle the crate and I explained that the harmonium had only cost about ten pounds. Mr Patel was adamant. "It is piano and is much more costly than ten pounds." I suddenly remembered that I knew one of the senior officers in the Customs and Excise Head Office in Dar es Salaam. I asked Mr Patel if he would let me ring his head office to speak to the Assistant Commissioner of Customs, who I had entertained on one of his visits to the Central Province. Mr Patel grudgingly agreed and remarkably I managed to get through to the head office, more remarkably still my friend was in his office and came to the phone. I explained the situation and told him the saga and the fact that if the harmonium was in a state from which it could be restored to some sort of activity I was going to give it to the church in Mpwapwa. He was persuaded and said let me speak to Mr Patel, which he did. Mr Patel's attitude changed immediately and he personally gathered together a team of labourers to transport the crate onto a lorry and get it to the railway station.

We all managed to get berths on the train and left Dar es Salaam by the evening mail. Dad was most impressed by the train and enjoyed a good dinner and was most interested in his coupe with its bed and very smart and clean bedding with mosquito net, washbasin, etcetera. I must say that the Tanganyika Railways were a model in those days and one could travel in real comfort and be looked after by very smart stewards and courteous officials.

We arrived back in Mpwapwa safely and the harmonium crate was manhandled off the train and onto our departmental lorry and was finally lowered onto the veranda of our house. I arranged for a couple of workmen from the workshop to come and open the crate which appeared to have suffered no damage whatsoever in spite of the vast amount of handling it had been subjected to over the last eight or nine weeks. The story was very different when we got inside the crate. The keyboard was lying diagonally across the bottom of the crate, the footpedals were broken off, the bellows were ruptured and much of the old Victorian carved woodwork was damaged. I was very glad that we had avoided paying duty on the instrument as a piano.

127

It was all most depressing. However, under the supervision of Dad and with the advice of George Phelps, a master at the school in Mpwapwa, Araldi, Venturelli and Sanpieri managed to get the instrument reconstituted. George was quite a good organist and it was a great moment when he sat at the 'console' and with a great flourish played the first part of Bach's Toccata and Fugue in D minor and the old harmonium responded remarkably well. And so, after all the vicissitudes, the harmonium was established in the new church in the village and it seemed to fulfil its function satisfactorily up to the time in 1952 when we left Mpwapwa finally.

During Dad's stay in Mpwapwa, which lasted for six months, he entered into the life completely and seemed to enjoy himself immensely. He began to irritate Kathy a little as he was somewhat critical and so put his spoke in most things from how to bring up his grandson, including the right way of putting on nappies, to certain aspects of running a household of African servants. What annoyed Kathy most was that he was invariably right. However, Dad was very popular with all and sundry, Europeans and Africans. One of the problems was that he was an inveterate pipe smoker and Kathy couldn't tolerate his sucking on a bubbling pipe and the constant stream of spent matches.

At that time, I had built a library near the laboratory to house all our books and records. I was given the funds to employ a librarian and Doreen Gorton, the wife of my Senior Technician Eddy Gorton, held this post. They went on leave soon after we had returned from our leave and so I asked Kathy if she would stand in temporarily as librarian for the period of the Gorton's' leave. She jumped at the chance as she thought it would give her a respite from the house with Dad around all day. Dad of course settled himself in the library and showed Kathy how to do the job. He decided that the indexing system was all wrong, and I know he was right, and he modified the whole system, making it much easier to use.

Vic Lovemore and his wife, Edie farmed a parcel of land some fifteen miles away from us in the bush. Tony, a young man who worked with them temporarily, brought some locally grown tobacco as a present for Dad. It was twisted into a rope and was in a coil about ten inches in diameter. Tony said that it was

128

necessary to give the stuff a good soak in concentrated molasses for a few weeks. Dad said that was no problem and obtained a large washing up bowl, white enamel with a blue border. This was half filled with a highly concentrated solution of molasses, the tobacco was immersed in it and Dad put it under his bed to mature. You can imagine what our houseboy thought when he was cleaning the bedroom! He must have formed an exaggerated opinion of the masterly size of Dad's bowels and an odd idea of the bedroom habits of this old European. Dad eventually tried to smoke the final product but even he had to abandon the effort describing the aroma as that to be expected if one suddenly came across a brewery in the middle of a glue factory.

Tony was the brother of Molly Bell, the wife of Rob Bell, at that time incumbent of the District Office. Rob's father was a bigshot in the Raj in India. Rob and Molly had lots of rows, which often ended in Molly flinging plates full of food at her husband across the breakfast table. Upon this Rob marched out and into the government District Office next door to take up his duties as the administrator of the district with egg and tomato all over his shirt front which he refused to clean up, leaving it as a sign of the intransigence of his wife. He was, on the whole, a good Administration Officer and they were both really charming to meet socially.

While Dad was with us, I had to go on safari to Nairobi. Whenever any of our people in Mpwapwa had to go to either Nairobi or Dar es Salaam there was always a big shopping list for various items that were unavailable in our bush situation. On this occasion I had a large list that included curtain material, items of furniture, motor engine spares etc. Dad asked me to purchase for him a silver cup and have it inscribed with the inscription, 'THE WILDE CUP'. When I brought it back he presented it to the Mpwapwa tennis players to be competed for each year. This, he said, was a 'thank you' for all the kindness shown to him during his stay in our community. I believe the competition was devised and the first award made before he left for his return to England. Some years later when the service became completely Africanised, I heard that the cup was in the keeping of the last winner, a member of the school staff. I understand that the holder took the cup home with him and I have no idea where it is now. It might come up for auction someday and if it does and I happen still to be alive and active I would be prepared to bid for it.

While recently going through various old papers in the course of sorting out material for these memoirs I came across a letter which had been written by my father while he was with us in Mpwapwa. The letter was to a cousin of mine who was somewhat older than me. He was a very amusing man who had become blind as a consequence of an accident while playing tennis. He was Percy Hall, the son of my mother's brother, Fred. Percy, even after becoming blind, retained his keen sense of humour and used to write letters and conversed in a flowery way assuming the attitude of a most important and aristocratic landowner. In this friendly intercourse with me, he assumed the title of Lord Snitterton. Apparently he carried on this farce with my father as well. I include below, a copy of this missive as it epitomises my father's sense of humour. My father's handwriting was always very good and legible so it is easy for me to copy this letter to Percy in spite of the fact that it was written on flimsy airmail paper and is rather well worn after all these years.

Mpwapwa, Tanganyika.
28th April 1949

My dear Snitterton,

I was somewhat disturbed to receive your last valuable despatch by surface mail. Surely a matter of such urgency should have been entrusted to nothing less than a diplomatic bag.

His Excellency the Governor would have been only too pleased, I know, to forward with utmost despatch, such an important letter from the seat of Government to me where I have now made my headquarters up country. In future, therefore, I beg of you that no consideration of finance even though the estate credits may be in such a rocky condition – should be permitted to delay your communications to me.

Regarding the valuable consignment you mentioned in your letter, apparently one of the escorting destroyers rammed the carrying vessel, catching her prow between middle C and C sharp. The results were disastrous and my staff has, in consequence, been busily engaged in reorganising the somewhat shattered cargo. Apart from a little flatness in the top register, broken pedals, ruptured bellows and considerably damaged Victorian cabinet making, the organ can be made to emit sounds recognisable, in a faint breeze, as to a certain extent chromatic. Timbre, in slight degree, remains.

I trust that the ferret and fox terriers have worked well and that the odd 8/- per brace is helping to swell the Snitterton coffers. I, for my part, am having trouble with marauding lions and as a consequence of failure of the rains and the carnivorous depredations and an unprecedented outburst of rinderpest, am contemplating selling off 6,000 head of my stock and funding the capital so realised, in a project for selling toffee apples to wandering Masai warriors who, contrary to what one would expect, stuff them through holes in their ears and noses and indulge in war dances nodding their heads violently at close range, in an endeavour to smash the toffee off each other's sticks. When success in this endeavour is attained, the warrior flings his spear at the nearest elephant and leaping into the air, utters a sound somewhat resembling the tribal word 'Conkers'. Some of my tribal retainers, by the way, on hearing of your world-shattering exploit, devised a new dance and gave a feast in your honour. The dance was somewhat like a bolero but performed on the head instead of the feet and the main dish was leopards' giblets fried in monkey blood and garnished with bristles from a porcupine's nasal septum. Your talking of home grown tobacco reminds me of a sample cured and sauced (Note the technical terminology) by Jack. I smoked it, he sniffed it and decided that the aroma was, rather that to be expected if one suddenly came across a brewery in the middle of a glue factory. Jack, unfortunately, got hold of your letter and has noted the 10/- debt. He has, however, as a special consideration, agreed to reduce his usual interest from twenty per cent to eighteen and a half per cent. I hope your Lordship and Lady Lucy are in the best of health and enjoying the nice weather I hear you are having in the good old country. It has just been our rainy season but we haven't had the required rain for a good crop. In some parts behind these hills it is grieving to see the crops going west and some of the farmers will lose thousands of pounds and some, perhaps will be ruined, so it's not the golden country some might think. I am very pleased to say that we are all keeping well at present, I am feeling very fit. Jack has had about three weeks of it, with a very bad attack of malaria and the sun caught him. He is now quite well again and pressing on with his work

We had a very nice Easter here; Good Friday a golf tournament; Saturday a tennis tournament. While this was on, your humble and a few others were preparing a good meal roasting two sheep on spits in the field opposite here. We had several campfires to cook pancakes and boil kettles and roast corncobs. We also had a bar and plenty of pastries, pies, corncobs etc. I cut up the sheep and everybody was walking or sitting on the grass with a chunk of mutton in one hand and a cob in the other. We had hurricane lamps all over the place. At about 9.30 we transferred the bar and lamps across the lane into our garden and had dancing on the lawn. We all had a good time and closed down at midnight. They all found their way home. Jack was at church about a mile away at 7 o'clock in the morning and we all went for the morning service and Jack read the second lesson. Monday I was invited to go with a party arranged by a Mr and Mrs Hornby, who are leaving here this week, to Lake Nzuhe at Kimagai. We had a grand time boating, bathing and roaming in the bush and what a lunch and tea- knife and fork do in the bush. Three chickens, half a boiled ham, all kinds of pies and pastries, salad, tea, coffee and bottles of beer. When returning home a great tree fell across the road and trapped the first vehicle. Luckily, no one was hurt and we had to find another way home. One car was left behind and someone from the lab brought it back the following day. We have had another lion roaming round here lately but he will have to make a kill before we are able to get him.

I hope you both will be able to have a nice holiday this summer. You couldn't slip over here for a few weeks by any chance, you would certainly hear some funny noises. We have all sorts of insects flying about, large and small. I shall be able to tell you all about it when I come home. I shall soon be seeing you I hope. Give my kind regards to enquiring friends.

With love from all to you both, I hope you keep well.

Love, Uncle Hillary.

A characteristic feature of life in the Colonial Service in Africa was the way in which social contacts were made with other expatriates in the Service. Hospitality was of great importance and there was nothing unusual about a complete stranger arriving on the station, unannounced, with his safari kit and servants. News of his arrival spread rapidly and one of the residents on the station would invite him in for a chat and then suggest that instead of pitching his tent somewhere, he should have his bed put up on the veranda and use the facilities of the host's house and table. His servants would be provided with accommodation in the servants' quarters and food would appear for them. On these occasions there would be a lively exchange of news of places and people, some of whom would be mutual friends. In this way friendships were established and when the visitor left, his host might never see him again but if their paths should cross again, the friendships so formed would be taken up again and further cemented. It is amazing how these casual contacts produced a sort of network of association that lasted for years and in some cases the friendships were lifelong.

In most departments the majority of the officers were moved from one station to another according to the exigencies of the duties of their department. Very few field officers and their families spent long periods in one station. Some had the job of moving house and office several times in one tour and so the housing provided was equipped with a basic allocation of furnishing. This conformed to what was described as Public Works issue and was controlled by members of the Public Works Department, usually designated as the PWD or as often frivolously referred to as the 'Piddle de dee'. Furniture was basic but adequate. Repairs of houses and their decoration was the responsibility of the PWD Officer assigned to the station or district and there were supposedly strict rules as to the periods between the relevant inspections and the appropriate repairs and decorations required. If some poor unfortunate PWD Officer was stationed where there were senior members of the administration or of other departments occupying houses, he was sometimes put into an invidious position of trying to maintain friendly social relations while having to consider bending the official rules. One of the jokes about the PWD was the idea that you could have your house decorated in 'any colour you want as long as it's buff'.

In my position as the head of the research section of the Veterinary Department I was stationed in Mpwapwa for the entire period of my service in Tanganyika. Not only that, but as I was in charge of all the works on the station and rose to the dizzy heights of the rank of Chief Veterinary Research Officer, the only moves I and my family made during our stay in Tanganyika were from one house to a bigger and more prestigious one. Also, the PWD was happy to leave the control and even the construction of buildings to us so that they were relieved of some part of their duties. The result was that we had a pretty free hand and as long as we had the funds and workers available, we could build as we wished. We even made our own bricks, firing them in our own kilns and obtaining the necessary fuel from the bush clearing operations that we were conducting in order to establish good grazing land. We blasted stone from some of the many outcrops of rock in our land and to this end I was instructed in the process and obtained my blasting certificate. Life was, therefore, very varied and there was never a dull moment.

There were also problems with lions killing experimental cattle and leopards killing sheep and goats. So life was interesting but we had to make our own entertainment, which sometimes resulted in hilarious occasions. I have written something about this side of our lives in tropical Africa in 'Wilde Tales from Africa'. Home leave was generous and in those days before flying became the recognised means of travelling around the world we came home on leave by sea and the voyage to the UK was a holiday in itself. We travelled in comfort, each trip being like a luxury cruise but more exclusive than the organised holidays of today. When we arrived in Britain we had to live somewhere. Some people were lucky and could stay with family but this was not necessarily a good thing. Others of us would travel around our own islands and in some cases see more of England, Wales, Scotland or Ireland than we might have seen had we lived and worked at home. Sometimes we might rent a cottage or take a trip to Europe or America. It was common to find that ones old friends after the first half hour drifted away. This was only natural as they had established new circles of friends and acquaintances. We did, of course, miss out on such things as films, shows and television, but I think that the richness of our lives in Africa among indigenous peoples provided recompense enough. Our return for another tour was another luxury cruise. In later years air travel became the norm and our cruising pleasures became things of the past.

In our early days in Tanganyika when we left our home in Mpwapwa for long leave, we didn't even lock the house doors but left things in the capable hands of our faithful and reliable cook, Sudi who stayed with his family in his accommodation across the compound and kept his eye on everything. True, we did hear on occasion that our house servant had been seen on a special occasion in the village in one of the Bwana's suits or one of the Memsahib's cardigans, but we let sleeping dogs lie. We always found everything in satisfactory order when we returned and a meal was ready for us, either in our own house or with friends. Later during our time in Africa, when we were in Nigeria and Kenya, things had deteriorated and burglary, mugging and theft with violence became more common. This is a sad commentary on the changes that have taken place in our lifetimes, not only in Africa but also throughout the world.

In our department, periodical meetings were arranged when senior staff came to Mpwapwa for discussions and the exchange of views. They were accommodated in our houses and, not only were the meetings of great value but the evenings provided opportunities for pleasant social gatherings and an *esprit de corps* was engendered. All the Veterinary Officers newly appointed from home, came to Mpwapwa on arrival in the Territory and it was my pleasant duty to give them a run down on the work that they would be expected to do and the diseases they could expect to encounter. Sometimes they stayed with us in Mpwapwa before being sent to a posting in the field but more often than not demands from the field were such that after a few days they were sent off to a station in one of the provinces where they were flung in at the deep end and presented with situations completely foreign to them.

When these officers came to attend one of our meetings, perhaps eighteen months or two years after being sent into the field, I was amazed by the way in which they had become confident and capable members of the departmental staff. They spoke with authority and with real expertise on subjects of consequence to their areas. They might have acquired specialist knowledge on the organisation of vaccine campaigns or the problems of disease control in their respective districts or of the best methods of salvaging hides and skins, their preservation and marketing and many other aspects of their work in the field. They had also gained an intimate knowledge of the tribal customs in their areas and how these impinged on their work in disease control and even, in some cases, they had learned sufficient of the local tribal language to assist them in their relationships with the stockowners. Two or three years previously when they were final year students they would never have believed that they would be handling the problems now facing them in their districts. It seemed to me the training we had in the British Veterinary Schools certainly produced graduates with flexibility and adaptability.

In Africa, the big chief of the territory was the Governor. We who didn't live and work at the seat of Government rarely saw and even more rarely met the Governor. While I was in Tanganyika the governor visited Mpwapwa once. When he announced that he was going to honour us with a visit everything had to be put into apple pie order. The great man was Sir Edward Twining and the Director, Bertie Lowe, escorted him up to the lab. I had to show him over the laboratory and its environs. It so happened that I had built, as cheaply as possible, a series of pens suitable to hold game and other wild animals, and I had working for me at that time Gerry Swynnerton, the Chief Game Warden. He procured for me, specimens of such animals as various antelopes and other herbivorous animals. There were many ideas at the time about the part played by game animals in maintaining foci of rinderpest virus, which could possibly seriously impede our attempts to control the disease in cattle. My work, in this respect, was unexpectedly successful. I even managed to breed some of the animals in my pens and we learned a substantial amount about their physiology and disease susceptibility. However, in one pen I had a young African buffalo. I felt that it needed a companion and so I put a young Zebu heifer in with the young bull. As I took Sir Edward round the animal compounds we came to this buffalo pen, I explained that the heifer was merely there as a companion for the bull. The Governor was most interested and he studied the situation for some moments and then said, "Does he pleasure her, Wilde?"

Later in the day, we had the honour of entertaining the Governor to tea in our house. James was about three at the time and he was trying to blow up a balloon with a singular lack of success. Finding his efforts to be of no avail, he came out of his corner behind the sofa and waddled over to the Governor and presented to him the recalcitrant balloon with the instruction, 'Blow'. Sir Edward was not amused and I picked James up and took him out to one of the servants who were hovering back-stage.

Horses were very rare in Tanganyika due to their susceptibility to trypanosomes and the prevalence of the tsetse fly carrier. Invariably, infection in the horse proved very serious and was usually fatal unless early effective treatment could be applied. In Mpwapwa we had established an area free from tsetse fly and so could keep a few horses. I acquired one when Bertie Lowe's mare, which had been served by a blood stallion (presumably in Kenya), was put in my care. I was present, supervising the birth and she produced a very nice filly, which Bertie allowed me to keep. I named the filly Judy and it grew well and as a two-year-old it was a very attractive animal. My Senior Technician, Eddie Gorton, was mad on horses. He had been involved with them in the army and undertook to school the filly. He was better at schooling horses than he was in his technical duties in the lab and made a good job of the horse so that for some years I rode around the station two or three mornings a week on my pre-breakfast inspection. I rode Judy until we left Tanganyika and sometimes Kathy accompanied me on a mule which we also had in our stables. For a brief period, we had a District Officer posted to Mpwapwa, who was keen on playing polo, as also was his wife. I, of course, had my pony and they obtained two others, lent me a polo stick and showed me the rudiments of polo. We had a few knockabouts with a puck on our primitive golf course. Unfortunately, just when I was beginning to be able to strike the puck to some effect, Chris was transferred to another station and my chances of becoming a polo player evaporated, never to be restored. This movement of the more junior Administrative Officers from station to station was common practice and in my eleven years in Mpwapwa we had many young officers occupying the 'boma'.

One of these officers, with whom we became well acquainted, was Dick Gower. He became a friend and was well liked on the station. He was a very keen sportsman and it was during his rather longer than most stay, that a football game was organised and I was dragged in to play. That was the last time that I ever played the game. Dick also organised a cricket match between the veterinary members and the rest of the station, including the school. The game was played on some rather rough ground in the village, which was scraped and stamped by the few prisoners that Dick had in the 'clink'. I've never been good at ball games but by some remarkable chance I was the top scorer on our side closely followed by Mr Sam, a burley Cape Coloured manager of one of our experimental farms. My score was thirteen. Needless to say, we lost, but the event enables me to claim the distinction of playing cricket against the man who was, later, to become the father of the popular and eminent Captain of England, David Gower.

Dick had quite a histrionic ability. This came to light when I organised a variety show in the bleeding hall at the lab. Dick did a one-man mime entitled on the programme, "the goalkeeper". It was quite hilarious, the goal posts being imagined and the goalkeeper alternating between complete boredom and manic activity. When the 'opposition' was obviously getting dangerously near, Dick mouthed frantic instructions at his team mates and when the crisis was over calmly retrieved his chewing gum from the place where he had stuck it on the imaginary goalpost. For this entertainment, I 'choreographed' a ballet entitled 'Ballet Insect'. In this the Good Fairy was Penelope Penworthy, otherwise known as Roy Egerton, our Workship Supervisor. Another rather ambitious item was the Indian Rope Trick that entailed quite a bit of hazardous acrobatics in the rafters.

Despite such light-hearted activities our official duties were not neglected. Some very fine work on the tsetse fly was done in Tanganyika. There are many species of the fly, *Glossina,* and each has its habitat in its own particular type of vegetation, climatic and physical conditions. These species demonstrated variations in predilection for species of the pathogen *Trypanosoma.* Some were more prevalent in forest, some in dry bushland, some in savannah. It was, therefore, possible to predict fairly accurately, the tsetse species likely to be of importance in any particular area. The vast amount of knowledge accumulated on this subject is the result of the difficult and arduous work put in by many workers in the fields of medicine, veterinary science and entomology in the areas where trypanosomiasis was rife. There are many eminent names in this field but I will only mention three here. Firstly Sir David Bruce who was the first to recognise the trypanosome as the cause of the disease, sleeping sickness in the human subject. Secondly Swynnerton, the father of Gerry who assisted me in my game animal work and whose name is perpetuated in the species, *T.swynnertoni*. Thirdly, H.E.Hornby, a former Director of my department and subsequently seconded to special duties during the Second World War. He, incidentally, was persuaded to come back to Mpwapwa from retirement in Southern Rhodesia, to take over my laboratory during my absence on leave.

I was involved in work on the use of trypanocidal drugs in the field and organised field experiments in an effort to reduce the losses due to this disease in cattle. One of these was in an area of bushland at Mkata in the Coastal Plain of Tanganyika. The idea was to see if cattle could be kept in good health in an area of varying fly density, which was partially seasonal, by means of prophylactic treatment. For this experiment I assigned one of the Afrikaner Stock Inspectors, Tom Bekker, to set up a camp in the area where we installed a large herd of cattle. A young new Stock Inspector Jim McNae who had just arrived in the territory from Manchester, was detailed by the Director to join the very bush-wise Bekker so that he could gain some experience. I would visit the scheme from time to time to see that all was going well and that the experimental plans were being adhered to. The area was some miles from the railway line at a point where access was possible. I travelled down on the coast mail train and got the train driver to stop at a point, which could be reached by the Land Rover with which our man had been supplied. When I arrived at the spot for the first time, he and the new recruit were waiting for me and they transported me to the camp where my tent had been pitched. The site was quite a good one and was dominated by a large thorn tree to the trunk of which a board had been nailed with the crudely painted sign 'Four Star Ranch. Sheriff's Office.' Above this title were four metal bottle tops nailed to the board. Tom said that I could have all my meals with them in what had been erected as a mess tent.

The meals were good and comprised mostly game antelope, which Tom had shot. The young recruit, Jim had taken to the shooting and camping adventure with delight. It was a far cry from being a schoolboy in Manchester. On the second day I was concerned to notice in the bottle of water on the table at mealtime, a considerable amount of wiggly activity. I asked where was the water supply. Tom explained that there was plenty of water in the pools, which in the wet season would be a running river but now were no more than a hippo wallow. "But surely," I said, "you are not drinking that untreated?"

"Oh no," said Tom, "we squeeze a lemon into it." I explained that while Tom might have gained some level of immunity from his childhood in South Africa, young Jim would be highly susceptible to all manner of diseases. I insisted on having all water for drinking boiled and this practice was instituted at least while I was in the camp. Jim informed me that after an unusual shower of rain, they had obtained their water from a series of elephant footprints. I adjured him not to drink any more water without having it boiled first. The experiment was concluded after several months and the results were very useful.

On another occasion the Administration was pressed to move the tribal people from a very highly eroded area of land at Kondoa-Irangi. The area was so badly eroded due to over stocking that it appeared like a number of miniature canyons and the cattle were beginning to die of starvation. Not far away to the east of the Bereku Ridge was an area of lush grazing on the borders of Masailand but this was covered with a variable density of bush which sustained the presence of three species of tsetse fly. The Department of Tsetse Research was engaged in clearing this area as a means of eradicating the fly populations therein. The Irangi people refused to move into this uninhabited area if they were not allowed to take their cattle with them. Had they done so in the conditions that were then extant their cattle would have died. The Administrative Officer of the area approached me to see if it would be possible to protect the cattle by means of some sort of drug regime. I agreed to devise an experiment designed to see if we could maintain susceptible cattle in the area being cleared, for sufficient time to permit the

Tsetse Research Department to achieve the eradication of the tsetse fly from the area. We carried out the experiment and showed that it would be possible to keep cattle alive and healthy for the period required. We found that prophylaxis could be effective but that it would be difficult and expensive to apply. It was decided as a result of our experiment that we could achieve the desired objective by routine observation of the introduced cattle and treatment with the drug of choice as soon as infection was diagnosed or was seriously suspected. To this end we agreed to train a team of local people in the taking of blood slides for examination at the nearest Veterinary Office and the injection of infected animals with the appropriate drug. It was a rather tedious job but it was a means of tiding over the difficulties of the tribe until the tsetse flies could be eradicated. Meanwhile, and over a period of several years, their old homeland could be given a chance to recover.

Before the war, Tanganyika attracted a large number of wealthy people from the west who visited the country and employed experienced hunters to take them on safari in the game areas. This provided a very lucrative business for a number of freelance hunters who set up camps and all the paraphernalia necessary to organise hunting expeditions for these wealthy tycoons. The hunters were known as 'White Hunters' and in addition to leading the safaris, some of them set up additional businesses that supplied all the necessities of hunting, including guns and camping gear. They also undertook the work of taxidermy, curing the skins of the unfortunate victims of the hunt and preparing rugs, carrosses and even stuffed specimens to be transported to their clients' homes, usually in America. When the war broke out, of course, this source of income came to an abrupt halt. The governments of the territories involved in this trade applied rules for hunting and issued licences from which substantial revenue was derived. Though this revenue was much diminished on the outbreak of war, licences were still issued for those inhabitants who could afford them. The White Hunters were now unemployed and were very ready to accept jobs as game observers and stock inspectors in government departments. The Veterinary Department of Tanganyika was prepared to augment its staff with these men who had a wealth of knowledge and experience of African conditions and the indigenous people so that we employed several of their number. They were mostly very colourful characters and were happy to give their services freely to any members of the service who were inclined to do a little hunting and who were prepared to buy the appropriate licences. Several members of my department took advantage of this situation purchasing an elephant licence and being taken on a hunt by the expert.

One of these hunters in our department, Basil Reel, was attached to the laboratory for a period, and had a reputation as one of the great elephants hunters. We did have a lot of trouble with the depredations of lions and leopards and Basil Reel was drafted onto my staff to help us to deal with this problem, for problem it was. The cattle we used in our work were of very little intrinsic value but as experimental entities they were of vital importance. Basil was a slightly built man but could maintain a fast walking speed for hours on end. His African assistants called him 'Bwana Tembo' (tembo is the Swahili word for elephant). He always carried a bottle of Phospherine as his means of keeping himself fit and in good health. Whether it was of value in this respect, I do not know but Basil swore by it. He often tried to get me to take out an elephant licence and let him take me out to shoot a big tusker, (Elephant ivory at that time was selling at £1 per 1lb.) I never would accept his offer. I would have hated to shoot one of those magnificent creatures. We did have to shoot the odd marauding lion or leopard, however, and Basil taught me how to flay and cure the skins. He often used to say that he would like to meet his end by being killed by an elephant but the poor chap died of cancer a few years after he left our department.

As a boy, I was a competent draughtsman and drawing was a hobby from an early age. When I arrived in Mpwapwa, I realised that there was so much colour that I should change my medium of pen and pencil and take up one of the painting media. Quite a few people whom I met were good artists including Rena Hornby and Rowena Culwick whose painting was under her maiden name, Rowena Bush. She was an excellent watercolourist and on occasions, when she accompanied her husband Theo on his visits to the lab, she very kindly gave me some tips. And so, I started to paint in watercolour. I later moved over to pastels and then, after a few years, I took up oils and I have painted ever since. I must have painted hundreds of pictures and still regard the art as my number one hobby. The subjects, of course, were all around us in Africa and many of my pictures have been taken to far distant parts by colleagues, friends and fellow Colonial Officers. My painting gave me a lot of pleasure and took up much of my spare time. I shall return, briefly, to this hobby later in this compilation of memoirs.

In 1950 Kathy was pregnant with our second child. As was the usual situation with the wives of officers in up country stations, there was no such thing as antenatal treatment. It was left to us to organise the arrangements for getting our wives to some suitable hospital at what we judged was the appropriate time. We were lucky in Mpwapwa, thanks to the hospital of the Groundnut Scheme. I was able to make arrangements with the staff of the hospital at Kongwa for Kathy to have one antenatal examination and to be taken there when she appeared to be coming into labour. The hospital was the most up-to-date in the whole of Tanganyika. It had on its staff eight consultants and was very well equipped. Apart from the Asian Sub Assistant Surgeons, very sparsely scattered European medics served the remainder of the territory. I had to take Kathy to Kongwa Hospital for a check up. Mona, the wife of one of my colleagues, Jim Buckley who was also a close friend, accompanied us on the trip. Mona was a plump lady who was always prepared for a bit of fun and on this occasion she didn't mind squeezing herself into the very limited accommodation behind the driving seat.

On the way back from Kongwa we had to cross a rather wide riverbed. It was the middle of the dry season and the crossing was about fifty yards of deep dry sand. I had to make a rush at it and unfortunately hit a large rock hidden in the sand in the centre of the riverbed. It was a disaster. The plug of the oil sump was sheared off and the entire oil content of the engine went into the sand. We tried to get the car out of the sand but, of course, we couldn't let Kathy in her pregnant state help out except by disembarking and so lightening the vehicle. Mona insisted on trying to help me to push but in spite of her weight we could produce no movement of the car. I had a spare gallon

144

of oil in the dickey seat and so I hacked a thick branch out of the bush and tried to whittle it into the shape of a plug and then hammered it into the sump hole. Tentatively I started the engine. My plug blew out and there was another patch of oil in the sand. We were now in real difficulties. The road was little used and we had about six hours of daylight left and we were 18 miles from home in thick bush. It was very hot and we had only one bottle of water. We sat in the sand in the shade of some thorn scrub and just hoped that some vehicle might turn up. After an hour or so there was truly, a godsend. A missionary on his way from Kongwa to the railway line drove up. He had to pass through Mpwapwa and so he would call in at our workshops and tell them what had happened. We had a long and uncomfortable wait and then, as the sun was sinking, along came Araldi and Venturelli in the laboratory lorry with a stout tow-rope. The two Italians were co-operators from Ethiopia who had been assigned to my surveillance for the duration of the war. They were great chaps and excellent mechanics and we got on very well together. With Kathy and Mona in the pick-up and me at the wheel of the Ford 4, I was towed back to Mpwapwa. Those who have ever travelled on African dirt roads in the dry season will be able to imagine the ordeal of steering in an open car being towed by a truck using a short towrope. By the time I arrived in Mpwapwa, I was indistinguishable in colour from the red of the road. As I steered through the village in the failing light the duka wallahs (shopkeepers) stared at me and asked among themselves "What red man was it, driving Bwana Wilde's motor?" Apart from the fact that the bath plug hole tended to get blocked up with red mud, a hot tub managed to get most of the dust off and restore me to a more or less normal colour.

It was the wet season in November when Kathy proclaimed that she had backache and was going into labour, just before midnight on the sixth of November. We called in Marie Egerton, who was the most experienced person on the station in the matter of childbirth. We had everything ready and loaded the car. Friends took care of James, and Gordon Read, known to all his friends as 'Kuku' because he was the Livestock Officer in charge of poultry husbandry, had the laboratory pick-up ready to follow us down the twenty-eight miles of mud road to Kongwa.

In the back of the vehicle he had put blankets, a mattress, cans of hot water and soaps, antiseptics, towels and everything else that we thought might be useful in an emergency. We started off knowing full well that the road would be difficult to traverse and that in parts there were washaways. With as much speed as we dared to take, we proceeded, managing to negotiate all the bad bits until we came to a point where the road had been washed away by a flash flood. All that remained was a jumble of boulders with a very steep drop into a rocky river bed. We searched around to see if we could cut through the bush at the side of the road and found a possible route, which required quite a lot of bush clearing so we set about it with an axe and a panga. As I remember the occasion, we were about six miles from Kongwa and the contractions were becoming more frequent. Marie was looking after Kathy, making her as comfortable as possible and giving her sips of hot drinks from a thermos flask. Gordon and I, working with the less than adequate illumination provided by two hand lamps, were hacking our way through the bush. Eventually we decided that we should try to get through the deviation. It was a bit hectic but I managed with the help of Gordon scrabbling about pushing in the mud, to get across. The pick-up negotiated the hazard more easily with its higher clearance. The rest of the way was muddy and unpleasant but we got to the hospital, greatly relieved and Robert Peter Havelock Wilde was born some hours later.

In 1951 we were in my third tour in Tanganyika and I was quite prepared to come back for a fourth tour when a suggestion arose from the USA that a research scheme should be set up to study the interactions between the African domestic animals and the plains game of tropical Africa. I suppose it was because of my work on the diseases of some wild animals, research which incidentally procured for me my master's degree, that I was approached through our department to organise a research programme and take over its direction. The plan was that a laboratory should be established at or near Ngorongoro on the edge of the Serengeti Plain. A team was to be selected and I was proposed as the leader. It was an exciting prospect but I had to think hard about it, as it would have meant my leaving the Colonial Service. However, it was proposed that when I went on leave, which was now imminent, I should go to the US to study, at various institutes, the latest techniques employed in virus research. I, therefore, accepted with, I may say, some apprehension. We packed up and left for the UK. We were able to leave all our household possessions in our house as the plan was for us to go back to my substantive job as Chief Veterinary Research Officer and from that post begin the organisation of the new research scheme. On arrival in London I was to report to the Colonial Veterinary Advisor in Whitehall. This I did and was ushered into the presence of Bob Simmons, who held the post and whom I had met when he was Director of Veterinary Services in Uganda. After the usual courtesies, Simmons said, "We are offering you promotion to the post of Assistant Director (Laboratory Services) in Nigeria." I was flabbergasted.

"What about the training in virus work which has been arranged in the USA?" I asked.

"If you accept the Nigeria post we have made arrangements with the US funding organisation to provide the training as it will be of great advantage to you in the laboratories in Nigeria." was the reply. Senior colleagues in the Service had advised me that if one was offered promotion it was not only wise to accept but very unwise to turn it down. The upshot was that I was appointed ADLS Nigeria on a significantly increased salary. I had entertained some apprehension about the game job, as it had not exactly been decided how the scheme was to be funded nor on what terms I would be employed. The information which I had received about the scheme was vague and I had no idea what say I would have in appointing staff or to whom I would be responsible except that I knew it was to be funded and run from America. I never found out about these factors and, in any case, the scheme was abandoned. Perhaps there were wheels within wheels and the idea was not supported in London.

The Colonial Office was agreeable to my going back to Mpwapwa after I finished my spell in the States, in order to be able to pack and consign our household possessions. I was to have my leave after being in America. The period of my training was to be three months. I had anticipated that it would be for six months but was more than happy to accept three months.

We spent a short time at Kathy's old home at Fylingthorpe

which is a small village almost contiguous with Robin Hood's Bay, six miles south of Whitby on the North Yorkshire coast. Kathy and I, accompanied by James spent a short holiday in Ireland, flying to the Isle of Man, staying there for a few days and then on to Dublin where we were met by Rob Lee and Joyce. Rob was a colleague who had come out to Tanganyika as a Veterinary Officer and was one of those whom I welcomed to the territory in my capacity as head of the laboratory. He was very much attracted to the research work and was later brought in to run the lab when I went on my first leave. Our short stay in Ireland encompassed a visit to Blarney where we kissed the Blarney Stone and a call on Bertie Lowe and Rita at their farm to which they had finally retired. Meanwhile, his Grandma in Fylingthorpe was looking after baby Peter. In November 1951, I left for the United States. I flew in a British Airways Stratocruiser calling at Keflavic and New Brunswick, terminating at Idlewild, NY. There I had to go through a prolonged and cumbersome examination by the immigration authorities. I was kept waiting in a cubicle for a long time and I began to fear that I would miss my plane to Washington. I detected a good deal of inefficiency and bureaucracy; however, I eventually passed muster and flew to Washington in a Convair.

My visit to the States saw me based in Washington at the United States Department of Agriculture and my work centre was in the huge building which was the headquarters of this august organisation housing its main Veterinary Laboratories. I had been booked into a hotel and was collected the following day by the Research Officer who was my base liaison contact. There then commenced a complex organisation of the work I was to do and the various research centres in which I was to do it. Details of all this would just produce a boring and unnecessary catalogue of laboratories and research workers and of journeys by train and Greyhound Coach as well as hotels and the people who were lined up for me to meet. Some of the places which made the greatest impression on me were, the Walter Reed Hospital where the virus being worked on was that of mumps, Cornell University Veterinary School where the work was on several virus diseases and Rutgers University where the most important thing seemed to be the 'grid game' *viz.* American football. My contact there was Professor Fred Beaudet, who was a most kindly and hospitable man. Fred was very keen on the game and was a great friend of the Chief Coach of the University team. The Coach was idolised by all the alumni and occupied a position at least as high as, if not higher, than the Principal of the University. While I was in Rutgers, there was a special meeting of the Alumnus Organisation as one of the needle matches was to be played the following week. Fred insisted on my attending the occasion and I was wined and dined lavishly. After the dinner, we all trooped into a large lecture theatre and waited for the proceedings to start. When the great company was comfortably seated the Chief Coach climbed onto the stage and to my astonishment and horror called the meeting to order and then said in ringing tones, "Friends, tonight we are honoured to have as our guest, Dr Jack Wilde from Africa. I think, before we screen the films we should hear what Dr Wilde thinks of the grid-game. Now Jack, let's have your views." I was dumbfounded but in order not to let my host down, I stood up and faced the serried ranks of very large men, any one of whom could have had me as a starter to the meal we had just eaten. I said that I had not been fortunate enough to see a real live game of American football but that I had seen it on the 'movies' and was intrigued. When I had been in New York and had found that about six pounds weight of the eight or nine pounds of the New York Times was devoted to the game I thought I should find out something about it. I was, of course, directed to Rutgers and very fortunate to be introduced to Dr Fred Beaudet who had brought me here this very night. After a few incursions into the realms of my ignorance I said that they would not want me to waste any more of their time but that I was as anxious to see the films which I had learned were to show the last filmed games of their next week's opponents, as they were. I thanked them profusely for their great hospitality and sat down. There was a roar of applause and quite undeservedly I received a standing ovation.

I visited the Naval Hospital at Bethesda and the University of Princeton where I met and stayed with Dick Shuman who had worked on rinderpest with an American team on an island in the St Lawrence River. At the suggestion of the USDA I went to see some of the great stock markets and a factory for the production of cattle feeds which had to be called 'chow' by order of the management. Any employee heard to refer to any of their products as 'foods' was promptly fined. While I was in the region of the Mississippi I took a day off and went to call on a brother of Kathy's mother, Uncle Willie who hadn't been seen by any of the family since he had left for America in the early part of the century.

Visiting the great stockyards of Chicago and Omaha was a testing experience. It was necessary to be in the yards on the catwalks at a very early hour in the morning. It was midwinter and the mercury was some enormous figure below zero. I wasn't equipped with suitable clothing and so I wore two pairs of pyjamas under my outer clothing. My veterinary contact thought that "real smart" of me, he had never thought of the idea himself but he would try it. Great numbers of cattle and other stock were bought and sold in a day and huge transport lorries were filled with the animals and I was told, they would be travelling all over the States during the next forty-eight hours. It occurred to me how vulnerable they were to a possible epidemic of some exotic disease such as rinderpest. No wonder the Americans were interested in rinderpest during the Second World War.

When I was in Washington I walked around the city at weekends. This is a most unusual activity, I believe, among the indigenous population, but it enabled me to see quite a lot of this extraordinary city. I went up the Washington Memorial by means of the elevator, an ascent of five hundred and fifty-five feet, and returned to ground level down eight hundred and ninety-eight steps. I visited the Capitol on the Capitol Hill and entered the Senate House, the Library of Congress and other parts of the Capitol complex. My walk took in the Jefferson Memorial, the Lincoln Memorial, the reflecting pool and the tidal basin. I stayed in the Houston Hotel and by the time I got back there I must have walked several miles. I managed to fit in a concert by the Philadelphia Orchestra under the baton of its Conductor, Eugene Ormandy. From my rather limited spending money, I paid four dollars eighty for a box seat, which was very uncomfortable, but it was worth it. The programme included Concerto for Orchestra in D Maj. by Handel, Chopin's No1

Concerto in E minor, Schuman's Sixth Symphony and Liszt's 2nd Concerto. The pianist was Alexander Brasilowsky. Later, when I was in Philadelphia, I was delighted to attend another concert by the Philadelphia Orchestra in its own concert hall, again conducted by Ormandy with Oscar Levant as pianist. On this occasion the programme included works by Sibelius, Gershwin and Tchaikowsky.

At the same time as I was in the States, a friend, Steve Barnet who was a Veterinary Research Officer in Kenya, was working for a spell with the eminent protozoologist, Taliaferro in Chicago University. I took the opportunity to visit him in the famous or notorious city where one of my most outstanding memories is of standing on an island in the middle of the Michigan Boulevard trying to cross the road. Obviously, I did eventually get across but at the time I entertained serious doubts of ever escaping from that traffic. I managed to make a short visit to Buffalo and crossed over into Canada at the Niagara Falls. The falls were spectacular as it was before a large part of the falls broke back to the position existing now. On my return to Buffalo I had to wait several hours for a train and it was viciously cold. I had nowhere to go apart from snack bars where I warmed up with coffee but one couldn't sit in snack bars for hours and so I went into a small theatre advertising a programme of 'Burlesque'. I had no idea what this might be but I thought it might be some sort of variety show. How wrong I was. I had never before seen such explicit stripping and sexy exposure. This certainly was an extraordinary experience.

When I was in New York it was the Christmas season so I had no official contacts. I think that it was the most miserable Christmas I have experienced either before or since. I was in a room on the twelfth floor of the Hotel Abbey. The room was warm, indeed overwarm, but I was feeling very unwell. So much so that I staggered into the street and found a doctor and was examined. He declared, rightly or wrongly, that I was suffering from virus pneumonia. Dr Politzer prescribed sixteen 250mg tablets of Aureomycin, one to be taken every four hours. He didn't give me a prescription but said that I could buy them over the counter at any drug store. I should encounter no difficulty, especially as I was a veterinary surgeon. I did have no difficulty in spite of my doubts and when the pharmacist found that I was a vet from England I could hardly get away from him as he had spent some time in the Boots Company in Nottingham, England. I still had to pay, what was to me, rather a large lump sum but then I hastened away through the freezing streets to my hotel room to start my course of treatment. I knew quite a lot about the broad-spectrum antibiotics and I was aware that large doses could cause rectal bleeding and in my case they did. I felt quite sure that I was not suffering from pneumonia and so stopped taking the tablets and just stayed in bed over Christmas. I began to feel better but was very hungry and so I put on the warmest clothing I could muster and went out to a drug store in the street and had a good bacon and egg breakfast.

I had two rather unpleasant experiences in that hotel. I was awakened one night by the noise of an awful row. It sounded as though some one was attempting to murder a woman. There were female screams and appeals not to kill her, I didn't know what to do. I couldn't locate the direction from which the noises were coming. They sounded as though they were next door or in the corridor outside my room. I tentatively opened the door but there was nothing to seen there. I decided that the noise might be coming from air conditioning vents. The noises stopped and I returned to my bed and sleep. Everything seemed quite normal in the hotel the next day and so I dismissed the event from my mind and put the whole thing down to idiosyncratic behaviour in New York.

The other episode occurred a few days after Christmas when I was sitting at the table in my hotel room writing some letters. I looked through the window, which overlooked a well between my part of the building and another part at right angles to it. A window cleaner was at work on the windows of the latter part of the building. He wore a belt to which were attached two straps, one on each side and each was supplied with a hook. The windows, which he was cleaning, were on the same level as my room, which was on the twelfth floor. As he finished one window he released one hook from a supporting hook at the side of the window frame, hitched it to the corresponding hook on the next window then released the second hook and quickly clipped it to the hook on the second window. As he did this, he swung his body across and his feet were then applied to the wall beneath the window frame. I was, to say the least, fascinated and at the same time scared stiff. I quickly reached for my camera but could not get a suitable view. There was, in the corridor next to my room, a door affording exit to the fire escape leading down to the yard far below. I thoughtlessly opened the door and stepped out onto the platform of the escape and the door swung to. The temperature was some degrees below freezing but I was in my shirtsleeves having been in my overheated room. It was impossible to open the door from the outside. I took the photo and then looked down at the vast amount of iron steps below me. I felt panic taking hold and peered around like a trapped animal. By good fortune, a maid in one of the rooms on my floor saw me and with great presence of mind she came round and opened the door from the inside. What a relief!

During my stay in New York I did another walk about and actually found myself in the Bowry and Chinatown. I was told that I was very ill advised to go to these places on my own. Like all tourists I went up the Empire State Building and looked at the Rockefeller Building and Wall Street. I attended Sunday morning service in the very large church in Fifth Avenue, which was a revelation to me. The sermon was preached by the Rev Leland Starke and what a good sermon it was. The collection was taken up by a vast body of about twenty sidesmen all clad in tail coats and striped trousers. When the offertory tray came past me I felt ashamed as I dropped my humble dollar into a mass of ten and twenty dollar bills.

I left New York and took the train to Iowa for my visit to Ames Veterinary School. There I was looked after by Professor Frank Ramsay and his family who made me very much at home. They insisted on taking me to their Square Dance night where I was taught the rudiments of this type of dancing. I didn't make a great success of the dancing but the evening was convivial and I felt welcome. I was most impressed by the fact that the Veterinary School housed in its midst, a large, spacious building which was devoted to sculpture, presided over by a most eminent sculptor, Christian Peterson. He produced some beautiful pieces of all kinds of subjects and the campus was enhanced by some of his massive works.

153

At the end of January I was alarmed by news from Kathy about Peter. Apparently the local nurse had given him an injection and it had caused a large and painful swelling in his leg. The local doctor didn't seem to me able to ameliorate the condition and said that things were serious. When I received another letter from Kathy saying that Peter seemed to be paralysed in the leg and asking me to come home at once, I made arrangements to fly back to England. I got to Idlewild Airport to find that my flight had been held back. Police and army were much in evidence and I learned that King George VI had died and the authorities were holding the plane back as the Duke of Windsor might want to fly to England immediately. Eventually he chose another route and we left for Shannon and London on the 6th of February. In London I stayed the night with my old friend Fred Bell and his wife, Margaret. Fred was then on the staff of our *alma mater*, the Royal Veterinary College. He was very interested in my views on the USA, particularly as he was due to make his first visit to the States shortly after mine. One thing that I commented on was the apparently universal need for people in New York, repeatedly to clear their throats rather noisily. I said that I had noticed this before I went to America in Alastair Cook's weekly 'Letter from America'. This was compulsory listening for me when I was in the UK. Fred told me much later, after he had done his visit to America, that when in NewYork he was in an elevator and found that the one other person in the lift was none other than Alastair Cook. In his usual forthright manner, he addressed his fellow traveller. "You're Alastair Cook aren't you?"

"Yes, I am indeed." was the reply. Fred, quite unabashed in the presence of this celebrity, went on to tell Mr Cook that a friend of his who had recently visited the USA for the first time had commented on the amount of throat clearing that went on in the very popular programme 'Letter from America'. Since then there has been a complete absence of the throaty noises in Alastair Cook's record making weekly letter on this BBC programme.

When I arrived home, I was relieved to find that Peter was improving and very shortly afterwards he seemed to be completely recovered. I think that when the nurse gave the inoculation she must have bruised a nerve without causing lasting damage.

I left for Tanganyika by air on the 12th of March. Kathy and the boys were to join me later. In Mpwapwa I was faced with the hassle of sorting out our possessions and packing up all that had to go to Nigeria. Several crate loads were consigned to Lagos via the Cape and then I made my sad farewells to our old friends and travelled to Dar es Salaam from where I flew to Nigeria, calling in at Khartoum and El Fasher, where we spent the night. Next day we flew to Maidugari where I first set foot on Nigerian soil.

CHAPTER 5

Nigeria

I arrived in Nigeria at Maidugari in March 1952. I flew by internal plane to Jos where I was met by Tony Thorne, Senior Veterinary Research Officer at the Vom Laboratories. At that time, Nigeria was divided into three regions, Northern, Eastern and Western. These were linked together as a federation with a Federal Government whose headquarters was based in Lagos, the country's main port and outlet to the sea. The research services were mainly a federal responsibility, the Veterinary Research Services being established in Vom on the Jos Plateau. The head of these services, answerable to the Federal Government was the Inspector General of Veterinary Services, with his Headquarters at Vom. The head of the Laboratories entitled Deputy Director of Laboratory Services was abbreviated as DDLS. Each region had its Director of Veterinary Services responsible for the veterinary field services in his region but relying on the headquarters for research and responsible to the Federal Government through the Inspector General. My position as DDLS was on the same level as the Regional Directors but responsible for advice and research aid to them. When I arrived in Nigeria, the Inspector General was Roy Marshall who had been head of the laboratories but was promoted to the top post when the previous holder, Bill Beaton, left to take up a post in East Africa. I gathered, over my first tour in Nigeria, that Beaton had been somewhat of a martinet not only in the Department but also on the station. I think that Marshall had suffered as well as the more subordinate officers.

This was the beginning of what proved to be the unhappiest

period of all my service in Africa. I did not really want the Nigerian job but I had heard that Marshall was a capable vet, was very well aware of the necessities of veterinary research and was well respected. I was, therefore, determined to give him every possible support and expected to have an interesting and fulfilling period of research. My expectations were to be dashed from the start. Firstly, Thorne had expected to get the post to which I had been appointed by the Colonial Office and was, therefore, resentful. Marshall made no effort to welcome me or, when they arrived a week or so after my arrival, Kathy and the two boys. Indeed, I had been in Vom for more than two weeks before I even met Marshall and this was in a situation where I was appointed as his number two. There were two large and imposing houses on the station, one for the Inspector General and one for the officer holding my post. The remaining staff houses were bungalows distributed along a ring road running round the station. These were occupied by my staff and the Head of the Veterinary School and his assistant. There was also a small catering rest house for visitors and temporary staff appointments.

I was accommodated, temporarily, in the rest house and when Kathy and the two boys arrived by air from the UK they joined me. I was told that my house was not ready for us. However, I went round to see the house and found that it had been virtually stripped of its correct quota of furniture. I discovered later that Marshall had given instructions for the furniture to be removed from our house and redistributed to other houses, including his own, which was lavishly furnished. Makeshift items such as wardrobes constructed of wooden frames and soft board had been fitted into our house leaving us with the very minimum of bush type furniture. Our heavy loads had not arrived from East Africa so we had to live virtually as though in a camp. We had no table, so that when we received our heavy loads we took our meals on a wooden crate covered with a bed sheet.

This treatment of any newly arriving officer, let alone one who was arriving as number two in the department, was completely incomprehensible to me. I was used to the traditional hospitality, which was the norm in all my previous experiences

157

in East Africa. It was a *sine qua non* in Tanganyika and indeed, in East Africa generally, that anyone arriving for the first time either as a new member of the staff or as a passing visitor was given a warm welcome and was helped generously and hospitably on arrival. This did not happen in my case at Vom. Some members of my staff did the best they could in the circumstances, but the dreadful inhospitality accorded to me, Kathy and the boys quite obviously stemmed from Marshall and his wife, a not very likeable type of woman. I could not understand this but over a period of time I think I arrived at a possible conclusion.

Marshall had served only in Nigeria and considered the Nigerian Service to be the cream of the African Colonial Services. I think that he resented the Colonial Office's appointment of an officer from the east as a slur on West Africa. There is no doubt in my mind that our veterinary work in East Africa was definitely in advance of that which was extant in Nigeria. The Vom Laboratories were well established and were perhaps the best in West Africa but in many aspects, veterinary work and field control lagged behind the developments which had taken place elsewhere. Indifferent work had been done since Marshall had been put in charge. In that time he appears to have done no recorded veterinary work at all. Any advances which had taken place, as far as I could ascertain, were due to the efforts of Tony Thorne and a few of his colleagues. I could quite understand how Thorne felt that he had been unfairly passed over but I suspect that the Colonial Office had realised that some new blood was necessary. Whether I was the one who could supply the necessary stimulus is a matter for others to decide, but I did my best in very difficult circumstances. It soon became apparent to me that Marshall did not occupy his office at all but that he spent the working day in an office which he had caused to be built onto the side of his house. It was explained to me that he usually left this 'bolt hole' at 4 p.m. and drove to Bukuru to consort with his tin mining friends at the club or managed to get in a few holes of golf on the Rayfield course. His private office was regarded by the staff in general as out of bounds. In my time at Vom, the only times when Marshall visited the laboratories were when he wanted a VIP visitor to be shown round the labs and to have demonstrated the scope of our research and the manufacture of vaccines.

As in most African tropical countries, rinderpest was of paramount importance and Vom had introduced the newly developed goat adapted virus vaccine, which, fundamentally, had made it possible to eradicate the disease from the East African Territories. When I arrived in Vom, the production of this vaccine had been set up by Tony Thorne and large amounts were being prepared and distributed to several West African countries in addition to those being used under our direction in Nigeria and the Cameroons. The way in which it was applied in the field left a lot to be desired. I have described earlier how our campaigns in East Africa were handled with the use of crushes and strictly controlled so that we could immunise millions of cattle in a year. I went out in Nigeria to see how the widespread immunisation of cattle was carried out in the field. I was appalled at the primitive nature of the method being used. No crushes were constructed. No holding pens were organised. The owners and a few locally employed labourers and Departmental assistants (dignified by the title 'mallam') caught beasts individually and threw them to the ground to inoculate them. The mallams then slapped a handful of dung on the backside of the animal as a crude method of identification and returned it to the herd. This was most unsatisfactory in many respects, the most important of which were that, at most, only a few hundred head of stock could be injected in a day and there was no certainty that the majority of cattle in any one area was immunised. This bore no comparison with the four to five thousand cattle dealt with in East Africa in a day with the disciplined organisation provided by a cadre of smartly uniformed Veterinary Guards and a team of trained Veterinary Assistants.

Regarding the financial administration of a laboratory such as that in Vom in any Colonial Service, cumbersome, time consuming and costly methods were common. In Nigeria the process of estimating for and obtaining funds was carried to extraordinarily convoluted lengths. I found that I was responsible for drawing up estimates of the finance required for the next year. This, of course, I had done in Tanganyika. One rarely obtained approval for the sums projected but in Nigeria, the methods were more complicated. I suspect that this was due to a considerable tendency in Nigeria for unethical use of Government funds. I found that I had first to submit what were called 'advance proposals' which were sent to the Treasury in Lagos. Mine, of course, had to go through Marshall who secreted himself in his office. He then passed them on to a European clerk who was styled 'Veterinary Secretary'. This functionary looked them over and gave his verdict to Marshall who then sent for me and relayed the 'Veterinary Secretary's' views as my instructions. I suggested that it would be a good idea if he, Marshall, looked over the proposals with me and that I might be credited with knowing what was required for the Laboratory under my control, rather better than a person whose only qualification for his elevated position was that he had been an AA patrolman in England before he was given his post as a lay secretary in the office of the Vom headquarters. Marshall, in a condescending manner, went over the proposals with me. He informed me that I had no chance of getting them approved as they stood, inferring that I had a lot to learn about such matters. However, if I insisted, he would forward them to Lagos. After the long delay, which was usual in the process of obtaining Government funds, my advance proposals were returned approved almost in their entirety. As can be well imagined, this did not make me any more popular with Marshall.

This insertion of advance proposals into the business of estimating and obtaining the necessary funds to carry on the work of a department obviously delayed the possibility of ordering and receiving the equipment so necessary for such operations as vaccine production. After approval of the advance proposals, modified and in some cases, markedly curtailed, one had to submit in the appropriate manner, the final estimates. All our very sophisticated equipment had to be ordered from overseas, primarily from the UK. By the time we had negotiated the specifications and price of the items, the prices had usually increased to figures higher than those entered in the original proposals and sometimes the details had been altered. The result was that we might have to transfer funds from some other section of the approved estimates, which complicated affairs

The authority, exemplified above, which Marshall had passed over to the Veterinary Secretary, was a bone of contention among the laboratory staff. This man was allowed by Marshall to exercise undue control over professional and technical staff; the administration of General Orders (for example, in such matters as travelling and subsistence expenses while on 'tour') and access to such services as those of the stores, without reference to the DDLS. He was given unseemly authority, which he was in no way qualified to exert.

In the government departments in East Africa, the day to day handling of finance was in the hands, largely, of Asian staff working under the supervision of expatriate officers. In Nigeria, where there was an upper level of Africans who were more highly educated than their counterparts in East Africa, most of the work carried out by Asians in East Africa was in the hands of Africans. This applied also in business, including that of the big overseas companies who had many branches throughout West Africa. Many more Africans held positions of responsibility and many constituted the professional classes in the disciplines of trade, law and medicine. In these professions it was possible to make big profits and there was keen competition.

However, corruption was rife and bribery pervaded all walks of life. I will give here a few examples of types of activities that were common in the system. I was told by some of my African friends, that poorer people in hospital were made to pay to the lower levels of hospital staff, small sums of money in order to obtain a mug of water or a bedpan. This especially occurred at night when the more senior officials were at home in bed. Such bribery was regarded as quite acceptable and there was a generally known expression for it. It was referred to as 'the customary gift'.

I have known African artisans and contractors who were employed on work by expatriates or companies, who asked their employers to pay them in cash and not by cheque. To cash or pay in a cheque, they might have to travel several miles to the nearest township with a branch of a bank, often by bicycle or on foot. Having reached the bank, the teller has been known to say that the transaction could not be carried out at that time for various spurious reasons. The poor chap with his cheque would be told to come the next day when, the same treatment might well be repeated. However, if a suitably large amount of cash was passed over to the teller, magically the obstructive reasons disappeared and the cheque was cashed.

Litigation was common and if an African wished to consult a lawyer, it was frequently necessary for the litigant to have to make a series of customary gift payments in rising value before he was able to have a consultation with the solicitor. The first was, as a rule, paid to the 'Mai Gardi' that is the watchman or doorkeeper. This would give him access to the outer office. The second might be necessary to see the Chief Clerk who would require his gift in order to assure access to the great man himself. Having achieved audience with this individual, he would be required to pay a first payment on the fee before the business could be conducted. Poor people were badly served, whereas the rich professionals or high up officials and expatriates received special attention.

Government officials were experts at finding loopholes in the legislation, which they could exploit to their advantage. I came to the conclusion that this was the reason for the very frequent amendments to financial orders which streamed out of Government so producing a burdensome bureaucracy which, in its turn generated more 'jobs for the boys' and elevated positions for the employees at headquarters. Returns could be demanded in triplicate. These were eventually regarded as insufficiently secure so that returns had to be submitted in quadruplicate, later in quintuplicate and even in sextuplicate. An allegation was brought to me by one of my senior African technicians that the Chief Clerk was demanding of him a proportion of his monthly wage, so that he could be assured of promotion to a higher grade. The implication was that the Chief Clerk would see to it that there would be no promotion if the monthly sum did not materialise. The Chief Clerk, of course, had no jurisdiction in this matter but the technician was not to know that. I had this allegation investigated thoroughly and it proved to be true. The Chief Clerk was suspended on full pay, pending the case being brought to court. This was a matter of about three months. When the case did come to court, I was called as an official witness and it was patently obvious that the accused was guilty. The

Chief Clerk, in his exalted position in society, was not without friends in the judiciary and the case was thrown out on a technical point due to the fact that the magistrate did not include in his transcript of the hearing, the fact that the accused had pleaded 'Not guilty'. The Chief Clerk was restored to his post immediately. In the first week after his triumphal return to the office he presented me with a request for compassionate leave so that he could visit his 'aged parents'. I discovered to my chagrin that according to standing orders I was unable to refuse the request.

When we transferred from Tanganyika to Nigeria, the difference between the two countries immediately became apparent. I have already indicated the differences in the populations and the relatively strong intrusion of the Africans into management and the professional classes in Nigeria. There were, however, marked differences in climate, topography and ethnological distribution. As I have said, the country was divided into three main regions, each with its own centre of government and its own predominant customs and tribal traditions. The Northern Region extended from the borders of the Sahara desert to the Central Plateau where the main town was Jos. The administrative centre was Kaduna, the common language was Hausa and the people were almost entirely Islamic. The southern part of the country was divided into two main regions, the Western Region being Yoroba and the Eastern Region being more mixed tribally but mainly Ibo. There was also a separate area of highland to the southeast, the Southern Cameroons. These regions brought Nigeria to the sea in the Gulf of Guinea. The Northern Region was mostly semi-arid, interspersed with spectacular rocky outcrops while the other regions were largely covered by tropical forest in areas of which cacao plantations flourished. Near the coast, the forest merged into swamps, lagoons and the estuaries of rivers.

Road safari in Tanganyika had rarely been interrupted by rivers of flowing water, except in heavy storms in the wet season. These torrents of water lasted only briefly during and immediately after flood storms and quickly reverted to their dry season form of sand rivers. By contrast, in Nigeria there are several permanent rivers, the greatest of these being the Rivers

Niger and Benue. These, in parts, are kilometres wide. Thus, safari in Nigeria is punctuated by river crossings, the smaller ones being by ferry and the larger by bridges. The railway running from the north at Kano to the sea at Lagos has to cross these rivers and where it does cross, the bridge serves not only the railway but also the road and so driving across the Benue at Makurdi, for example, one has to traverse a long road/rail bridge. It is, of course, obvious that some means must exist, of making sure that the motor car and the train are not on the bridge at the same time, particularly if they are travelling in opposite directions. Signalling methods are operated on the long bridges but on the shorter ones, it is imperative that the motorist makes sure that a train is not approaching either from before or behind. One has to accept that the train has right of way. Failure to concede this on the part of the car driver invariably ends in disaster. This rarely happens but the experience of one of our servants provides a salutary lesson. Dodo was riding his bicycle to Jos with, precariously balanced on the carrier, a large bundle of colanuts destined to be sold by his wife in the market. Like most cyclists in Africa, Dodo had a superior attitude towards the road and the fact that there might be other vehicles requiring to use it. He was in the middle of the short road/rail bridge on the road to Jos before he noticed a large monster belching smoke and steam approaching the other end of the bridge. His reaction was unusually prompt. He leapt off the cycle and flung it and the nuts and himself over the parapet into the river. I understand that he got an awful pasting from his wife for the loss of the colanuts.

The river crossings by ferry were very variable, hardly any two being similar. The simplest of them were based on the idea of lashing together two canoes a few feet apart by means of poles and securing to the poles a decking of planks. The vehicle to be transported had to drive onto this decking and then, its brakes, if any existed, were applied and the ferry was heaved, by hand, across the river by means of a rope or chain anchored to a tree trunk on each side of the river. Some of the more substantial ferries were based on a pontoon contraption hauled across by a winch and chain.

Safari by road provided a variety of adventures but amazingly, one heard of very few catastrophes. There were some tarmac roads but most journeys were over rather rough murram surfaces, often with plenty of potholes. I bought for our safaris, a long wheelbase Land Rover which was, I think, the first of its kind to arrive on the Plateau.

On one safari we were driving from Enugu to Mamfe along a rough mud road passing through areas of cacao plantations. We traversed the beautiful Cross River on a larger than usual ferry. Incidentally, this was the stretch of the river used as the location for the making of the film, 'Sanders of the River' featuring Paul Robeson. We arrived at a small river that crossed the road. This was spanned by the semblance of a bridge that, unfortunately, was devoid of decking. The planking, which presumably belonged to the bridge, lay scattered in the road and amongst the surrounding bushes. I presumed that the bridge had been damaged by a flash flood and got out of the car to investigate. Suddenly there appeared from the surrounding forest, a group of Africans. I pointed out to them that there was virtually no bridge to drive across and how were we going to get to Mamfe? "Not to worry Master," said the obvious spokesman, "we will soon fix it." In a matter of five minutes the planks were in place and I drove across after I had distributed a liberal sum of money to the stalwarts for their kindness in helping us on our way. Before we reached the next bend in the road, James, who was in the back of the Land Rover drew my attention to the scene we had just left. There was the helpful gang in the process of scattering the planking around in the haphazard arrangement that had prevailed on our arrival. One must acknowledge the ingenuity of the local inhabitants for devising this method of producing an income.

Vom was a government station situated on the Jos Plateau, some eighteen miles from the township of Jos. It was, essentially, the Federal Veterinary Headquarters and was populated almost entirely by government employees. A small portion of the government land of Vom had been allocated to the West African Trypanosomiasis Organisation which had established its research centre there. This was entitled the West African Institute for Trypanosomiasis Research, (WAITR) and its laboratories and staff accommodation lay about quarter of a mile from the Veterinary Laboratories. There was a very friendly co-operation between the officers of the two organisations. The Director of WAITR was medical Colonel Hugh Mulligan who had worked on malaria in India and had gained a prestigious reputation in tropical protozoology.

The Veterinary Laboratories and ancillary housing occupied an area inside an extinct volcano. The altitude was approximately, 4000 feet and so, the climate was, by West African standards, very pleasant and even, at certain times of the year, quite cool. Whether or not the volcanic association had anything to do with it, Vom seemed to attract very severe and spectacular thunderstorms. Indeed, meteorologists visited Vom in the course of their studies of electric storms. Deaths from lightning strike had been recorded and in some of the violent storms items of electrical equipment were damaged. On the whole, however, Vom was, climatically, a very attractive station and was visited by many from the hotter areas as a 'hill station' very popular for local leave and as a respite from the heat of other areas of West Africa.

Social activities in Vom centred on the Club that had a tennis court and a snooker table. The latter was purchased and installed at great expense, the money being raised by the members who bought interest free redeemable bonds. During the time I spent as chairman of the Club Committee, I remember that at each meeting, an invariable item on the agenda was 'Repayment of Snooker Table Bonds'. We organised entertainment and ran a bar. An entertainment, which I produced, was a rather ambitious variety show. The music was supplied by a bunch of gramophone records, which Tony Thorne had recently acquired and these were started and stopped by the dexterity of one of our members crouching behind our improvised stage. One item was a ballet, based on the one that I had produced in Mpwapwa. I gave it the same title, Ballet Insect. In it, the fairy wore a tutu and hobnailed boots, a pair of wings and carried a fly sprayer as a wand. I borrowed a trumpet and mimed the trumpet part in the popular tune, 'Cherry Pink and Apple Blossom Wine'. People were amazed, as they didn't know that I could play the trumpet. Nor did I. Nevertheless, the show was an acclaimed success and helped to pay off some of the snooker bonds. Four miles away, on the road to Jos, was a large

166

and very active club, which was heavily subsidised by the very large consortium of tin miners at Bukuru. The main company was the ATMN, the Amalgamated Tin Mines of Nigeria. This club had a swimming pool, a large bar, sporting facilities including golf, a large auditorium used for stage shows and cinema presentations and a well-patronised restaurant. As a result of our variety show the committee of the Bukuru club invited us to perform some of our items on their stage for one of their big entertainment nights. My trumpet 'solo' was among the selected items and was well received.

Bukuru was the centre of the very important tin and columbite industry and a characteristic of the area was provided by the huge machines called draglines, which literally walked over the land like prehistoric monsters, tearing out great quarries. In these quarries, the tin and columbite were washed out of the spoil by powerful jets of water. Many of these quarries became artificial lakes, which attracted waders and other species of aquatic birds. After my time in Nigeria, I believe that a club was formed for sailing on one of the artificial lakes, which resulted from the activities of the draglines.

About three miles from Vom was a hospital established some thirty years before our arrival in Nigeria. This was run by Dr Barndon and his wife who had come out to the country as medical missionaries. Dr Barndon was a theologian but also was qualified in medicine and engineering. The pair was dedicated to the health and welfare of the Biroms who were the native inhabitants of the Plateau. At that time, the Biroms were part of a primitive tribal group which were designated 'Pagans'. They were not Hausas but had probably inhabited the north of Nigeria long before the Islamic Hausas had infiltrated into the area. With the advent of more sophisticated Africans, some ethnologists suggested that the original inhabitants had been pushed back into the more rocky and inhospitable areas where they maintained their ancient lifestyles. When we were in Nigeria, the female Biroms were unclothed except for a variable type of grass skirt or G-strings from which depended leafy twigs, small grass mats or iron rings. The males were mostly completely naked except for a cover made as a suitably shaped basket woven from grass and which was worn on the penis. The Birom houses were round thatched huts scattered in groups in almost inaccessible places in the rocky outcrops on the Plateau. These people existed on a most primitive diet and slept on benches of hardened mud with a hollow underneath in which grass could be burned to provide some sort of heating. They appeared to have little in the way of textiles. When self-government came into being, nakedness in public was made illegal and I hope something was done to improve the standards of living and education of these people.

Dr Barndon's Vom Mission Hospital, by virtue of its situation, catered mostly for Biroms. These people were not used to seeing, let alone entering, solid brick buildings and Dr Barndon adapted his hospital to this characteristic of these primitive people. His clinic and theatre were solidly built but where one might expect wards, there were rows of Birom huts. These provided living accommodation for the patients and their families who used the huts as they would their village homes and here they cooked and lived looking after the patient who received visits from the medical and nursing staff who provided the necessary treatments. One section of the hospital was devoted to sufferers of leprosy. No payment for treatment was demanded but grateful patients helped to sustain the hospital by bringing gifts of produce from their cultivated plots.

Sunday services were held in the Barndons' living quarters and people from Vom were always welcome. Rob Lee who was appointed as head of the parasitology section of the lab and was a handsome bachelor, was particularly welcomed by the nurses of the hospital who were, of course, all dedicated Christians. On one Sunday evening, we went over to a service and Rob tagged along with us. All the ladies just about fell over each other to get to the harmonium to play Rob's favourite hymn. When they asked him what his favourite hymn was he was somewhat disconcerted since he hadn't any particular hymns in mind but he rose to the occasion and said, somewhat diffidently, "Be thou my vision". At that there was a subdued argument among the ladies to determine who was to play this hymn. The one who found the music first promptly pushed herself onto the stool and started to play.

To shorten the distance from the mission to the more populated areas, Dr Barndon had built two bridges across a ravine. They were a form of suspension bridge, the decking being supported from heavy steel cables slung from sturdily built stone arches at each side of the ravine. These arches were of such a size as to allow vehicles up to the size of a family saloon car to pass through. One of the commonest vehicles on the roads was the 'mammy wagon' which was the local equivalent of a bus, carrying large numbers of passengers and various types of load. These could not get onto the bridge and had to go the long way round. To drive across in a normal car was a frightening operation as the decking consisted of transverse heavy planks attached between two heavy cables. These rose up like a wave as the vehicle proceeded to move forward.

Another tribe represented in our area was the Fulani. These people I would describe as the counter-part of the Masai in East Africa. They are nomadic pastoralists and depend for their livelihood on their cattle. The women of the tribe make butter from their cows' milk and sell their butter as balls floating in a gourd of milk. The physiognomy of these people is much more aquiline than that of the Bantu Africans. In this tribe the initiation ceremonies of the young men coming to manhood bore a parallel to those practised by the Masai. The ceremony was called 'The Fulani Beatings' and was officially banned by the British Administration as it often caused severe injuries to the participants and sometimes there were fatalities. Kathy and I were privileged to witness one of these ceremonies. We were invited very confidentially to the tribal village, to arrive soon after dawn. We were allocated seats among the elders and when I asked for permission to take photographs, the permission was freely granted.

Briefly, as we saw the ceremony, it went as follows. Each year as the young men approached the time for taking a wife, they were selected for initiation into the manhood of the tribe. The people gathered in the appropriate venue and the elders took their places on their stools. A passage, clear of people, was demarcated in front of the elders and on each side of this passage the senior men of the tribe were lined up, each man being in possession of a stout stick about three quarters of an inch thick. The candidates for initiation were then led along the passage holding with outstretched arms, above their heads, a stick or long antelope horn. The candidate at this stage had a sponsor at each side. Each sponsor had a stick with which to fend off the efforts of the men along the sides, who attempted to strike the young man across the chest or belly. Not all the attacks were successfully fended off and the candidate usually took some painful strikes. This, however, was just the beginning. When all the candidates had passed through, their sponsors abandoned them and they had to walk through the passageway alone and unprotected. The men at the side at this stage aim their blows with even greater ferocity. Some of the candidates have, tied to their stick or horn, a small piece of mirror. The idea of this is for the young man to be able to see that there are no tears in his eyes. It is during this phase that serious damage can be caused. There have been cases when the spleen or liver has been burst and the candidate on such an occasion will almost certainly die. The excitement and even frenzy of the candidates can be such that they expose themselves a second time to the ordeal. It is accepted that those who show the greatest bravery will have the choice of the most attractive of the nubile women. I wonder if, since self-government has been established, this custom still flourishes?

Wherever one goes in Africa, dancing will be encountered. Tribal dances are a basic part of African culture. The dances vary with the tribes and some are very complicated, requiring a high degree of expertise, others are simpler and even pedestrian. Some require a considerable amount of energy and physical strength. The types of dance also are associated with matters of importance to the tribe such as harvest or matrimony or, as I have described above, initiation into manhood. Not far from Vom there was a tribe called the Miangos in which the dancing was very disciplined. In all my experience of tribal dances I have never seen such precise dance movements. These were based on skilful drumming. The drums varied in size but were made from hollowed out pieces of large tree trunks over the ends of which were stretched animal skins. The drumming and dancing were in the same class as some of the military movements seen at military tattoos. Bound round the legs of the dancers, all male, were plaits of grass, which were virtually strings of little grass boxes, which contained seeds or small pebbles. As the feet were stamped on the ground they made a swishing sound which was synchronised with the drumbeats. Another local tribal dance was made up of high leaps into the air followed by falling to the ground, landing violently on the buttocks. This dance was, indeed, painful to witness.

There were some traditional ceremonies of which the worst that came to my attention was the ghastly 'horse beatings' practised by some Ibo tribes in the south. When a man attained a certain status in the tribe, he had to establish his position *vis a vis* his peers. To do this, he would have to purchase a horse. Horses did not live in the southern regions of Nigeria because of the prevalence of trypanosomiasis in the forested areas of the south. The horse, therefore, had to be purchased in Northern Nigeria and walked great distances to the tribal home. When it arrived, possibly now suffering from the debilitating disease caused by the trypanosomes, the ceremony was arranged and all the tribal people of importance were invited and sustained throughout the period of the ceremony. On the day set for the festivities, the poor horse was brought into the middle of the area set aside for the activities and was then beaten with clubs persistently until it dropped dead. The host thus attained the appropriate status of 'a one horse man'. If he achieved more wealth, he might then perform a repeat performance in order to attain greater prestige in the tribe. Some affluent tribal members purchased two horses at once slaughtering them both in the one ceremony. I was appalled when one of my very senior, and well-educated Nigerian staff, came to me and asked for special leave. I asked him what was the purpose of his taking leave. He told me that his father was performing the horse beating ceremony. I asked him how he, as an educated man, could condone such activity. He said that it was essential in his tribe and he, as the eldest son must take part in the ceremony. When he reached his father's status in the tribe, he also would have to perform his own horse beating.

While we were in Nigeria, the time came when some sort of formal education for James and Peter was necessary. A lady did run a small school in her house at Bukuru for pre-school and first year primary children but it was not particularly what was required for our two boys. Mrs Early, the wife of one of my

171

Senior Technicians had been a primary school teacher and she was prepared to take James and Peter as pupils in the mornings of weekdays and so this introduction to school was arranged. I dropped the boys off at Early's house on my way to the lab in the morning, and picked them up on my way home for lunch. It was a very good arrangement and Mrs Early was very helpful in starting the boys off in their education. There is an amusing anecdote from this time. While waiting for me to pick the boys up at lunchtime, Mrs Early used to read them some little stories. One day as lunchtime approached, Mrs Early asked the boys what story they would like her to read. James said that they would like the one about the king who was so mean that he would not go to the lavatory. This proved to be the story about the king who was described as 'so mean that he would not spend a penny'. There were other children on the station so that there were some parties and picnics and minor adventures. It is fortunate that our boys suffered no serious illnesses from these forays into the bush and on the riverbanks where we went for the odd picnic. Later, we discovered that in some of the places we could have been exposed to onchocerciasis (river blindness) carried by Culicoides midges and some years later Lassa fever virus was found in an area that was not far away.

A feature of the wild life of the Plateau of Nigeria was, and I suppose still is, the extraordinary viciousness of the wild bee population. Many deaths of animals, and even human beings, were recorded as resulting from multiple bee stings while we were in Nigeria. These wild insects were notorious for their unprovoked attacks on cattle and human beings. A swarm settled in the roof of our house and during daylight hours, members of this group would attack anyone moving in our front garden. This became such a painful nuisance that the man we employed as a gardener could not do any jobs in the front garden where his work had to be suspended. Visitors to our house were warned not to leave their cars but to wait at the foot of the patio steps until either I or one of the servants, protected by a mosquito net, went down to the car. The visitors then leapt swiftly under the net and were escorted indoors. This was a most unpleasant situation, several friends receiving the odd sting so that I decided I would have to do something about it.

It was very difficult to get at the hive as the only way I could approach the underside of the roof was by leaning outwards from the upstairs veranda. This was such a hazardous procedure that I attached a rope from a roof timber to my waist to support me. By this means in the darkness of the evening I managed to spray a good deal of Gamexane into the roof space hoping for a result. Fortunately the operation was successful and the next morning the floor of one of the rooms which had a boarded up fireplace in it, was covered with dead and dying bees to a depth of about two inches and we were left in comparative peace.

Soon after I was established in Vom, there was a vacancy for another research officer for work, primarily on parasitology. I was fortunate enough to be able to get my old friend, Rob Lee appointed by the Colonial Office to this post. Rob had first come out to Africa in 1946 when he was appointed to Tanganyika. He worked with me for some months and was then transferred to the field where he had a lot of experience in the provinces principally dealing with outbreaks of rinderpest and other epizootics. He was really research minded and began to take a keen interest in the many parasites of which there were large populations in the livestock of the country. Unfortunately he contracted a lung infection and had to have hospital treatment back home in Ireland. Because of his illness, he had to leave the service and when he recovered he specialised in animal parasitology so he was the obvious man to fill the post in my lab in Vom. I was delighted when he was appointed to the post and welcomed him to Vom in 1953. He was a great asset to the Nigerian service and produced some good work. He married Joyce during his first leave from Vom and stayed in Nigeria for some years after I left and returned to East Africa. He went back to Dublin where he became a lecturer in parasitology in Trinity College and finished up as Professor of Veterinary Parasitology and Dean of the Dublin Veterinary School.[*]

Another important addition to my research staff was Walter Plowright, who had been working in Kenya and was transferred

[*] Destination 5 Memories of an Irish Veterinatrian by Robert P Lee 2003 Morrigan Co. Mayo, Ireland. ISBN: 0 907677 029

to Vom during my period as Head of the Laboratories. He had already made some very important contributions to veterinary virological work, primarily on rinderpest. I was very pleased to have him on my staff and did my best to create the conditions necessary to permit him to follow up his virus work. His arrival made it important for us to have more sophisticated equipment for virological work and so I converted one of the rooms in the main laboratory into a positive pressure laboratory. This was a rather difficult job, as it involved sealing the room in such a way that the air entering it had to pass through very fine bacteriological filters. Entry to the room had to be through a double door arrangement which allowed air to pass out of the room only and permitted no entry of air except through the filters. I don't know whether the room was very satisfactory but it did permit Walter to start his work on the rinderpest virus that later became so successful. However, my rather clumsy effort was soon superseded by the introduction of the new positive pressure cabinets which are now to be found in all laboratories involved in pathological research. After some preliminary work in Vom, Walter returned to Kenya to direct virus work in the newly erected East African Veterinary Research Organisation laboratories at Muguga about ten miles from the Kenya Veterinary Headquarters at Kabete. He became a very eminent scientist in the virological field and has been the recipient of many honourable awards which include Fellowship of the Royal Society. I feel honoured myself to have been helpful to him in a very small way in the early part of his career.

Our Land Rover was excellent for safaris on the very rough murram roads of Nigeria. It came in very useful when Marshall retired and I assumed the duties of the Inspector General in an acting capacity. It was, at this time when the Queen and Prince Phillip made an official visit to Nigeria and Kathy and I were invited to a royal garden party in Lagos. We decided to make the journey by road so that I could see some more of the country over which I now held some responsibility in veterinary affairs. One of the mechanics in the laboratory workshop was due for leave and as his home was near Lagos he came to see me to ask if he could have a lift in the back of our Land Rover. I agreed as he was familiar with the car and would help me with its maintenance should we encounter any trouble. Moreover, much of our journey would be through Yoruba country and since he was a Yoruba, of course, was at home with the language. We left Vom one very hot day and descended from the Plateau onto the plains. By evening we arrived at Makurdi on the Benue River and pulled into the rest house. We found a little shade near the rest house wall and began to unload our night luggage. Momadu, our mechanic, could lay out his mat and sleep in the truck. I noticed an awful stink like the smell of putrid meat. I couldn't locate the source. I told Momadu that he could unroll the canvas sides of the Land Rover's cover so that he could be protected from prying eyes and wandering hands. The source of the stink was immediately revealed. In the rolled canvas, Momadu had put a piece of meat to take to his family, as meat was not easy to come by in his home village. The package, wrapped in a scruffy piece of brown paper was crawling in maggots, which were scattered around, as the canvas was unrolled. We had to get some disinfectant to clean up the mess and dispel some of the stench. Our journey was resumed on the following morning when we crossed the long road rail bridge over the River Benue and with a night stopover in Enugu we arrived safely in Lagos where we enjoyed the hospitality of the Pathologist in charge of Lagos Hospital whom we had met in Vom and who had invited us to stay. After the garden party I looked over the Lagos Veterinary Office where the Veterinary Officer in charge was Bill Brewster. The posting to the Lagos area was not a popular one and so the incumbent had to make the best of it. Bill had acquired a little rather dilapidated stone building on Tarkwa, a small island about half a mile offshore. He had the place cleaned up and arranged for camp equipment and cooking facilities to be installed together with the services of a cook. We had a very pleasant weekend there where the cool sea breezes made a wonderful release from the heat and noise of Lagos. During that weekend we were surprised to hear that the Queen's party was to spend a day on the island having lunch at the Governor's Lodge on the other side of the island. When she arrived, she was greeted by large numbers of the people from Lagos spending the weekend relaxing on Tarkwa. They were all in scanty beachwear as, indeed, were we. Unfortunately, we couldn't enjoy more than

175

a weekend in this pleasant spot as I had to be back in Vom for official business by the following Thursday. The journey back was without untoward incident until Wednesday afternoon when we had just crossed a river by ferry and were travelling slowly along a track which was a network of deep potholes among stones and sand. Suddenly, the front end of the vehicle dropped with an ominous thud and crack. The engine mounting had broken. The situation was serious. There was no noticeable habitation about and it seemed that we were stuck. By amazing good luck a motorist came towards us from the direction in which we had to go. He informed us that a few miles ahead there was a trade centre but they were on holiday and he didn't know if any of the staff were there. Trade centres were institutes set up by government for the training of African artisans in such subjects as building and mechanical engineering. I managed to find a piece of bush timber and jam it in such a position that I could drive the car ahead very slowly and with infinite care. We got near to the gates to the centre and tried to find someone who could help. By what seemed to be a miracle, the first house we tried was open and in the garden, a European was slumbering gently in the shade of a mango tree. I approached him and he woke up. I explained our predicament and he said he could help. He directed us to a workshop where he opened up and, of all things, disclosed a welding outfit. He was the only member of staff on the centre, all the rest were having a special holiday. He was an expert welder and he fabricated a bracket, which he welded onto the chassis so that it would support the engine sufficiently to permit us to travel with care and at slow speeds. You can imagine how grateful we were to this benefactor and how lucky we were to be able to proceed on our way. By this time it was getting dark and so we proceeded slowly until midnight when we arrived at the beginning of the escarpment that led up to the Plateau. We had a Primus stove in the truck as well as some sausages and a loaf of bread. We wakened the two boys and started frying. James and Peter thought it was a great adventure. Our supper eaten, we started to creep our way up the escarpment and without further trouble arrived home in Vom, very tired and very relieved.

When Marshall retired and left Nigeria, he made no attempt

to carry out normal procedure and did not even give me any advice as to the functions of the office in which I was to act until a new head could be appointed. He handed over all confidential papers to the so-called Veterinary Secretary who also was given the keys to confidential files. This was quite reprehensible and indicates the kind of person Marshall was. Nevertheless he was appointed Veterinary Adviser to the Colonial Office where his incompetence could be extended to all veterinary services throughout the Colonial ambit. It was soon after Marshall left that I received a letter from the Secretariat requesting my recommendations of any of my officers for honours. Previous correspondence on this subject was in the confidential files and I asked Blythe for the necessary files to be opened. He was inclined not to let me have the files saying that they were confidential. I pointed out to him in no uncertain terms that I was now in office and that all confidential matters would be in my hands and not his. When I examined the previous correspondence I found that Marshall had never recommended any member of the staff for an honour and, as far as I know, he never received one himself. I recommended two members of staff, one for a CBE and one for an MBE Both were awarded. I also found that several members of the staff had been listed for Coronation Medals. There was a letter from the Resident drawing Marshall's notice to the fact that he had omitted Wilde's name from his list and so he, the Resident, had put my name among his recommendations and so rectified the omission. Coronation medals were awarded to almost all civil servants including the most junior. This example of small mindedness is an indication of the unpleasant atmosphere in which I had to perform my duties.

During the year in which I was acting head of the department, the post of Inspector General was changed to that of Director of Veterinary Research. A year after I had assumed charge, I received a hand written letter from Marshall, now Veterinary Advisor to the Colonial Office, saying that he expected that I would be disappointed as I had not been promoted to the substantive post but that it had not been his decision. He implied that the decision had been made over his head and that the new DVR would be Ian Taylor, who was being transferred from Uganda. Some years later, when I was on an official visit to Australia, I met Bob Randall, who had been Director of Veterinary Services, Uganda. Taylor was in his department in Entebbe when Marshall visited him from the Colonial Office and asked his permission to offer the DVR, Vom job to Taylor. Randall told me that he was delighted, as he was quite happy to get Taylor out of his department. At first, Taylor turned down the offer on the very cogent grounds that he had never made any vaccines in his career and he expected he would not be welcome in a laboratory one of whose main functions was vaccine production. However, Marshall persisted and eventually returned to London with Taylor's acceptance. So much for Marshall and his integrity.

When Taylor arrived in Vom I received him and helped him to settle in. I accompanied him to Lagos and Kaduna and introduced him to the Government and the officials who would be of importance to him. He thanked me for being so helpful, indicating that he had been very apprehensive in the circumstances, thinking that I might have refused to help him in his job. His actual words were rather more colloquial.

Some years before this, a building project had been planned and started, I think originally, by Beaton. It was to provide a headquarters for the Department of Veterinary Research and comprised an office for the Director and his staff with a library and all the appurtenances of a prestigious headquarters. It had a purely administartive function and when Taylor arrived it was nearing completion. Most of us had not taken much interest in it and had casually noticed the progress of the building work. We had built a new bacteriology lab, designed by me, and a rabies laboratory designed by Tony Thorne. I had also obtained the funds to have made in the UK and shipped out to us, a mobile laboratory. It was a first class small laboratory with provision for bacterial and virus work with sterilising apparatus. It could be plugged into mains electricity when it was visiting a site where this existed but it had its own generator that was capable of producing sufficient power for all the functions of an advanced laboratory including air conditioning. It was designed with the object of making possible advanced investigation on the spot in the field in any area of Nigeria. However, Taylor's first priority was the completion of the Director's office and the ordering of a suitable carpet. I was relegated to a table in the corner of the library. When he had settled in he consulted mostly with the junior members of the staff and I heard of his decisions from these members. I found, one day when I wanted to consult him over a matter of policy that he had 'gone to London on official business'. I therefore made the decision to apply to the Colonial Office for a transfer to another territory.

Shortly after this the Governor General, Sir James Robertson visited us. Taylor escorted him round the new building and the laboratories. As he was leaving the building, Sir James sent for me and said, "I am going to visit the WAITR laboratories and I would like you to accompany me in the car." When we were seated in the back of the Gubernatorial Rolls, Sir James told me that he had heard that I had applied for a transfer. He assured me that he could see how unpleasant was my situation but he said, "I would like you to stay on. This man Taylor has no idea of how to manage this department. He obviously does not have the necessary knowledge of Nigerian conditions and the work of this laboratory." He then repeated how he fully understood my difficulty but he would deem it a personal favour if I would withdraw my application and try to exercise my influence on the running of the department. I acquiesced. The Governor said, "Thank you, Wilde, I'm grateful to you."

After a month or so I found that I was not kept in touch with the affairs of the Department and had to rely on messages sent to me by junior members of the staff whose company Taylor seemed to cultivate. I was not consulted on the research or vaccine production programme and might as well have not bothered to visit the lab but stay at home and pass my time in whatever pursuit took my fancy. I explained the situation to the Secretariat and I was offered the post of Deputy Director of the East African Tsetse and Trypanosomiasis Research Organisation based in Uganda. Shortly afterwards I received a letter from John Ford, the new Director of that organisation, saying how delighted he was to have been offered me for the post and he hoped I would accept. I did accept and there followed a very cordial correspondence between me and John Ford. My tour in

Nigeria was ending and so we packed up and were booked on the SS Apapa, Elder Dempster Line, bound for Liverpool.

The day of our departure was a sad one. Most of the expatriate staff and a great crowd of the African staff and our own domestic staff were at the station at Bukuru. Some of the African staff were in tears. As the train pulled out there was a rush for the cars and the crowd who could find places in the cars posted away down the road to the road rail bridge on the way to Jos and there they were waving us off from the roadside. I have to admit that we were emotionally affected. When we arrived in Lagos, we stayed in a hotel for the few days we had to wait for the sailing. It was then that a remarkable thing happened which was to affect the whole course of the rest of my career. Communications in Nigeria and between Nigeria and anywhere else were completely unreliable. Telephones didn't work and telegrams took days and sometimes weeks to reach anywhere overseas. The postal service was subject to delay and was unreliable. Amazingly a letter from the UK addressed to me and which I assumed had arrived in Vom after our departure, was readdressed to me at the hotel in Lagos and delivered to me in the hotel the next day. I never heard who had readdressed it as no one would have believed that a letter sent to us in transit in Lagos could possibly ever find us. However, it did find us and it had come from the Veterinary Director of the Wellcome Foundation in London. In it Dr Montgomery wrote that he heard that I was leaving Nigeria. He had heard a rumour that I was taking up an appointment in Uganda, in which case the proposition he had in mind might not interest me. The Foundation was looking for some suitable person to build a research laboratory in Kenya for work on the possibility of finding a cure for East Coast fever. In any case, he and his colleagues would be very pleased if I would visit them when we arrived in the UK.

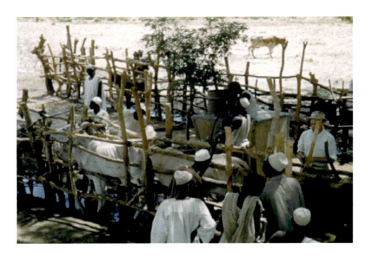

A locally made cattle crush. Dr Ian Macadam supervises collection of blood samples from Borani cattle.

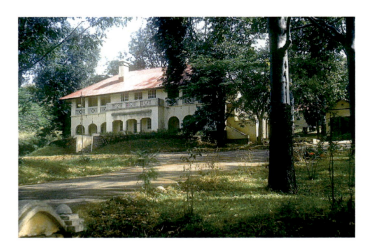

The house in Vom.

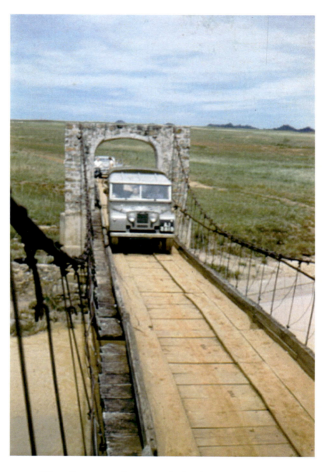

Veterinary work – travels in the Land Rover.
Dr Barndon's Bridge.

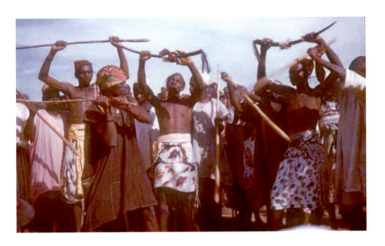

Fulani Beatings.

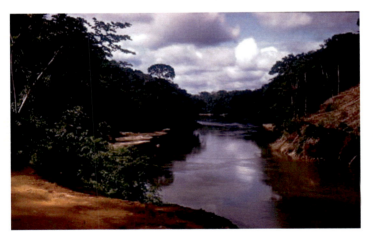

Cross River from our rest house – the film 'Sanders of the River' was made here.

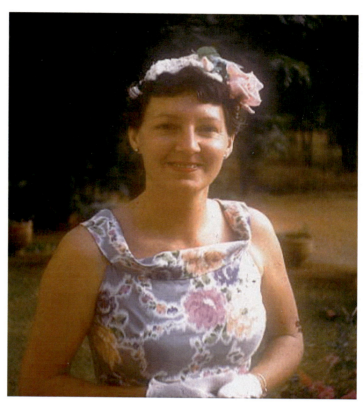

Kathy – An official occasion.

There were only four hands aboard for this virtually inland trip and all were lost. I received this news in the newspaper at home. The report included a photograph of the trawler partially submerged but with the funnel and the top of the wheelhouse above water.

Sometime later I had the opportunity to go out with a drifter from Lowestoft. I had met the skipper in Whitby where he was in charge of a smart private yacht. He invited me to Lowestoft and I took the chance, one weekend, to see the difference between drifting and trawling. We were out in the North Sea for only about thirty-six hours but it was sufficient for me to learn how the great lengths of drift net were positioned and how the herrings caught in the meshes of the nets were retrieved. To my mind this kind of fishing was much less exciting than trawling there being long periods when the ship was just rolling with the engines shut off.

My friend the skipper was Charlie Sansom. He insisted on my staying as a guest in his house. He had a daughter called Edna who must have been four or five years my senior. She was quite a pleasant girl and seemed to think I was all right although I didn't share her great enthusiasm for attending boxing and all-in wrestling matches. I think that Charlie and his wife were afraid that Edna was getting perilously near to being 'left on the shelf'. They treated me with great friendliness and plied me with massive and very nourishing meals. It was fairly clear to me that I was qualifying in their eyes as a suitable prospective son-in-law. I was invited to go to their home whenever I liked. I did go down for the weekend on a few occasions but our relationship didn't flower and I withdrew my attentions with discretion and that was the end of that.

Before I finished my course at Imperial College I went to the Plymouth Marine Laboratory to take the Easter Course. It was very interesting and instructive involving collection of specimens in the Salcombe estuary and in other coastal situations and examination of numerous marine species in a very well equipped laboratory. The instructors were excellent and the company formed of students from several universities was pleasant and convivial. The laboratory possessed a small inshore fishing boat named 'Gamarus' and also a small trawler. In the latter we made a trip to the Eddystone lighthouse so that I was able to see the area from which my scallops came.

One memorable incident that remains firmly in my mind from my last year in Imperial College was the destruction of the Crystal Palace in 1936. We, in the Dramatic Society, were rehearsing Priestley's 'Laburnham Grove' in the evening, when someone remarked on a bright light in the sky over to the south. We all took a look and realised that there must be a big fire somewhere in South London. When we were told that the Crystal Palace was on fire we thought someone was pulling our legs. "How can a structure of glass and steel burn?" we asked ourselves. The news next day, however, confirmed the rumour. The fiercest of fires demolished the whole structure with the exception of the two towers.

It was also around this time that the rumblings of a national upset over the demands of the new king, Edward VIII, to be permitted to marry an American divorcee, Mrs Simpson, were making themselves felt. The press became full of reports of a grave breach between the King and the Prime Minister, Stanley Baldwin. The views of important people, including Winston Churchill and many other politicians, were a daily feature of the press. The new king had attracted a lot of sympathy from the working classes by his activities in visiting some of the more run down parts of the country and talking to the coal miners, particularly those in Wales. The nation was divided. My student friends and I became embroiled in heated arguments over the issue. My feelings were very strongly against the king. Large sums of money had been spent on the education of the Prince of Wales in order to prepare him for his duties as the future king. All this he was now prepared to throw away for his right to marry the wrong woman. It was hard luck on him but my view was that he had to sacrifice his own desires in order to fulfil his duty as monarch. He should have regarded it as his overwhelming destiny. His abdication came to me as no shock and I welcomed the accession of King George VI. He, of course, proved remarkably brave in taking up the mantle which was virtually forced upon him.

The aforementioned play by Priestley was memorable for me in another respect. I was playing the part of the uncle from

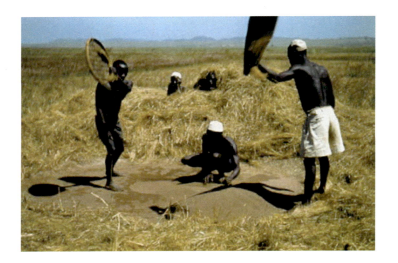

Farmers winnowing crop.

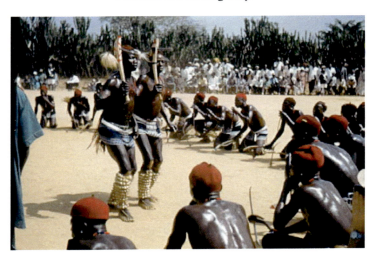

Miango Dancers, Northern Nigeria

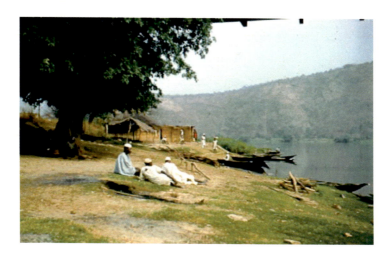

On the banks of the River Niger

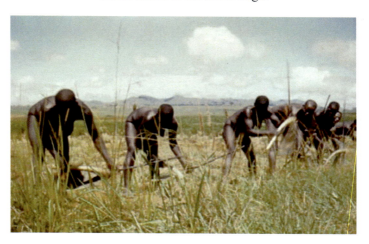

Nigerian Farming

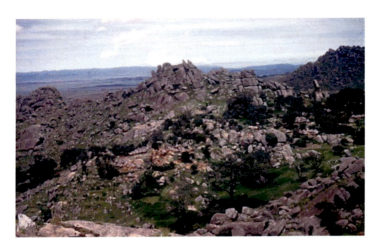

Birom villages in rocky areas

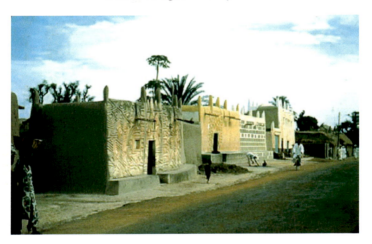

Street in Bukuru

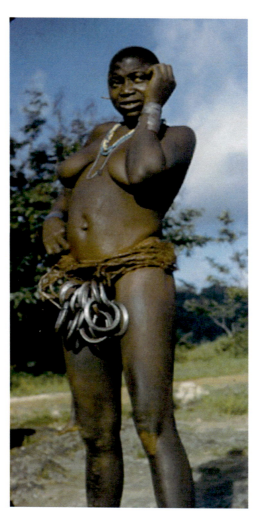

Birom Nigerian woman with ordainments

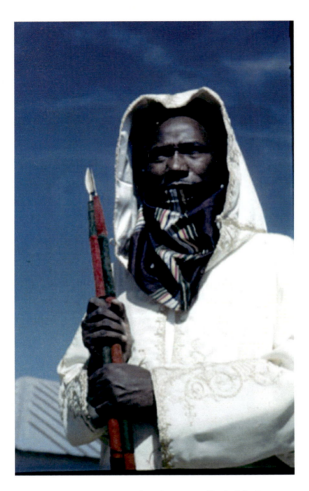

The Sardauna of Sokato, a tribal chief

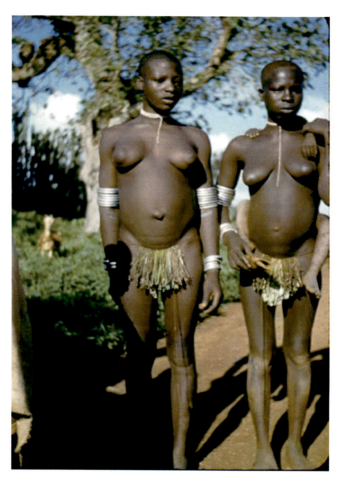

Two pagan women with babies on their backs

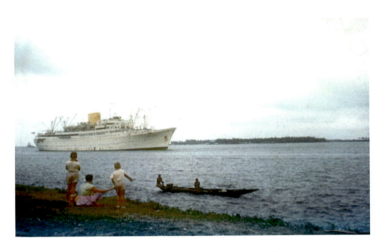

Home leave – watching the ship arrive in Lagos

CHAPTER 6

Kenya

Before leaving Nigeria I had purchased a Vauxhall Velox car to be delivered to us when we arrived in Liverpool docks. Rather to my surprise the car was waiting for us on arrival so that we were immediately mobile and drove across the Pennines to Kathy's old home on the Yorkshire coast. When Kathy and the boys were settled in with Kathy's parents I contacted Dr Montgomery at the Wellcome Headquarters in Euston Road and went to London by train. I attended at Euston Road for an interview with Dr Montgomery and Tim Evans, his Number Two. Tim I had met before when he was Director of Veterinary Services in the Sudan as he had visited Nairobi to attend meetings, which I also attended when I was in Tanganyika.

The meeting was very friendly and it was explained to me that the company, the Wellcome Foundation wished to set up a research laboratory in Kenya with the primary object of carrying out research on the cattle disease East Coast fever. At that time, there was no known means of therapy for the disease and the company considered that this might be a rewarding area of research aimed at finding a cure for the disease. I was, of course, very well acquainted with the disease having been actively involved with it in Tanganyika. It was a formidable prospect. The literature on East Coast fever, especially from South Africa, was voluminous. Since the beginning of the century some extraordinary experimental work had been recorded, particularly in a massive search for a means of artificial immunisation of cattle. No one had been able to crack the problem and the names of those who had tried were famous in the field of tropical veterinary research. They included that of Sir Arnold Theiler, who was responsible for the discovery of the protozoan parasite, the cause of the disease, which was named *Theileria parva* after Sir Arnold.

I pointed out this significant factor that, of course, was not news to Monty or Tim. They explained that this was the very reason for their interest. Wellcome had been a pioneer in the field of immunology and was also in a unique position to provide and experiment with whole ranges of chemotherapeutic compounds which had never been applied to many of the protozoan diseases including malaria The Board of the Foundation had decided that this field of enquiry was one in which they should take an interest. It might be fruitful or it might not but it had been accepted as worthy of a try. To say that I was apprehensive when I recalled the great names, which had tried and failed is an understatement. I was offered the post of head of this effort in the field of protozoan research. The conditions and remuneration were attractive. It is difficult for me to explain my reactions to this offer. I had been a member of the Colonial Service for some seventeen years and had just accepted a senior position in another quite prestigious research organisation. I felt like a non-swimmer hanging onto the bar at the side of the swimming pool, afraid to strike out into an unfamiliar environment.

Before I left Nigeria, a new condition of service for expatriates had been introduced in view of the change over to self-rule in the country. It made provision for officers in the service to retire early without forfeiting pension rights. The main condition, however, was that six months notice had to be given. I asked Dr Montgomery when they would like me to make my decision. He said that it would be as soon as possible if not earlier. I pointed out that I would need to give the service six months notice which would mean that I could not be free before the end of my leave. This would mean that, according to the regulations, if I resigned, I would have to forfeit my entire earned Colonial pension. Dr Montgomery decided that he would get the Company to approach the Colonial Office and see if the six-month requirement could be waived. As it happened, this approach was made and the Colonial Office consulted the

Governor General of Nigeria, Sir James Robertson – none other, and he promptly agreed that in my case, which he understood fully, I should be entitled to my Colonial pension. I therefore agreed to accept the Wellcome post. I became a member of the staff of the Wellcome Foundation Ltd.

I now had the sad duty of writing to John Ford to explain that I would not be joining his organisation. I felt very badly about this and put my position to him fully. He wrote back and congratulated me and said he fully understood the situation and agreed that I could not possibly turn down such a good offer. Later experience entirely confirmed this view and so I have to thank Marshall for the best move that I made in my career. Working for the Foundation was just in another world. They were marvellous people and were ideal employers. After a short holiday, I went to London to get experience in all the departments of the Company from the extensive modern laboratories at Beckenham, the experimental farms at Frant which were under the supervision of Sam Hignet, the pharmaceutical factory at Dartford and the huge Head Office in the Wellcome Building in Euston Road where were housed the Wellcome Library and Museum and the Wellcome Laboratories of Tropical Medicine directed by Dr Len Goodwin, who was to become a very good friend in later years.

I had long discussions with the Chief Accountant of the Company over the matters concerning funding and the employment of staff both professional and local. I discovered that the Foundation, in collaboration with the Government of Kenya, had obtained a parcel of land of about a hundred and twenty acres not far from the Kenya Veterinary Laboratories, on which we were to build our laboratories. I suggested that I be authorised to build some houses for me and my family and other permanent senior staff. This met with some dubiety. It would be a new departure for the Company to own houses and for overseas employees the custom was to rent houses or maintain staff in hotels. I pointed out that the running of a laboratory in tropical Africa was very different from employing sales staff. Indeed it was hardly likely that suitable housing would exist nearer to the lab than Nairobi. Such housing would be very expensive and in my opinion it was essential that my senior staff and I would, as it were, have to live on the premises. There would be animal houses and grazing cattle, which would require constant care and supervision, and further, during research, one cannot adhere to office hours and it would be necessary for me or other reliable staff to be available day and night. The fact that the area would be very vulnerable to raiders and other thieves, particularly as at that time, the Mau Mau were still active, should be taken into account. My views were accepted and were certainly supported by Tim Evans who had served in Africa.

While I was undergoing an indoctrination course, I was staying in the West Kent Hotel in Bickley, not too far from Beckenham where I had to spend a lot of time with the scientists with whom I would be in contact when the work in Kenya commenced. Christmas was approaching and the weather was very cold. I did some shopping for Christmas presents for Kathy and the boys. I aimed to drive back to Yorkshire about two days before Christmas and on the evening before my intended departure I packed all the presents in the boot of my Velox before I went to bed. I had been feeling pretty ropy all of the last day I spent in Beckenham and thought I must be incubating a cold. I had a poor night and in the morning I felt very ill, so much so that I thought I should see a doctor. The lady who owned the hotel sent for the local GP who came into my room and immediately asked me if I was sunburned. I said I might be but it shouldn't be obvious as I had been home from Africa for several weeks. He examined me and said I was very jaundiced. He said that I must go into hospital immediately and he rang for an ambulance. I protested, saying that I had to drive to Yorkshire that very day. He said very firmly that I was not driving anywhere and so I was packed off in an ambulance to Farnborough Hospital where I was put to bed in an isolation ward. This was in a very cold, wooden hut with workmen outside using a pneumatic drill but I was too ill to worry. Dr Montgomery called to see me and kindly agreed to let Kathy know that I would not be home for Christmas.

It took several days of tests before I was finally diagnosed as having virus hepatitis. I was very ill indeed, so much so that I thought I was going to die. I asked Dr Montgomery, who visited me nearly every day, to organise with the Crown Agents that they would commute my Colonial pension so that Kathy would have some funds to keep her going. Monty laughed and said that there was no need to think such morbid thoughts. I was not allowed to get out of bed except to use the commode and when I was taken in a wheelchair to the X-ray department. The nurse who took me shoved my chair like a bat out of hell. I think she was a Swede. The route was along rough paths through the hospital grounds with awkward steps here and there where she shot me off the seat and onto the path. I was on a strict diet of glucose and water. Each morning I was presented with a large plate piled high with powdered glucose and a large jug of water. This had to be imbibed in the day. Tim came to see me often and he was visibly appalled to see the conditions in which I had to live. He suggested that he should get the authorities to transfer me into a private room in the hospital main building. But I was too ill to face any change.

However, this state of affairs lasted for a month. I had, at the end of that time improved a little but I was still not allowed to get out of bed on my own and take any exercise and I was still on the glucose/water diet. I had naturally lost a lot of weight and my muscles hung down like half-filled bags of fluid. Hepatitis is a very depressing illness and my depression was exacerbated by the constant thought that having just employed me the Foundation would sack me, as I could not go ahead with the work for which I had been taken on. While I was in this very depressed state, I received a letter from Head Office telling me that a stateroom had been booked for my family and me in the SS Llangibby Castle, which was due to sail shortly. Of course, this was an impossibility for me and through Dr Montgomery, the booking had to be cancelled. Having for years had to rely on bookings made by the Colonial Office and the Tanganyika and Nigeria administrations which were all apparently hard to obtain, I was all the more worried but Dr Montgomery assured me that the travel department of the Foundation was not the least worried. Another booking would be made for a month later when I should be able to travel. The difference in attitude towards ship bookings made by Government and the Foundation could, perhaps be attributed to the fact that Government went for the cheapest berths while the Foundation booked the top class of

185

stateroom for their employees. While I was still confined to my bed in the hospital I received the information that a stateroom with *en suite* facilities and an ironing room had been booked for us in the SS Kenya Castle, Union Castle Line, sailing from Southampton in March.

Towards the end of January, I persuaded the doctor in charge of my case to let me leave the hospital and go home to Yorkshire where Kathy had been struggling to keep things, including the two young boys, on an even keel on her own. The doctor gave me strict injunctions. I could not drive myself and when I got home, I was to go to bed immediately and send for our GP to see me and keep a strict watch on me. On no account was I to do anything strenuous for several weeks and then I was to take things very gently. I was informed that I had almost certainly lost about half of my liver and must never donate blood to the Blood Donor Service. I had visions of life ahead as a frail invalid bound for an early demise. My one hope was that I should be fit to do a job for the Wellcome Foundation before having to throw in my cards. I made arrangements for a driver from the AA to drive me to York where Kathy's brother-in-law, Reg Wood could take over and drive me to Robin Hood's Bay.

The driver arrived at the hospital early on the 21st of January and I was discharged and helped out to the car and packed in the front passenger seat swathed in blankets. I'm told that I looked like a frail little old man. The driver was a very pleasant woman, called Mrs Stalper. The journey to York was uneventful and I was reunited there with Kathy and the boys and driven to Robin Hood's Bay where I was put to bed, quite exhausted. On our previous leave, we had helped Kathy's older sister, Nancy, a hospital Matron in Lloyd's Hospital, Bridlington, to purchase a house in Robin Hood's Bay so that she would have a place in which she could live when she retired. Her retirement was about ten years away but as Kathy's original home in the nearby village of Fylingthorpe was proving too big for her mother and father, we helped them to move into Nancy's house that was equipped with more modern facilities. That is where we stayed on one or two of our leaves.

Shortly after I arrived from hospital, Kathy's father was taken ill and had been collected by ambulance and taken to

Scarborough Hospital. The ambulance arrived at midnight when the ground was covered with ice and snow. The driver had no mate and so I had to get out of bed and help stretcher Kathy's father down the stairs, through the garden and into the ambulance at the gate. I don't think I was any the worse for the experience. Tim Evans had impressed on me the value of yoghurt as a help towards recovery from hepatitis. Accordingly, I started taking a daily pot of yoghurt. Slowly my health improved and I became able to take short walks but I was extremely weak. The boys, of course, were delighted to have me back with them, especially as they had a second lot of Christmas presents that had been left by Father Christmas for them with me when I was away in hospital.

We were booked to sail on Wednesday the 6th of March. The Wellcome people wanted me to visit them for a few days before our departure for a final briefing with the Chief Accountant's department and also for me to have discussions with Bob Kennedy, the Chief Engineer at Dartford. He was to give me advice on such matters as planning and materials and how to deal with architects. I was still feeling far from well and was distinctly weak and a little light-headed. However, we packed our luggage into the car and left Robin Hood's Bay early one cold wintry morning and set off for London. Kathy was driving for the first part of the journey but when we approached the Midlands and the roads were very icy and dangerous, I took over. Our progress was slow and darkness fell while we were still in Lincolnshire. Somehow or other, we found ourselves in Melton Mowbray. The town seemed to be in darkness but we found The Bell Inn, drove in and took a room for the night.

That was one of the worst nights of my life. The bedroom was cold and I couldn't sleep. I felt terrible and I was sure that I would not be able to drive on the next day and so my career might well come to an end. In the morning I took some aspirins and rested on the bed while Kathy and the boys had breakfast. I managed to dress myself. Kathy was rather frightened and the boys were miserable. Curiously Kathy doesn't remember much about the night but she does remember seeing on the bar of the inn, when we went in, a small silver jug on which were inscribed the letters K.E.W., which, of course, were her initials. We managed to get our things packed up and in the car and we moved off with me driving. We arrived safely in Kent and stayed at the West Kent Hotel where I had been staying when I was taken ill. I began to feel better and in the following few days I managed to get to all the meetings that had been arranged. The financial business was covered in the accounts department

The Chief Accountant almost made me laugh by asking me what funds I would require to cover expenses on board the ship. I said that I wouldn't require any as everything necessary except drinks was provided. Drinks, in any case, I would not expect the company to provide and in my particular case I had been warned by the hospital doctor not to touch a drop of alcohol for six months at the very least. This did not bother me, as I am a very moderate drinker even on a liner where all drinks are very cheap. The Accountant said that it might be a good thing if I had a drinks party for the Captain and the Senior Officers and any prestigious passengers who might be aboard. Also, when we went ashore at any ports *en route* the occasion might arise when I might be inclined to entertain local dignitaries. What a world of difference from the penny-pinching methods of the Government who would only refund a taxi fare after all details had been substantiated and then would demand a receipt. I began to realise that I was now representing a world-renowned commercial company and would be expected to act accordingly. I never did get into the role of a business executive in the accepted sense and although I was to have to do a lot of entertaining of influential people in my time with Wellcome, I never abused the privileges accorded to me

A point that caused me some concern was the car that I had purchased as an overseas purchase and as such, had to be shipped overseas. Originally it had been purchased before we left Nigeria with the arrangement that it would be shipped to Uganda where I had expected to be going. I asked the accountant for advice as to what I should do about this transaction. "No problem," he said. "We will purchase it from you and ship it out to Kenya as your company car." I was quite astonished but it was an easy way of fulfilling the legal Customs and Excise obligations and so we agreed a price and then the Company took over all the details of shipping the car out to Kenya. My high opinion of the Wellcome Foundation was, by now, firmly established.

Soon after we had gone aboard the MV Kenya Castle and were settling our selves in our stateroom, the Chief Steward knocked on the door and came in. He enquired if everything was in order and when I assured him that it was, he informed us that there were forty-five cartons of yoghurt in the cold room and would I like them to be brought to the cabin daily. I was not very familiar with yoghurt and the various ways in which it could be assimilated with the diet in those days and so I agreed to have the cartons delivered to our accommodation each morning. Throughout the voyage I consumed one or two cartons of the stuff every day, just spooning it out of the cartons and not liking it very much. Nowadays, I take my home-made yoghurt daily, mixed with my cereal at breakfast. The daily dose of undiluted sour commodity would have been much easier to stomach if I had adopted the same method at breakfast on board. I was still very weak and had to take things very gently. I did not drink any alcohol on the voyage but confined my drinking to tonic water. This was no hardship really, but when travelling at sea I do enjoy a John Collins at lunchtime and a pint of bitter in the evenings but I found the regimen quite acceptable.

It was while we were sailing along the African coast in the Indian Ocean, that a telegraph message was received and brought to me with the sad news that Kathy's father had died in hospital. I had to break the news to Kathy and, needless to say, she was very distressed. At this time a Scottish Presbyterian Minister, Robin Keltie, who was a passenger on board, heard the news and came to our cabin to offer his help and friendship. He was on his way to take up the post of Minister of the Nairobi Presbyterian Church and he became a good friend of ours in Kenya. We often visited him and his family at the manse and he frequently called on us.

The sea trip certainly helped me to recuperate and I was much better in health when we arrived at Mombasa after a very pleasant voyage. Keith Clarke, who was the Wellcome rep for Kenya, met us off the train in Nairobi. The Nairobi firm of Dalgety then handled the Burroughs Wellcome business. Keith Clarke operated within this agency with a small administrative staff headed by a pharmacist, George Strachan, who was an employee of Dalgety's. All these people were most helpful to us and did everything they could to make us welcome and comfortable. Initially we had been booked in at the Devon Hotel and the first few days there made it possible for us to find our feet and settle in. I did have the advantage of being familiar with Nairobi having visited the city several times during my service in Tanganyika. George Strachan and his wife, Betty were due to go home on leave and they very kindly offered us the use of their house while they were away. We accepted their offer gratefully and, being able to stay there for a period of several weeks, helped us to find our feet and enabled me to work myself gently into the job of organising the preliminary planning before building could be considered seriously. The Company had found a Senior Technician, called Jack Ford and he came out soon after we had established ourselves in the Strachans' house and we found a house for him between our land at Kabete and Nairobi. Ford was elderly and his wife was a problem. She was a constant complainer but we managed to keep on an even keel.

My first priority was to look at the estate which we were taking over and decide what to do with it. It comprised one hundred and twenty acres of abandoned coffee farm with the typical red soil of Kikuyu land. Some coffee trees remained but the majority of the land was covered with rough scrub and overgrown grasses. A large area on the north side was swampland, which in the dry season became a rather hard pan. The access to the land was off the main road from Nairobi to the Rift Valley and was little more than a mud track. Labour was required to do a lot of clearing before we could consider the siting of the laboratory buildings. At that time we were in the tail end of the Mau Mau rebellion and almost all the pool of Kikuyu men was either under restriction or just set free. I could only employ local people who had forsworn their oaths and had official certificates to authenticate them. There was no difficulty in obtaining suitable labour, as the people were anxious to get a wage so that they could support their families. I therefore, got Ford to take on labour as required and agree the terms of employment and wages. I knew that I would need ample grazing for the many cattle, which I would have to purchase and feed for our experimental work.

A start was made on the clearing of scrub and I showed the labourers how to make haystacks in order to provide a supply of feed for the initial cattle to be purchased. The African farmers did not generally practise conservation of fodder, which was abundant in the wet season, for use in the dry season. It became possible, as the bush was cleared, to consider the locating of the laboratory buildings and the choice of sites for the houses for staff. Contact was made with the architect, who had been chosen by Dr Montgomery when he had visited Kenya to arrange for the establishment of a Wellcome laboratory in Kenya. That had taken place before I was engaged for the job. The architect was Dick Polkinghorne, a partner in a well-known company of architects in Nairobi. Together we worked out the plans for the laboratory and ancillary buildings and the dwelling houses. Dick was a very pleasant chap and we became good friends. The only matters over which we had any differences were of a minor nature of no fundamental importance. In the early stages of our co-operation, the main difficulty I had with him was having to restrain his natural desire to add a lot of fancy details while I, still retaining some of my old civil service parsimony, insisted on basic functional necessities. On one point I did give way and that was to allow Dick to make provision for an ornamental pond and fountain outside the main entrance to the main building. Dick pointed out that when the contract was completed, such a prestigious establishment as 'The Wellcome Research Laboratory (East Africa)', would have to have a suitable opening ceremony when bigwigs from London and Kenya and the rest of East Africa and even, perhaps, the USA, would be present. In his opinion it would be necessary to have at least one feature to show that an architect had drawn up the plans.

The final plans were sent to the Wellcome offices in London for the comments and approval of the Company. They were received with favour, but it was decided by the Board, under the Chairmanship of Sir Michael Perrin, that the Chief Engineer of the Dartford factory should come out to Kenya to have a look at the site. So it was that Bob Kennedy came out to visit us, to go over the plans and see what he thought of the situation. Bob was an engineer and was inherently doubtful of the capabilities of architects but he was grudgingly approving of the way we intended to do things. He made a few minor suggestions but otherwise recommended that we call for tenders from building contractors and go ahead. Bob, unfortunately, died of cancer before the work was complete and so I was pleased that during his visit, I took him on safari to Treetops, which he thoroughly enjoyed.

There followed months of activity on the site. The Strachans returned from leave and we moved into the Devon Hotel but I had no intention of staying in a hotel six miles from our land at Kabete. To me it was too expensive and too far away. During my career I had always lived on the job, as it were, so that I was continuously available for any contingencies that might arise. I made enquiries about a possible temporary form of housing that could be erected for us on site. I found a half of a hut, which had previously provided accommodation for WRAC personnel in Nairobi. A Sikh builder had subsequently used it as a cement store and he was quite pleased to sell it. I got the contractors, who had been chosen to do our building, to dismantle it and erect it in the bush on our estate. It was rough and the floors were impregnated with cement but Kathy soon had them sparkling, a modicum of furniture installed, and we moved in. I had local people build a round, mud hut nearby which was thatched and divided into two halves. One half constituted our kitchen in which we installed a solid fuel Aga stove. The other half made temporary quarters for our cook and house servant. I then bought a Bedford lorry for the transport of stock and materials. The question of water supply presented a problem. I installed a tank outside the wooden house from which a pipe carried water to an improvised bathroom in the house. A forty-five gallon drum mounted over a wood fire provided hot water. A local African with a ramshackle pick-up truck transported the water in old oil drums every day.

The Mau Mau rebellion was drawing to a close but still, on the advice of the police, I procured a handgun for Kathleen. This was for her protection and that of James and Peter when I could not be present. We were, at that time, living in our wooden house in the middle of the bush on our estate. We were pretty isolated and paradoxically, I had taken on, among my other employees, some ex Mau Mau detainees for the protection of our developing establishment. These were styled 'Night Watchmen'. They armed themselves with vicious looking pangas and I am sure that any stray people wandering around the site at night would have been at grave risk of losing some part of their anatomy. It came to my knowledge that on our estate there was an old, ruined farmhouse, which until very recently had been used by the Mau Mau as a staging post for active members of this illegal organisation. During the digging of the foundations of our house we found a simi, the double-edged sword used by the Mau Mau for unmentionable atrocities. I also discovered that the land between our house and the laboratory buildings had been the site of a violent battle between the Mau Mau and the police in which eighteen people had been killed.

As it happened, however, the only interlopers we experienced were a few rats that ran along the tops of the wooden walls, which were open to the exterior at that stage. Occasionally the rats visited us at night, running along the bed heads. Later we procured two dogs. One, Prince, was a crossbred Doberman Pincher and the other was a pedigree Dalmatian whose registered name was Flik of Kirconnel. He was always called 'Flick'.

Dr Montgomery, on his preliminary visit, had obtained the agreement of the Nairobi City Council for us to tap into the Nairobi water supply, the main supply of which passed down the road at the entrance to our estate. I looked into this and decided that it would not be satisfactory for several reasons. Firstly, it would be very expensive; secondly, I would have no control over whatever was added to it in the way of purifying agents; thirdly I would not be able to rely on a constancy of supply, as breakdowns, bursts, failure of supply and other eventualities would be beyond my control. I therefore, found a water driller and consulted him. It was, thus, that I met Alf Richardson, a South African hydraulics engineer who had set up his own drilling business in Kenya. He came to Kabete and looked over our land with a practised eye and said that there would be plenty of water under our area. Accordingly, I asked for an estimate for the drilling of a borehole and the installation of a pump, which would be adequate for our future requirements. He gave me such an estimate and allowing for contingencies such as having to bore more deeply than originally calculated, it came to something in the region of £7000.

I was still so affected by my early experience of asking for funds from government with no hope of getting them that I was appalled by this, which appeared to me to be a huge sum, so that I hardly dared put the proposition to my bosses in London. However, I plucked up courage and composed a detailed letter to head office and posted it off by airmail. Imagine my delight and amazement when a cable arrived about four days later not only authorising me to proceed but suggesting that perhaps, I had underestimated the cost. They had, therefore, put at my disposal a sum of money twice that for which I had applied. I began to realise that I must put behind me the days of pinching and scraping that had prevailed in my civil service period. Suffice it to say that my loyalty to the Company knew no bounds and if they had said that it was necessary for the best progress of our work that I should stand on my head for half an hour each day, I would have done it without demur. However, this eventuality did not arise, nor was it likely to. My main contact on all matters concerning the development of the laboratory and the lines along which we should plan the future research was Tim Evans and we got on together without the slightest hitch.

The water supply was of first importance and so I authorised Alf Richardson to start boring. His lorry with all the paraphernalia for drilling deep boreholes arrived at the entrance to our estate on the main road. There had been a lot of rain and so, within thirty yards of turning off the tarmac onto our track, the heavy vehicle was bogged down and immovable. It took two days of hard work by a gang of my labour to dig the lorry out of the mud and get it onto a ridge of red coffee soil where we had provisionally decided to site the lab buildings. The drill rig was set up and drilling commenced. The rate of penetration varied and on occasion progress was very slow, because we had come against a stratum of hard rock. I had a lot of worries but Alf seemed unconcerned. We struck water at about three levels. These were what Alf called aquifers but he said the yield was not big enough and we would find better and more abundant water eventually. He was quite right as we found a supply, which satisfied him at a depth of four hundred and forty-one feet. A submersible pump was installed and the water supply was found to be more than adequate. We erected a temporary tank on a structure built of bush poles cut down on the estate and provisional reticulation was installed to take water to all the important points on the estate with special consideration for the imminent building operations.

We now found ourselves in the midst of a hive of industrial activity. The contractors employed local people for the unskilled labour. Most of the digging and transporting of soil and hard core was done by local Kikuyu women. Overall supervision on site was in the hands of an Asian fundi (Swahili for a skilled artisan) who was designated Mistri. His name was Manji and he was an amusing character. I found myself involved with building supplies and on occasion I had to drive into Nairobi for emergency supplies when the builders ran out of some essentials such as nails, screws, and such other items as I could get into my car. One evening when Kathy and the boys and I took a walk round the site before dark, an activity which became quite a regular routine, I discovered that the levels of concrete laid that day in the spray race, which was an essential for our future work with the cattle, were all wrong and would have necessitated complete break down and rebuilding. I decided to do the break down before the concrete set and so, as darkness fell, Kathy and the boys and I were all involved in a frantic breaking down of the concrete and re-levelling using shovels and shuttering and wheelbarrow and trowels. We finished by moonlight. Fortunately there was a full moon. Amazing to relate, our levels were correct and when the workers arrived in the morning they could proceed with the construction of the spray-race as though nothing had been wrong. I made my views very clear to Mistri Manji.

Work continued reasonably satisfactorily, or at least as satisfactorily as one could expect. Dick Polkinghorne made regular visits and supervised the works. On odd occasions he ordered some of the work to be knocked down as it was not up to the specifications, and made the builders put the matter right, but on the whole, I was very satisfied with the rate of progress. Our house was the first building to be completed so that I could move the family into reasonable accommodation 'and I could concentrate on the planning of the research, which lay before us. The first twelve months of our time in Kenya were very busy and fairly hectic. There was all the setting up of a nucleus of staff, African and expatriate. I started exploring the sources of cattle for the research and the necessary equipment for the laboratory. Microscopes, autoclaves, surgical instruments, fundamental reagents, office equipment and books and all the hundred and one items that were vital to the smooth running of an organisation such as was now my responsibility had to be ordered either through our agents in Nairobi or through the headquarters in London.

I selected from our African employees, a few individuals who had received a secondary school education and we started to train these men in the basics of laboratory technology. The senior of these was a member of the Luo tribe, Benjamin Okaro, who became a very responsible and competent senior technical worker. At the end of his first tour, John Ford went on leave and decided not to return to Kenya. He was in his late sixties and also I think he was probably forced into retirement by his wife, Hilda, who was not an easy woman to get on with. I was not sorry to see her go. She didn't like Africans and she was constantly coming to me with petty complaints. We were very fortunate to find Ford's replacement on our doorstep, so to speak. This was Bill Macleod, who was employed as Senior Technician in the East African Veterinary Research Organisation at Muguga about fifteen miles distant from Kabete. Bill had been the technician in the Pathology Department of the Royal Veterinary College when I was a student. He was a first class technician and became a most important member of the staff of our laboratory. His wife, Ivy, was a welcome addition to our little expatriate community and eventually became our bookkeeper.

I took onto the staff, some European girls who had finished their schooling in the Kenya High School for girls. Bill trained them in the fundamentals of Veterinary Technology and they became invaluable. Sadly, of course, they married and left Kenya and we had to take on replacements and train them. In our second year, the Company wrote to me saying that they had found a very promising vet who had lived in Kenya where his mother and father were the resident officials at the Limuru Golf Club. Would I be interested in taking him on? Of course I was most pleased to do so and Duncan Brown joined us. He was a very bright scientist and became a first class colleague in our work. Duncan was a keen and very good rugby player and was an important member of the Kenya Rugby Club.

In the first eighteen months of our time in Kenya, our finances were in the hands of the Wellcome agents, Dalgetys. The arrangement was not very satisfactory as the accounts were always delayed and I had no reliable information about our position and so I suggested that we should send all our accounts directly to Beckenham, where our finances were controlled. Ivy Macleod, who was now living with Bill in one of our houses, had done some bookkeeping and was only too pleased to be taken onto the staff. She proved to be a most conscientious and capable worker. Our returns went out to the financial section, in Beckenham, monthly and they were always in apple-pie order and always on time. Our colleagues there complimented us on the clarity and promptness of all our accounts and so this made matters easier for us.

I started the preliminary exploratory work before our laboratory was much more than a patchwork of foundations. Thanks to the kind hospitality of Howard Binns, who was the Director of the new East African Veterinary Research Organisation (usually referred to as EAVRO) who allowed us to use some of his accommodation and helped us with the supply of some cattle. We were able to work out a *modus operandi* for our main avenues of research as a result so that the least possible amount of time was wasted while our buildings were going up. Concurrently, the land was being cleared to produce adequate grazing for our experimental cattle and an acaricidal spray-race was installed so that all our cattle could be kept clear of ticks and, at the same time cleanse the estate of these parasites. This was of paramount importance as the disease we were working on was only transmitted by ticks. When the building work was completed, our establishment consisted of the main laboratory with a separate *post mortem* room, a thirty-foot high water tower with a large capacity tank and reticulation to all parts of the work

197

and residential areas. There were three newly built bungalows and the original, now much improved, wooden house which my family and I had inhabited in the early stages and these were augmented by three houses on the edge of the estate which had belonged to the contiguous Kenya Veterinary Department and which the Company had permitted me to buy as homes for senior staff. I had also built a block of four houses for senior African staff and these were occupied with pride by those who were selected for the top technical and artisan jobs.

At first it was not easy to obtain expatriate secretarial staff and I had to make do with a few temporary secretarial ladies, but eventually I was able to employ a permanent secretary who had worked in the Veterinary Headquarters and soon settled down as my personal secretary. Her name was Mavis Watts and she stayed in my employ for several years. In the early days of what became generally known as WRL (EA), I was preparing the ground for the research to be done and making sure that the facilities and staff necessary for the work were in place.

In the original planning, building and equipping, of course, the primary reason for the establishment of the Wellcome Research Laboratory (East Africa) was the study of East Coast fever in cattle. This disease is caused by the protozoan parasite *Theileria parva.* The disease is geographically confined to East Africa, and a few other contiguous countries. The disease had, earlier, been a scourge in South Africa but had been eradicated there by means of a drastic policy of slaughter of all infected cattle. At that time, the state of our knowledge of this killer disease was very incomplete. The epidemiology and transmission were strange but intriguing. The disease was only a problem in areas where ticks of the species *Rhipicephalus appendiculatus* were common ectoparasites. The intricacies of the disease, its transmission, clinical characteristics and high mortality rate formed the background on which it was my duty to explore all possible aspects of East Coast fever. As the Wellcome Foundation Ltd. conceived the whole project, it was natural that we should look for a means of chemotherapy and the possibility of producing an immunising agent.

Our work proceeded at a reasonable pace and our concentrated efforts were rewarded by a considerably increased knowledge of the parasite and the animal cells, which formed the obvious habitat in which it exercised its pathogenic attack. Our effort, based on the knowledge then extant, was initially concentrated on the testing of anti-protozoal drugs. The most obvious ones to start with were those that had proved effective against malaria. These and their analogues and new substances being produced in the Wellcome laboratories in England and America were studied with respect to their anti-protozoal properties. Their availability in suitable quantities for experiments on large animals was, of course, a restricting factor. We developed and refined our methods of testing and it soon became apparent that we had to go further into the cellular pathology of the disease and its immunology. Our work, therefore, became diversified and our resources including staff, required expansion. From time to time, members of the Wellcome staff, both veterinary and medical, were sent from Beckenham and Frant to spend periods working under my direction and providing ideas from their specific expertise.

A Swiss medical graduate turned up, quite fortuitously, in Nairobi and she came to see me with a view to getting a job, as she wanted to stay for some time in Kenya. Her speciality was cytology that, of course, fitted into our schedule very well. The Company gave me permission to employ her and so Dr Lotte Hulliger joined our team. I built an extension to our laboratory in the shape of a special cytology and tissue culture laboratory, and soon the work was opening up possibilities for exciting cytological and immunological exploration. I had, for some time nourished the idea of swinging from using animals for tests to the use of tissue culture. This change has since, played a large part in experimental chemotherapy and immunology. Workers in this field came out from the home laboratories to work with us for periods and then returned to their own labs taking materials and expertise with them. It was at this time that my own personal work took me into a close study of the haemocytosis (production of blood cells), associated with the immunology of East Coast fever and the effects of drugs on the cells of the bone marrow and blood. This work led to my being awarded a Doctorate of Philosophy of the University of London.

The Government of Kenya had established a regulatory

body with the responsibility of setting and maintaining professional standards within the veterinary profession. This Veterinary Board was based on the lines operated by the Royal College of Veterinary Surgeons in Britain, and I was appointed as a member. The new Director of Veterinary Services, the first African to occupy this post, was the Chairman of the Board. Applications for the right to practise Veterinary Medicine and Surgery were received from people qualified in many countries in the world and it was our duty to determine whether or not their qualifications were up to the standards required by the Kenya Veterinary Board. Many of the qualifications offered for acceptance were from countries or Veterinary Schools of which we knew nothing and so it was part of our job to obtain information about these qualifications and assess their acceptability or otherwise. This was quite a difficult operation and I carried out much of the investigation. The Chairman was Ishmael Muriithi, a Kikuyu man who had qualified in 1964 in Edinburgh and he gave me full support in maintaining our standards in Kenya. I remained on the Board until I left Kenya in 1970 and I received a very appreciative letter from the Minister of Agriculture, thanking me for my services on behalf of the profession in Kenya.

We did establish a branch of the British Veterinary Association in Kenya, of which I was a member and served for a period as its President. We held annual meetings to which we invited representatives of the profession in Tanganyika, by now, Tanzania, and Uganda. Sometimes veterinarians visited us from the Sudan and from countries south of Tanzania including those that had replaced the Rhodesias and Nyasaland.

Another aspect of the work at Kabete arose when it was realised that the very efficiently run dog section of the Kenya police might well be exploited for the testing of new drugs for the Company. This led to my appointing John Berger, a veterinary surgeon practising among the farmers of the Highlands of Kenya. He became our parasitologist and made a most salutary contribution to the Company's work on internal parasites.

An interesting episode occurred after I had become established in the new laboratories. I was approached by an official of the CSIRO of Australia to see if I would be interested in going to the Yeerongpilly Laboratory in Queensland to Direct Research on tick-borne diseases of livestock. I was offered my flight to Australia and all travelling and accommodation expenses and it was pointed out that if I didn't want the job when I had seen it, there was no obligation to accept. I didn't feel very enthusiastic but I took up the subject with my bosses in London. They said I should accept the invitation to Australia and see what the post entailed as it could be regarded as an honour for the Wellcome Foundation and me. If the prospect attracted me on closer inspection then they would not stand in my way. I don't think they were trying to get rid of me as we had the best of relationships. So I went to Australia. I must say that the CSIRO gave me right royal treatment and I was flown all over the eastern seaboard of the continent. I met some most pleasant people in all departments of the organisation and the universities and veterinary and medical laboratories. Among those I met was the very man who had been Director of Veterinary Services in Uganda when Marshall visited him to persuade Ian Taylor to accept the job of Director of Veterinary Research in Vom, Nigeria.

However, there were aspects of the post in Queensland that didn't appeal to me. These were mostly associated with the administrative aspects of the position, particularly as the CSIRO was in the process of transferring Yeerongpilly activities to a new site where these would be incorporated into a larger agricultural and tick-borne organisation where it had been decided that the overall directorate would alternate annually between the Director of Agricultural Research and me as Director of Tick-borne Diseases. I could foresee considerable risks of bureaucracy and friction. I felt very embarrassed about declining the offer. They had all been so hospitable and kind to me. Fundamentally the job could not compare with the one I was already in. My loyalty to Wellcome who had been wonderful employers was too strong for me to leave and I certainly have never regretted the decision.

One thing of outstanding interest, which came my way when I was visiting Dr Tatchell in Brisbane, was his method of obtaining saliva from ticks in order to examine the infective particles that would be injected into the mammalian host at feeding. I introduced this technique into our work in WRL (EA). I also demonstrated this technique to a couple of newly appointed research workers in the EAVRO labs. They published work on this technique without acknowledgement to me or to Dr Tatchell.

I think that my colleagues, Duncan Brown, John Berger, Lotte Hulliger and Bill MacLeod constituted a good team and the work we started has, directly or indirectly, provided a sound basis on which more work has been done to produce salutary results. Some of this work has been done in the Wellcome Labs and some in other organisations including the Centre for Tropical Veterinary Medicine, a part of the Veterinary faculty of the University of Edinburgh. John Berger, sadly died of a heart attack some years ago and Duncan Brown has this year retired from the valuable work he has been doing for some years in the CTVM. Lotte returned to Switzerland and when I was last in touch with her, she was working in the laboratories of the Geigy Corporation. The WRL (EA) buildings and estate since africanisation became complete have been turned over to support the commercial activities of the Wellcome Foundation. I am not sure if they are still being used since the merger of Wellcome with Glaxo.

I have dealt with the technicalities of our work with, perhaps, more detail than is desirable in an autobiography such as this, but I feel that the time I spent with Wellcome was such an important part of my life that it is, I think, necessary to the narrative. The work we did in Kabete was all recorded in reports, which were in the archives of the old Wellcome Foundation. I did draw a lot of the work together at the suggestion of a colleague and it is published in Advances in Veterinary Science. Vol.11 1967, pp 207-259 under the title, 'East Coast Fever'.

During our period in Kenya, great advances were made in many parts of the world in research on the virus diseases. In human medicine, advances in the use of vaccines against poliomyelitis reduced this disease markedly throughout the world. The Wellcome Foundation was one of the active organisations in this field. Tissue culture came to the fore in this work and the Foundation workers were involved in the trials of different lines of culture cells. They wished to try out new sources of these cells and I was asked to supply kidney cells from vervet monkeys for some experimental work in connection with polio immunisation. I organised this production of renal cells from monkeys and despatched the material to the laboratories in London. The logistics were exacting and tissues were sent, express to London, a process that involved strict time and temperature programmes. The work imposed a strain on our expertise and limited facilities and I was pleased when the scheme was abandoned because of the risks of transmitting unwanted exotic viruses with the tissues.

I was also asked to help two eminent medical researchers, Drs Foy and Kondi who were involved in work on the anaemias and certain deficiency diseases of man in the tropics. Foy and Kondi had been working for many years in various parts of the world and were highly respected for their researches into human diseases, supported by the Wellcome Trust. In Kenya, they worked in the laboratories of the Kenya Medical Department situated in Nairobi. They were, naturally interested in the establishment of the Wellcome Research Laboratories (EA) and we became good friends. Their research in Kenya depended on their obtaining clinical material from the Nairobi hospitals. This was necessarily restricted and so Foy took the step of building a unit for the breeding of baboons in association with the Kenya Medical Research Laboratories. This unit was remarkably successful and a thriving population of baboons was achieved. My function in this outfit was to act as surgeon in order to expose the various parts of the alimentary tract from the stomach to the colon. Kondi was the anaesthetist. I had never, before, done any surgery on primates but basing my approach on the work I had done on dogs, cats and cattle, I developed a method of opening and closing the abdominal cavity of the baboons, which was speedy and caused the least possible damage. I never lost a baboon under this surgery, with one notable exception, but on about three occasions had to give the 'kiss of life' to a large dog baboon due to respiratory collapse under the anaesthetic. The exception was once, when an eminent expert on the surgery of baboons visited from England. He had brought with him a special instrument, rather like a trephine, with which, he affirmed, entry into the alimentary tract was facilitated and closure was easy. He had brought for our use an adhesive with which closure of any wounds, including those of the gut, and the muscles and skin, could be effectively and rapidly completed.

Dr Foy asked me if I would be prepared to do the laparotomy for this eminent visitor and he would demonstrate the sampling of alimentary contents and closure of the wounds with his special instrument and adhesive. I agreed and we went ahead. I opened the abdomen and exposed the intestine, whereupon the 'expert' went to work. I am sure he had never done such an operation before. His instrument was ghastly and when he produced his adhesive – I am sure it was an early version of Super Glue – his gloves, the delicate peritoneal lining, any muscles and connective tissue got tangled up in strings of glue and withdrawal of his fingers caused nasty tears of any tissue with which he came into contact. I was of the opinion that the visitor had never used these things before and had come out to the baboon unit, of which many people must have heard, in order to 'give it a try'. I was deeply distressed and incensed. I insisted on destroying the baboon while still under the anaesthetic. I never heard of this man again. I should think he was only too anxious to leave Kenya and forget the nastiness of his visit to Nairobi. Foy and Kondi were as appalled as I was and the man's name was not mentioned again in my presence.

The work of our laboratory was expanded to take in other *ad hoc* investigations including some more advanced chemotherapeutic research on anaplasm species in the bovine animal. This was another tick-borne disease, which occurs widely throughout tropical countries all over the world. In Africa, the pathogen, *Anaplasma marginale* is ubiquitous and in native cattle causes little serious disease. The indigenous cattle are usually infected in the calf stage when little pathological effect is manifested. The problem arises when improved or exotic cattle are introduced as older animals. Then the pathogen can cause serious debilitating or even fatal disease in fully susceptible cattle. There was, at that time, no known specific therapy. It was, therefore, of importance that such a therapeutic agent should be found and made available for the treatment of expensive introduced stock. Our work was to test various possibly chemotherapeutic substances, which could be made available by our chemists in the home laboratories. The initial problem was to find animals, which were sufficiently susceptible to act as indicators of the presence of the parasite in their blood in numbers, which could be recognised as increased, or which could be determined by some sort of measurable clinical reaction. We visited several farms, which practised tick control by means of dipping and where a fair proportion of the calf crop would be sold. Provision of suitable test animals appeared to be almost impossible. It was decided therefore, to purchase young indigenous calves which we would splenectomise and which would then act as indicators of the presence and proliferation of the parasite and thus could demonstrate the effect of any drugs applied. The operation caused no noticeable set-back in the growth and well being of the calves which were well fed and cared for and could grow on to maturity after the tests had been completed.

We did a great deal of work on this *Anaplasma* screen and it contributed considerably to the knowledge of the disease and the production of drugs of value in combating anaplasmosis. Incorporated into this programme later, came a chemotherapeutic screen against babesiosis, another tick borne disease, generally known as redwater in many species of animals and occurring in temperate climates including the United Kingdom, as well as in tropical and sub-tropical countries.

We had been working on East Coast fever for some four or five years when a delegation of veterinary research scientists came out from the Glasgow Veterinary School to assist in the establishment of a faculty of veterinary medicine in the newly formed University of Kenya. The faculty buildings were erected close to the laboratories of the Kenya Veterinary Department at Kabete. It was accepted that the group would take up various research projects in the course of establishing the faculty. As might well be expected, the problems presented included the subject of East Coast fever. The group, under the direction of Professor Ian McIntyre, came to see me to find out the situation regarding our work. None of the group had previously had any practical experience of East Coast fever and so ten of the visitors assembled, at my invitation, in my office, where I explained the work we had done and the proposed future projection of our research. Of course it was not for me to consider that we had any exclusive right in this field. I told them of our ideas for the further plans in the pursuit of either a curative solution or the development of a practical means of immunisation. I agreed to supply the Glasgow team with some of our infected ticks and expressed the hope that our mutual co-operation might speed the arrival at a successful conclusion. Unfortunately, there was no reciprocal collaboration. The Glasgow team, of which members had enjoyed some lucrative association with one of the well-known pharmaceutical houses on the subject of a vaccine for a parasitic disease caused by the parasite *Dictyocaulus,* were well versed in publicity. Soon the local press was publishing optimistic articles about the problems concerning East Coast fever about to be overcome, now that a powerful team of scientists had come out to do research on the subject.

We had produced some very promising guidelines for the further work on East Coast fever but I realised that it would cost the Company a lot of money to fund the work that would be necessary if we were to continue along the lines that I had visualised. The Food and Agriculture Organisation of the United Nations was very interested in the subject and I realised that FAO was considering a programme of research in this field. I took up this aspect of the situation with my superiors in the Foundation and pointed out that even should we be successful in producing a remedy for the disease or a means of immunisation, it would not produce a financial return of any significance for the Company. I am quite sure in my own mind that the Foundation had realised this from the start of our project. I believe that they had mainly been interested in establishing a research presence in East Africa and that any success would have been a bonus for the Company and a prestigious aid to the East African countries, The business side of the Foundation had already established trading companies in Kenya, Tanganyika and Uganda, with boards of directors of which I was one in each company with an overall manager, based in Nairobi. Indeed, a small factory had been built in Nairobi for the processing of some Wellcome products for which there was a reasonable market among the populations of East Africa.

To cut a rather complicated process short, I made proposals, which virtually could have made my post in the Company redundant. The FAO set up a research group to work in the EAVRO laboratories along the lines, which had been established by us. They offered Duncan Brown and me, research posts in the scheme. Duncan accepted but I did not. The Foundation was, as usual, most generous to me and offered me the support necessary for me to continue the programme on which we were engaged for as long as I wished to carry on. I was at this time also Director of the Wellcome Laboratories for Research on foot-and-mouth Disease, which had been built as a joint project with the Government of Kenya near the airport at Embakazi.

Time for our home leave was approaching and so it was suggested that I should discuss the future of WRL (EA) with the directors in London. I put the whole situation to them in detail and also the fact that our two sons had now left East Africa, James to enter the RAF and Peter to take up a place in medical school. In addition, Kathy's health had been causing us some concern over the previous four or five years and she had suffered some horrendous surgery in Nairobi. It was decided that I should return to Kenya for another tour and draw the work programme to a conclusion and concentrate on getting the foot-and-mouth disease work which had suffered from several set-backs, especially financially, into the 'black'. The development of the research and production at the WLRFM had gone ahead to the extent that the Government of Kenya had initiated a programme of control and possible eradication of foot-and-mouth disease from the country. Splendid work on the isolation and growth in tissue culture of the important strains of F&M virus had been done by the research team, of which outstanding members were Tony Garland, Chris Schermbrucker and Ruth Simpson. The whole enterprise was a joint effort between the Kenya Veterinary Department and Wellcome. My job was to give every possible help to the production by administrative and financial organisation so that the experts could forge ahead with the production of the most effective of the appropriate vaccines. New stainless steel culture tanks had been installed and enough vaccine to support the commencement of a countrywide campaign was produced. Later, this was not enough and much larger tanks were installed to meet the rising demand for vaccine. The whole operation became financially viable for the first time since its inception. To those of us who had been intimately involved with this scheme from the start, the success was a credit to those who had devised the enterprise and redounds to the credit of the workers, who had overcome many obstacles and who can be regarded as the advance guard in the large scale production of successful vaccines against this hitherto very damaging disease

Sir Michael Perrin, Chairman of the Wellcome Foundation, came out to Kenya accompanied by his wife to look at the work we were doing on behalf of the company. It was, of course, part of my duty to make all arrangements for this visit and to ensure that all went smoothly. He was particularly interested in the Wellcome Laboratories for Research into foot-and-mouth Disease. The company's success in this project was of great importance for the possible future development of an important worldwide programme. This virus is one of the most infective of all viruses and work on it can only be carried out in laboratories with the strictest regimes of quarantine. Our laboratories had been built with the most rigorous attention to precautions against any escape of virus out of the laboratories and against entry of any extraneous pathogens. Among other restrictions this meant that all workers in the labs and any visitors had to divest themselves of all clothing and pass through showers before entering the quarantine area. Dressing rooms were provided on the outside and on the other side of the showers. Sterile clothing was provided which in our case, as Kenya is a hot country, comprised of T-shirts, shorts and tackies (like tennis shoes). These were kept in sterile packs and provided in an inner dressing room. I made all arrangements for Sir Michael's visit. On the phone, Chris Schermbrucker asked me what sort of a size was our visitor's girth. I said that I thought it was about the same as mine. He was about my height and I had always regarded him as quite slender.

We duly arrived at the labs and I advised the staff that we were on our way through. When we arrived in the inner changing room there was Sir Michael's sterile pack awaiting him and I opened it for him. Then he tried to don it. It was far too small. I hadn't realised that Sir Michael had quite a pot. I had to open the door to call Chris and ask him to bring a pack of two sizes larger. In came Chris with the larger pack followed by the senior male staff and so our illustrious guest had the staff introduced to him in a state of nature, in which I still was myself. He took it in his stride, donned his quarantine clothes and strode into the labs. After the Chairman had completed the official part of his visit to our Kenya set up, Kathy and I took Michael and Nancy on a safari, which included a game camp on the Tana River where we were housed in tents and then to the Coast where they enjoyed the Indian Ocean and lived in a palm thatched hut a few yards from the sea. Peter who was on holiday from his university accompanied us and became official photography instructor to Lady Perrin and also introduced our guests to the delights of snorkelling on the coral reef.

During the last home leave, mentioned above, Kathy and I looked around for a suitable house to purchase as a *pied a terre* that would provide a home for the two boys for their leaves and vacations, respectively. We felt also, that while it would not be necessarily where we would wish to live when we finally left Africa, it would provide us with an entry into the property market when we came to live in Britain. It was a wise decision. We settled for a bungalow in the village of Sleights near to Whitby.

During our last tour of service in Kenya there were lots of complications, not the least of which was a very serious series of operations suffered by Kathy. I will go into this later. One good thing which happened, was that I was visited in my labs by Sir Alex Robertson, Professor of Tropical Veterinary Medicine in the Royal (Dick) School of Veterinary Studies of the University of Edinburgh and Director of the Centre for Tropical Veterinary Medicine. Hearing that I was in my last tour in Kenya, he offered me a research fellowship in the CTVM to be in charge of the section of Protozoology. I accepted the offer without hesitation. Tim Evans had retired from his position in the Wellcome Foundation and Dr Montgomery had died. A committee had been formed after a wholesale reorganisation of the Foundation, to liaise with my unit in East Africa. This committee was put under the control of Alex Thompson, Head of anaerobic bacteriology at Beckenham. He knew nothing about our work in the field of protozoology and was apparently imbued with the importance of committees and his position as chairman. The former happy relationship was lost and typical committee bureaucratic methods were instituted, which meant delays in the making of decisions and publication of results and more tortuous methods of reporting and organisation. The whole atmosphere had changed and I was glad to be retiring. I was informed that when I left my post, Paul Capstick, who had been briefly on the staff of the Kenya Veterinary Laboratory, would replace me. Paul was a virologist of some repute and so it was clear that our ECF work was to be brought to a close.

Of course, life in Kenya was not all work, I had a family and we had to live. James and Peter had to be educated and we had to take part in the social life of expatriates in Kenya. Kenya was, of the three East African countries, the most European orientated and was certainly the most advanced part of the Africa in which we had lived. There was a large and influential farming community inhabiting the so-called 'White Highlands' and unlike the position in Tanganyika, the veterinary services had been strongly influenced towards the maintenance of a healthy European livestock population. Indigenous flocks and herds were, of course, also catered for in the country. The Kenya Veterinary Department research and vaccine production establishment was much more advanced in its capacity and personnel than the corresponding departments in Tanganyika and Uganda. Several large international companies maintained branches in Kenya and European farmers had established herds and flocks of very high quality exotic animals. An annual agricultural show was mounted and the stock shown included specimens which would have been highly placed in the big agricultural shows in Britain. The time of our arrival in Kenya coincided with the development of tarmac roads on many of the more important routes.

My interest in painting flourished in Kenya where there were many artists and there established a very active society, the Kenya Arts Society. It was through this association that I met and became friendly with many amateur artists among whom Joyce Butter was outstanding. She was really a professional who had studied art in London and was a brilliant portrait painter. She was very helpful to me and gave me some very useful instruction in my oil painting. She was a larger than life character and was regarded by many as officious and dictatorial, especially by women. I got on with her very well and made light of her rather demanding attitude. Kathy had her reservations. She considered that she just put on people like me who were expected to accept her ideas and do her bidding. Her husband, John, was the financial advisor to the Government and his signature appeared on the Kenya bank notes. I first met Joyce when I was elected onto the committee of the Kenya Arts Society (KAS) of which she was President. The Society had a studio and ancillary rooms near to Government house. Here we employed a teacher who acted as a general executive and manager of the Society and also ran classes for members and especially for young promising Kenyans several of whom aspired to winning scholarships to art schools in Britain. A few years after I joined the KAS, Joyce resigned from the office of President and I was elected to the post in which I served for about five years.

One of our functions was the mounting of our own annual art exhibition and the setting up of a very prestigious annual exhibition on behalf of the Esso Oil Company. This was an open exhibition attracting entries from all over East Africa. The venue for the exhibition was the City Hall in Nairobi where we usually had in excess of four hundred pictures to hang. An independent committee, whose chairman was the Managing Director of the Esso Company, judged the exhibition and picked out the picture that was deemed the best. This picture was used as the calendar for the Esso Company for the following year. The prize was quite an appreciable monetary sum and a large amount of free petrol. I forget the actual figures but there was very keen competition. I entered a picture each year and with my fourth entry I won the second prize. The following year I received a highly commended certificate but in 1963 I was awarded the first prize with a painting entitled, 'Beach Trader'. This success gave me, I think, more satisfaction than any other that I have achieved.

It was about two years after this win that I became

President of the Kenya Arts Society and took on the responsibility for mounting the exhibitions. In this I was assisted by Joyce Butter and several other members including Mrs Benn "Benny" and Gwen Streets, who had previous experience of the work. With several KAS and Esso exhibitions under my belt I became fairly competent in the matter of mounting art exhibitions. On one memorable occasion, when we were in the City Hall working on the Esso exhibition, there was a terrific rainstorm. It was reported that 5inches of rain fell in about two hours. When I came out ready to go home, I found the water lapping up the City Hall steps and I had to wade, knee deep onto the pavement and round the corner to where I had parked my car. I was appalled to see my Citroen with the water level up to a height above the middle of the doors. I had to wait some time to allow a little lowering of the level before I could open the door. Of course, the water rushed in and flooded the vehicle to a depth level with the seat. I didn't really hope for the engine to start but it did and also, the mechanism, which raised the car suspension in that model, operated and the car went up and the water rushed out to the level of the bottom of the door. In those cars there was a deep well so that the pedals were all under water. I started to move and joined the traffic creeping along the main streets in deep water. Even a gentle change of speed caused a rush of water splashing up under the dashboard and back over the seat and up my trousers. When, very gingerly, I arrived at a bit of road high enough to be only an inch or two under water, I stopped the car and bailed and mopped as much water out as I could and then drove the six miles home, still with the water sloshing around my feet. Needless to say, the vehicle had to go into the Citroen workshops to have a complete dry out, particularly of the engine compartment. The interior of the car stank for weeks, well into the hot season when it dried out completely.

Two members of my KAS committee were architects and our treasurer was a judge of the high court, Gerald Harris. I was President of the KAS for five years until we left Kenya in 1970. Joyce Butter and her husband left Kenya at the same time as we did. Her husband accepted appointment as financial advisor to the ruler of one of the Trucial States. I was most touched and highly honoured when the KAS gave a dinner party for Kathy and me and jointly for Joyce and John and presented us with presents. I received a very lovely book 'Africa' by Emil Schultess and an Arab door lock from Lamu. This was most welcome to me as I had taken a great interest in Lamu and had made something of a reputation in painting Arab doors as subjects. Once, when in Lamu on a visit, I had bought an old Arab doorway and some pieces of carving that are, together with the door lock, in our house to this day.

James and Peter started their formal schooling in Kenya, going first to the Westlands Primary School. Peter was exceptionally bright as a pupil and so he, together with a friend, was pushed up two years so that when they moved on to the Prince of Wales public school Peter and James were in the same year. The school was only about a mile away from our estate but when they started we signed them in as boarders. They hated it and especially the archaic system of the school authorities putting the discipline into the hands of senior prefects who seemed to be encouraged to dispense corporal punishment. We, therefore, agreed to their becoming day pupils and they remained as such until the end of their schooldays. James was never academically inclined but Peter completed his sixth form years as a prefect and both of them left school in 1967 and came to England with us when we took leave in that year. James joined the RAF and started his training and Peter made enquiries of medical schools in England and Scotland, and although all were prepared to give him a place they made it a condition that he should wait until he attained the age of eighteen before he would be permitted to take up his studies. He was a few months under seventeen. However, he pressed on, trying more of the schools until Liverpool University Medical Faculty offered him a place.

When Peter was still twelve and James, fifteen, one of the teachers at the Prince of Wales School, Hugh Cowey, planned a climb of Mount Kilimanjaro by a large number of schoolboys. Our two boys were keen to join this adventure and I was approached to see if I would be prepared to act as leader for one of the groups. I agreed to take the youngest group as this would be the one in which James and Peter would be included. Dr Lotte Hulliger who was then on my staff agreed to lead another group if she could also include her live in partner, Ruedi Schenkel. As a result of my previous experience on Kilimanjaro I had very firm ideas as to how such a climb had to be organised. Cowie was a very energetic young man and he fixed up all the logistics and timing of the ascents. He established tented camps, one near Peter's hut at 12,000 feet and the second at the foot of the main peak, Kibo at about 16,000 feet. He organised the times allotted to each group and the arrangements for the feeding at each camp. He made a very good job of it and spent several days at each camp, also taking a group of the older boys up to the summit.

When climbing at high altitudes one of the first considerations is clothing. The temperature falls very markedly as one reaches heights of 8,000 feet and more. This fall, of course, is greatest as evening becomes night. I had impressed on the boys in my group and their parents the importance of wearing several layers of warm but fairly loose clothing. Even so, some of the members of my group had tighter clothing than was advisable and this applied most importantly to the hands and feet. Two pairs of woolly socks are very good but not if they have to be squeezed into tight boots and the same applies for tight gloves.

We travelled by coach from Nairobi across the border into Tanzania via the great north road and then through Arusha to Moshi. Thence we were driven in a Land Rover up a rough road through the fields of maize and coffee to a place called Marangu where there are two hotels that specialise in making arrangements for tourists and others wishing to essay the climb of Kilimanjaro. Hugh Cowie had made an arrangement with the owners of the Marangu Guest House for us to have tents in the grounds so that we could avoid the expense of staying in the Guest House itself. Indeed, there would not have been enough rooms to accommodate all of us. The proprietors supplied our meals and made us very welcome. We spent one night in this camp and on the following morning, after a good breakfast, were taken in the Land Rover up a rough track in the forest to our first camp of the climb that had been set up at what was known as Bismarck's Hut, at an altitude of about 6,000 feet. From here we set off on foot through the rain forest among the huge trees with vast buttresses at their bases. We were, at first, within the sound of running water as the clear water from the melted ice of the peaks cascaded down to the hot plains below us. As we gained height, the tall forest trees gave place to the giant heather, which comprises trees of up to twenty feet high. From this scrubby forest we emerged onto the open highland, very similar in general appearance to the moorlands that I knew so well in Derbyshire, but this moorland was liberally sprinkled with everlasting flowers. The atmosphere was clear and we had glimpses of the two peaks of Kilimanjaro, the nearer, minor peak, Mawenzi and the major peak, Kibo. We now had a long trudge rising to ridges and then plunging down to streams that crossed the path and then rising again to the next ridge, gradually increasing our altitude until at about 5p.m. we reached Peter's hut which is at about 12,000 feet. Here, near the banks of a crystal clear stream, Hugh had sited our tent and soon a cup of tea was ready for us and very welcome it was. The boys were hot and sweaty and James took off his boots and socks and jumped into a shallow part of the stream. He soon jumped out as the water was literally melted ice. He swears to this day that his feet have never been normal since. Around the stream were clumps of giant ragwort growing up to twelve feet high and lobelias of up to nine feet. Night fell rapidly and the temperature with it and we were soon pleased to eat a hot stew and get under blankets in the tent. We were all tired and slept fairly well but the brilliant sunrise had us up and out of the tent to enjoy the view of the dazzling white clouds below us and the clear view of the peaks ahead. We had a good breakfast, enjoyed by most but some of the boys were beginning to feel a little queasy on account of the altitude.

We started to climb slowly round the base of Mawenzi and up to the saddle. I insisted on the march being made slowly with periodic rests to allow for some degree of acclimatisation. All went well as we reached the saddle between the two peaks. This area has a moonscape type of appearance. The saddle rises as a gentle slope along a path of shale interspersed with larger rocks, a rather tedious prospect. Away in the distance, some six or so miles before us was Kibo hut. We occasionally caught a glimpse of the sun's reflection on the tin roof of the hut but for a long time we didn't seem to get any nearer. Soon the clouds formed around the summit of Kibo and suddenly it was no longer visible. We reached the hut soon after 4p.m. and found that a tent had been erected and a couple of guides had prepared mugs of tea. They had prepared some soup and a hot meal but most of the boys were not in eating mood. I encouraged them to take some soup and then we all settled down in the tent well wrapped up in blankets and tried to sleep, but not before I got them to take off their shoes and socks and rub Vaseline liberally into their feet before replacing their boots. The camp was roused at about 1a.m. and more tea and soup were prepared and dispensed by the guides and then slowly, I encouraged the boys to get all their warmest clothing and their boots on and we crept out of the tent into an atmosphere at about twelve degrees below zero.

Some yards from the Kibo hut is a lonely looking corrugated iron contraption that surrounds a long drop. This must certainly be the highest permanent loo in the whole of Africa. Those who could endure the prospect of removing as little clothing as was necessary did so with trepidation, the corrugated door swinging noisily in the bitterly cold wind. The night was pitch black and at about 2 o'clock the senior guide appeared with a storm lantern and signalled that we should now start the final climb.

I had drilled into the boys' heads that they should climb slowly and rest after every few steps and that when they did rest, they must on no account sit down but rest on their sticks - each boy had a spiked stick. The path was fairly gentle and firm for the first quarter of a mile or so but then it became interspersed with very loose scree and four or five steps between rests were about reasonable. During the first three hundred feet we experienced very cold hands and feet, but as dawn approached, we came up to the 'caves', really an overhanging rock shelf. Here I ordered a good sit down rest and then after another hundred or so feet upwards, one of the boys complained that he felt too sick and couldn't go further. This posed a problem. We couldn't leave him at this point alone and to send him back to Kibo hut with the guide would leave me with the rest of the boys with no flexibility of action if any of the others proved unable to continue. I had a good look at the boy and gave him a tablet against altitude sickness and told him he would now be all right.

216

We started tentatively again and then the sun came up in all its glory. In a few minutes we were divesting ourselves of our outer garments and feeling almost uncomfortably warm. The boy who had felt sick soon seemed to recover and so we carried on to Gilman's point, which overlooks the ice wall of the crater, all the boys highly elated with their success. Cloud began to build up and so I decided we should make our way back to Kibo Hut. The return down the cone was greatly enjoyed as it is easy to scree-ride down much of the declivities. However, the weather degenerated into a cold mist, which then became a snowstorm which was fairly heavy by the time we reached Kibo Hut. It had been my intention to carry on to Peter's hut when we came down from the peak but had we done this the boys would have been soaked as would the bedding which we had to take with us. I therefore decided to stay in the tent at Kibo and go all the way to Bismarck's, a trek of about thirty miles the next day. This is what we did and while all the boys were very tired by the time we arrived at Bismarck's, where the Land Rover was waiting for us, they were all very happy, and were delighted to receive the everlasting flower garlands which the guides made for them between Peter's Hut and Bismarck's. None of them needed any rocking when we got back to Marangu.

When our boys were at the Westlands Primary School I sat on the parents' committee and met a well respected teacher, Mrs Allen. We became friends with her and her husband Vic de V.Allen. Vic was a dedicated worker for an organisation called the Association for the Physically Disabled of Kenya (APDK). I became very interested in this charitable institution and went to see what it was doing. The functions included the helping of disabled people either to overcome their disabilities or to be trained for useful and rewarding work that could help them to make a living and restore their self-respect. The majority of the people helped were Africans with little or no means of support but there were among them several of the poorer and less able Asians. Many of the patients were, of course, children and they received special treatment that included schooling while they were receiving physiotherapy. The APDK had a building in which were offices, a physiotherapy room and a schoolroom. In addition, on the edge of Nairobi there was a workshop where disabled adults were trained in various skills such as joinery and boot making. The organisation also supported a ward in the Mater Miserichordia Hospital where the APDK patients could receive proper treatment and nursing by medical staff and the nuns.

I was invited to become a member of the management committee of which Vic was chairman. I was very pleased to accept the invitation and agreed to help with fund raising. The secretary/manager of the APDK was a very active lady called Jo Cowley, who did a tremendous amount of work and really kept everything running smoothly and efficiently. She was, of course, a voluntary worker as were all the other helpers. Vic Allen was always ready to do any extra work that was required. He had served in the Kenya Police for many years and had retired some years before we knew him, when he was a very senior officer. He was involved in the case of the murder of Lord Errol in the days of the rather disreputable 'happy valley'. Vic showed us the spot where the police found the car with Lord Errol's body in it. I enjoyed working with the very pleasant people who formed the committee and did such things as designing Christmas Cards and getting them printed for sale. The Association had a stall each year at the annual show of the Kenya Agricultural Organisation and at one of these I gave the APDK one of my paintings that was put up for raffle and made £700. I was active with the APDK for several years but when Kenya became completely independent under Jomo Kenyatta, things became difficult as the business of work permits was applied to charities so that Jo Cowley lost her voluntary job and an African had to be appointed in her place, and of course, had to be paid. Vic was replaced by an African who was quite an educated and pleasant fellow but he did not have the know-how and also had to make a living as well so that things deteriorated. I was asked to stay on the committee and I did in order to help the new chairman. The initiative and energy were no longer there so that our funds diminished and much of the work had to be abandoned. I do not know what happened to the APDK after I left Kenya, but reports of affairs in Kenya that come to us are depressing.

One of our great pleasures in Kenya was provided by our visits to the Coast. In our early days the main roads in Kenya were made of mud that, in parts, was reinforced by the addition of crushed termite mounds. This material gave a little more substance to the road surface but in the wet season all mud roads were reduced to churned up slush. Road travel was very hazardous in wet weather. In the dry season the main roads tended to powder with wear and in the main roads corrugations were developed by the speed of the traffic. This phenomenon, combined with the thick clouds of red dust, made motoring very unpleasant and dangerous. Between Nairobi and Mombasa on the coast were about three hundred miles of this kind of road. We always tried to take our coast holiday when the road was at its best, when the journey, while hot, was otherwise good from the driving point of view. We had some very pleasant holidays on the coast with miles of clean white sand and the Indian Ocean at twenty degrees Celsius or more. We stayed at various places along the coastline from small hotels to hired beach houses. We snorkelled on the reef and sailed in the native fishermens ngalawas, outrigger canoes made from hollowed-out logs. Kathy says she has never enjoyed lobster thermidor as much as those I cooked in our beach hut. Nowadays, most TV viewers are familiar with the brilliant fish we used to watch on the reef but the goggling produced for us magnificent views.

We used to go from time to time to the various game parks, Tsavo, Serengeti, Amboseli and others. We became members of the Nairobi Game Park so that we could go out there at any time without having to pay high entrance fees. So we could go for an hour or two as the sun was beginning to set and sit and watch the cheetahs getting ready for their evening hunt. We saw great changes in some of the areas where herds of elephants altered the nature of the vegetation. Some areas which I remembered from my early visits to Kenya, as heavily wooded and dense bush, became denuded of trees by the time we were about to leave Kenya, indicating how the elephant herds could convert woodland to savannah in their search for fodder.

At the Jomo Kenyatta Hospital, a new room was being constructed to accommodate a cobalt bomb for treatment of Africans suffering from various forms of cancer. The hospital committee decided that it would be a good thing to have a mural painted on the internal walls immediately facing the apparatus so

219

that patients could see something to relieve their nervousness at being in what, to the African peasant, must have been frightening isolation and a fearsome piece of apparatus. After considering several ideas, the Matron, Miss Lil Richmond, approached me as she had seen some of my pictures in exhibitions. I was asked to meet her and Doctor Gregory, the Chairman of the committee, to give them some ideas and to let them know if I would execute the mural. When we met, we agreed that the pictorial presentation should be something that would be familiar to untutored patients who undoubtedly would be frightened by their strange surroundings when under treatment. The doctor suggested, as I thought, the unsatisfactory idea of a wall full of butterflies. I, diplomatically, suggested that this subject would not be very familiar to African peasants and put forward the theme of scenes from village life. Lil Richmond supported this suggestion and I was asked to do a few sketches for scrutiny by the committee.

The upshot was that I was asked to paint the mural on the inner wall of the treatment room and this is what I did. I judged that the patient lying on his or her back with some part of the body under the rotating emiter would have, in view, the upper part of the facing wall and the part of the ceiling immediately adjacent to the top of the wall. Accordingly, I designed the village scenes along the top half of the wall and made the ceiling section into an African sky. As soon as the wall and ceiling were rendered and painted white I started up. I had a limited time in which to complete the work since, as soon as the room was ready and the apparatus was installed, this addition to the hospital was to be opened by the President, Jomo Kenyatta. I could only work on the mural on Saturday afternoons and Sundays and so I had to get my skates on. I was hard at it on a Saturday afternoon when I received a message from the hospital that I was required at home. I expected to find Kathy ill or some such emergency and so I jumped into my car and hurried home.

I was amazed to find, when I arrived, that our son, James, who was now in the RAF, had turned up at our house. It transpired that he was stationed in Bahrain and the RAF were flying some training flights of Hercules planes across Arabia to Kenya. James, while being a very junior aircraftsman, had managed to inform the Senior NCO who was drafting the crews for the flights that his mother and father were living in Nairobi. The NCO was not inclined to believe him but James managed to overcome his doubts and he got the ride. Two complete crews formed the compliment of the flight and James was included. When the plane arrived in Nairobi, James and the other most junior member of the crew with whom he had struck up a friendship, got leave from the officer in charge and took a taxi out to Kabete. Kathy, of course, was to put it into the vernacular, 'gobsmacked', but was overjoyed to see her son and so a message was sent to me and I was of course also overjoyed. We promptly got in touch with the rest of the two crews and invited them out to a party. They arrived with a crate of drinks and a good time was had by all. The plane could not make the return journey until a spare part could be procured and so we arranged to take all those who wanted to go to the market in Nairobi and then on to the Nairobi Game Park. The men bought souvenirs at prices brought down to reasonable levels by me and thoroughly enjoyed the visit to the Park, seeing lions and other exotic game. James's stock had gone up to the extent that he was given a 'clutch' in the cockpit and flew the plane, in a manner of speaking, across Arabia.

We did our major shopping in Nairobi or at Westlands where an active shopping centre with a large petrol station and banks had developed but we were lucky enough to have, not far away, a duka (shop or general store) where we could buy most of the day to day supplies. It also incorporated a sub-post office where our mail was delivered and petrol pumps from which we obtained our motor fuel. A family of Kojah Ishmaelies, of whom the boss was Kantilal Patel, owned the duka, and his two brothers assisted in the daily work of the business. Dadubahai, the elder of the two ran the post office. They all lived with their families in the building that housed the duka. Like most of the Asian tradesmen in East Africa, they were always most obliging and would go to great lengths to make sure that their customers had what they required. If an item was not in stock, they would make every effort to find a source and get it as soon as possible.

We were good customers at the duka and from time to time, the Patels would invite us and some of our associates to a curry meal in the evening. The women of the families did all the cooking in typical Asian manner in the back quarters of the duka. Only the males joined us for the meal even though our party invariably was half-male and half-female. The women of the establishment ate after the males and guests had finished. We always got on very well with the Patels and also many of the Asian business people in the bazaar in Nairobi where we purchased such things as furniture, textiles and other household goods. Some of the shopkeepers became good friends and we were invited to their houses and some of them came to visit us. We purchased a lot of electrical items including such things as tape recorders, highly unusual at the time. We became friends with the owner of a very up-to-date electrical goods shop in Nairobi. He was Richard Desai and his very pleasant wife was called Daisy. I could rely on Richard to see that whatever I bought in his shop was the best and most reliable article of its kind.

Our period in Kenya was very interesting and, in many ways, rewarding but it was marred to a great extent by the trouble suffered by Kathy, surgically, during our thirteen years at Kabete. The trouble started with abdominal discomfort and pain which was treated by our GP. Temporary remission occurred but was followed by a repetition of the trouble. Our GP, Dr Brian MacShane, suggested that a gynaecologist should see Kathy and an appointment was made with a Mr Preston who said that my wife was probably suffering from endometriosis and should have a hysterectomy. Accordingly the operation was arranged and Kathy went into what was then the womens' department of the European Hospital in Nairobi. I well remember Brian MacShane saying that this was probably the answer to Kathy's problem and that she should be 'a new woman two weeks after the operation'. Things didn't live up to this prophecy and I found Kathy in bed in the hospital with a catheter in situ. I was present when the surgeon came round to see Kathy and I asked him why the catheter was necessary. He admitted that there had been an accident during the operation and a vesico-vaginal fistula had been made. That meant a hole between the bladder and the vagina, through which the bladder was leaking and that until it was repaired, Kathy would have to be permanently catheterised.

I asked how soon he could make the repair. He told me that we would have to wait for three months. I was appalled and said that he must do the repair immediately or I would call in another surgeon to make good his mistake. He said that the tissue of the bladder wall was of such a nature that it would be difficult to repair until it had had some months to settle. The operation was, incidentally, being paid for privately. I said that my wife was not going to suffer the discomfort and indignity of having a catheter up her urethra for months and demanded that the repair was effected immediately. Mr Preston reluctantly agreed and the operation was arranged for a few days later. When Kathy was back in her bed in the ward, I was present when Preston visited her again. He explained to me that the operation had been very difficult and that it had been necessary to insert a titanium suture into the tissue of the bladder wall in order to make the closure secure. He said that the suture might become permanently buried in the tissue or it might work its way out and have to be removed.

When she was discharged from the hospital, Kathy was not feeling very comfortable. Pains recurred in the lower abdomen and these became so bad that I had to take her to see the GP. Antibiotic treatment was prescribed and this had to be repeated at intervals when the symptoms recurred. Matters became so bad that Kathy would suddenly jump when a sharp pain occurred in her bladder region. This was very frequent when we were travelling in the car. Brian was consulted again, in fact on several occasions, and he began to think that Kathy was imagining these pains. He suggested that we should go and see Preston again but Kathy refused to see Preston or any other surgeon. She complained that the pain was very bad at urination and Brian tried treating for cystitis. There was temporary remission but when the pain recurred, eventually, we had to resort to the injection of local anaesthetic up the urethra several times a day. At last things became so intolerable that in desperation Kathy agreed to see Preston again. After examination by him he said that there were caruncles in the urethra and that they should be removed. Another operation was arranged. When she was being wheeled into the theatre, Kathy wrote on a piece of cigarette packet, a note that she asked the theatre sister to give to the surgeon. It read, 'Mr Preston, there is something there and I want to see it'.

Amazing to relate, Preston seemed to have come to the end of his dissimulation as, when Kathy came to in her bed after the operation, there was a small bottle of formalin on her bedside table and in it was a full curved surgical needle, with a broken eye and, by now rusty. The news of this had spread through the hospital and it caused a lot of speculation as only a few months previously, one of the local surgeons had been sued for leaving a swab in the abdomen of a patient. His Medical Defence Insurance had had to pay £60,000 damages. I met Preston once more at Kathy's bedside. He seemed to be very down in the mouth. I said, "Mr Preston, we all make mistakes and you have made a big one now. All I ask is that you make sure that Kathy recovers fully." I intimated that I did not expect a bill. He said that he was very grateful that I was taking that attitude and hoped Kathy would now make a complete recovery. I had no desire to make money out of a surgeon's mistake but there is no doubt in my mind that Preston's actions and explanations had been most reprehensible and deceitful. He had not informed our GP or anyone in the hospital that he had broken a needle and left it in the bladder. Had Kathy not indicated that she knew something was there, who knows what Preston would have done or said?

Unfortunately that was not the end of the matter. This botched operation was the beginning of a whole series of troubles for us. I can say with some confidence, that these continued to cause problems and miseries for the rest of Kathy's life, that is more than thirty-five years after the first operation. While we were still in Kenya there was a series of painful upsets for Kathy leading to more operations and treatments. She suffered several attacks of pain in the region of the left inguinal fossa. These were mostly due to the development of abscesses in the region of the bladder. The episodes were often accompanied by bouts of constipation and were very depressing. It was while one of these attacks was being suffered, that we had arranged to go for a short break at the Coast. It was Easter, and Peter was on holiday from university with us. We drove down to Mombasa where we were to stay in a friend's house on Nyali Beach. We arrived there in the late afternoon and Kathy was feeling so ill that she went straight to bed. I decided that if things did not improve overnight, we would organise a flight to London and have Kathy properly treated. Wellcome would have been able to get her into a suitable hospital.

The morning dawned hot and sunny. Peter suggested that Kathy should take a walk into the sea that was, of course, beautifully warm. She agreed and we, all three, walked slowly down the beach and into the warm water. I supported Kathy on one side and Peter on the other. We slowly entered the sea and moved down the sloping beach until the water came up to Kathy's chest when she suddenly said, 'The pain's gone'. It was quite like a miracle, but it was most probably because the pressure of the water had caused an abscess to burst. When we emerged from the sea, pus and blood were pouring down Kathy's legs. When we returned to Nairobi, after the very satisfactory weekend break, Kathy went into hospital and had the remnants of the abscess cleaned up. Unfortunately, the abscess syndrome recurred on several occasions until, once more, Kathy had to go into hospital again. This time it was thought that surgical interference was called for. Incidentally, Mr Preston had left Kenya and not long afterwards, we heard that he had died. The surgeon who was brought in to the problem was a Mr J.A.S.Green. I give here a transcript of Mr Green's report.

"This lady has had a long history of pelvic infection following a hysterectomy ten years ago after which a vesico-vaginal fistula developed. This was repaired but later she had chronic pelvic pain and micturitional symptoms, relieved by the removal of a foreign body.

In 1969 she began to get abdominal pain again and there was a discharge of pus from the urethra, which relieved her symptoms.

A barium enema done some few months ago showed some spasm of the descending colon but nothing else. The appendix did not fill.

I first saw her on the 20th January when she gave two days history of lower abdominal pain, rather worse on the right than on the left. Temp. 101F and there was

225

suprapubic tenderness and tenderness in the right iliac fossa. I thought it probable that she had an inflamed pelvic appendix and on the 21ˢᵗ January opened the abdomen through the old lower midline incision. It was found that the appendix was normal and it was removed. She had had a hysterectomy and the tubes and ovaries were not identifiable.

The lower sigmoid was the site of an inflammatory mass, the affected part being just to the left of the recto-sigmoid junction. No diverticula was (sic) seen in the rest of the sigmoid. Clinically it appeared to be either diverticulitis or an inflamed carcinoma. However, I decided to do nothing more on this occasion and simply closed the wound without drainage.

On the 28ᵗʰ January I sigmoidoscoped the patient but was not able to pass the instrument further than fifteen cms. As the sigmoid colon was too adherent and bound down. A barium enema was then done which showed a ring constriction of the sigmoid, carcinoma being considered the likely cause'.

At this point I received an urgent telephone call asking me to attend at the hospital. By the time I reached Kathy's bedside, Mr Green and our GP, who had been to see her, had left the hospital and I was given a message asking me to visit Mr Green's consulting rooms. I went there immediately and had a discussion with the surgeon. Kathy had told me when I had just seen her, that she had been told that she had a cancer of the bowel. She asserted that she was sure that she did not have a cancer and I must say that with all her history and her general condition, I was inclined to agree with her. All the symptoms we had seen and/or experienced pointed in my opinion to the 'mass' mentioned by the surgeon being due to a constant insult to the tissues for a period of fifteen months by a broken surgical needle.

When I met Mr Green in his consulting room that morning, he explained the position as he saw it and assured me that a further operation was necessary. He said that it might be that I would prefer to take Kathy to London for the operation but that if I was satisfied to let him operate he was prepared to do so immediately. I gave my views on the possibility of the 'mass' being an exuberant growth of inflammatory tissue due to the long-term presence of the surgical needle. He saw my point but said that he thought it would be wise to do a hemi-colectomy and he described the operation with drawings of what would have to be done. I agreed to his opening up Kathy's abdomen again and operating as he saw fit as he knew the situation and I felt it was much more expeditious than having to start the whole process again after what would be a very uncomfortable flight to London and then having someone new to start the whole procedure once more.

Mr Green's report continues;

'After preparation with Thalazole and streptomycin for several days I reopened the abdomen on the 4th February up to the left and above the umbilicus. The mass was now larger and adherent in the left iliac fossa, and on freeing it a small abscess was opened. A left hemi-colectomy was done with anastomosis with the transverse colon to the upper rectum just below the sacral promontory. There was no suggestion of any metastases in the abdomen and liver and glands were clear'.

The pathologist's report was as follows;

'The colon showed no evidence of malignancy, diverticulosis or colitis. The muscular wall was thickened and there were large masses of chronic inflammatory cells outside the muscular layer, although there was a slight infiltration into the muscle also. No amoebae or schistosome ova were seen and there was no cause for the inflammatory condition observable.

When last seen, Mrs Wilde was in good condition and her bowels were working satisfactorily.

No clear diagnosis of the cause of her colonic lesion has been made, but it is presumed to be some form of non-specific granuloma'.

Signed J.A.S. Green. FRCS

I have described this episode in our lives in factual detail as it is so expressive of the obvious effort of one consultant to avoid the exposure of a colleague's mistakes and neglect even to the extent of being very economical with the truth. We hear of these examples of incompetence and even dishonesty and read of them in the press but this was what happened to us and it was common knowledge in the hospital and among members of the public. Fortunately, Kathy survived, but her healthy life was damaged irrevocably by this botched surgery and incompetent treatment. While she suffered mentally and physically for several years and also suffered subsequent surgery and treatment that might well be, at least in part, attributable to the series of episodes described above, our quality of life as a family was fundamentally damaged.

In our Tanganyika years I had developed a modest interest in Persian carpets. This started when I was in Dar es Salaam where, some of the dhows from Arabia came in with piles of rugs aboard and these were for sale. One of our Departmental Veterinary Guards was well known in the port and he was prepared to buy some of these rugs for any of the up-country members of the Department. I asked him to choose a few for me and paid him for his services. I obtained about three or four of the rugs which seemed very nice to me at what also seemed to be reasonable prices, since the dhows brought over what were the rather cheaper lines, mostly Shirazis. These are knotted on wool warps and wefts and do not wear as well as the more expensive types. However, they are usually brightly coloured and looked fine on the concrete floors of my bungalow. When I returned, a married man, after my first leave, I also purchased a large Indian carpet, pale blue in overall colour so that when Kathy arrived the place looked quite homely. On subsequent home leaves when we travelled by sea through the canal, I bought the odd Persian rug in Aden when the ship stopped there. When we went to Kenya, the rugs went with us and were a subject of conversation among our friends. Dick Polkinghorne, our architect, was a collector of Persian rugs and carpets and owned some that I admired. It came about that one evening as it was getting dark, Kathy and I were beginning to close up for the night when an old Ford Popular trundled down our rough road and pulled up outside the veranda.

We were a little apprehensive about strange arrivals at this time of day. The door of the car opened and a tall gangling Pakistani extricated himself and approached. He announced that he had been advised to call on us by Mr Holkingponk, who was one of his customers, and was a connoisseur of Persian carpets. One can imagine our doubts in these circumstances. Itinerant carpet sellers the world over are automatically suspect and one like this man, in the rapidly darkening evening in the uninhabited bush and at a time when every one was particularly security conscious, was obviously a shady character. However, he announced himself as Ahmed Mir and displayed a notebook with lists of names among which was that of Richard Polkinghorne. He said that he only called on people who had been recommended by his customers as prospective Persian carpet collectors. We had apparently been described as such by Dick Polkinghorne. Apprehensively, I agreed that he should show us some of his wares. He dug an armful of rugs out of the back of the Ford and came indoors. In the light of an oil lamp these were laid out on the floor. They were rather mediocre Shirazis and I dismissed them, saying that we already had some of these on our floor in the bedroom and that if he had nothing better we would not be buying. At this, he immediately brightened up. "Ah, sorr," he said, "I see you want good carpets."

He bundled his existing rugs back into the car and reappeared with some more. They were beautiful, all having cotton warps and wefts and with tight knotting. We sat together on the pile of rugs while he extolled the knotting, the patterns and colouring with enthusiasm. He would roll out a rug and then stand back and declare, "There you have a diamond on thee floor, sorr." He would turn the carpet over and run his fingernail across the knots and pronounce in flowery terms on the colours and designs. Intermittently he struck matches and endeavoured to light a briar pipe clenched between his teeth and in his excess of enthusiasm forgot the burning match until it burned his fingers. Then the match dropped onto the carpet or the floorboards and was promptly stamped out on whatever surface was beneath it. "Let me see your Shirazis," said Ahmed Mir. We brought them in. "These are not for you, sorr and Memsahib, they are too common. Let me have them and I will pay you for

229

them against any that you might buy from me." Thus, we bought our first quality Persians. We selected two Kashan rugs and let Ahmed have two of ours for a reduction in price on the Kashans. At the conclusion of our transaction we asked Ahmed if he would like a cup of tea. "No thank you. I will have a leetle whisky." So began a long friendship with a most pleasant and amusing man whose visits were always hilarious. Sometimes he would arrive with a stack of pans of curry which he had made for us and which were all so generous that when he had left, we had to distribute the food to our friends and even the night watchmen.

Through Ahmed Mir, we began to amass quite a lot of beautiful Persian rugs and carpets. His stories and anecdotes were always a great source of fun and we introduced him to several of our friends who enjoyed his visits as much as we did. He was straight in his dealing and he could be relied on for the quality of the carpets he sold. His 'daddy' as he said, had a carpet factory in Pakistan and he used to go there from time to time and bring back fresh stocks of real Persians together with a proportion of Pakistani wares. At that time there were regular carpet sales by auction in public buildings and hotels and Kathy and I would often go to them. They were usually on Sundays. At one of these, we saw and liked, a Persian runner that we thought might be useful for the bedroom corridor in our new house. I put in a bid and got it. The next evening along came Ahmed. "I saw you Sorr at the auction and you were bidding! You paid one hundred pounds for a runner. My God, sorr, it was jonks!"

Some four or five years after WRL(EA) was established, Alf Richardson, the driller, came to see me and asked if I would like to put some money into an enterprise which he and a friend, Kitch Morson were about to launch. It transpired that in the bamboo forest near to Kitch Morson's farm they had sunk a borehole and struck gas. The gas was carbon dioxide and the pressure was so great that the drill had been blown high into the air when it broke through into the gas. The background to this was as follows. Kitch's father had owned a coffee farm at Limuru and through the forest some six miles or so away, he had a sawmill. It was his practice to leave home in the morning and do a day's work at the mill and after 4p.m. come back home through the forest. He made the journey on horseback. Some way on his journey home he regularly stopped at a spring where bubbles of gas came up from the bottom of the pool. The gas was carbon dioxide and so, taking out his hip flask of whisky he had a tot, adding the bubbly pool water as his soda water. The old man had been dead some years when Kitch had the idea of boring at the point in the forest so well patronised by his father, to see if the gas was available in commercially viable quantities. He therefore put the idea to his friend, Alf Richardson, and they agreed upon a plan of action.

Kitch would cut a road into the forest to the spring where his father had invariably had his homeward tot. Here it was assumed that there would be gas underground and so Alf would drill at this spot. The idea simmered for some time until Alf's work was a bit slack and the pair of them started the operation. When they struck the gas, as mentioned above, the pressure was intense. They managed to put in a liner and capped the hole. They had chemical and pressure tests done and it was determined that they had tapped a very big supply of chemically pure carbon dioxide. They considered what to do and eventually decided to float a company to market the gas. Further up the Rift Valley there was a company called Carbacid, which, at that time was the sole supplier of carbon dioxide to the whole of East Africa.

Various people, including me, were approached to be founder shareholders, and a company was formed with five of us plus Kitch and Alf as founder members. Kitch and Alf held the majority of the shares and the remainder were owned by the rest of us. I was invited to be a Director. I put this proposition to my company at home and they were quite agreeable as the post would be non-executive and should not take up much of my time. Wellcome left the decision to my discretion. I was apprehensive at first, especially as I had never before sat on a company board and the whole thing was a novelty to me. However, I thought it might be interesting and certainly would be a new experience and so I accepted. It was very interesting and exciting. I was taken to the site and had a demonstration of the great power of the gas under pressure, when the cap valve was opened. The jet of gas literally screamed into the air with frightening volume. When large rocks were thrown into the jet stream they were cast aside like feathers. A factory was built near the borehole and machinery to fill gas cylinders was installed.

Meanwhile, of course, the news of our venture spread abroad and Carbacid which had, up to now, held the monopoly of the supply of carbon dioxide gas in East Africa, began to get worried. There developed a cat and mouse activity with Carbacid trying to get us, now called Kagwe, to sell out to them. We had reason to believe that the pressure of gas in the Carbacid boreholes was diminishing appreciably and their supplies might be coming to an end. It appeared that their company was having difficulties in maintaining supplies to their customers. They made a silly offer to buy us up, pointing out that whereas we had no experience of the process of extraction and methods of distribution, they, Carbacid, had a well established network of customers and a fleet of the necessary transport to maintain the business.

There followed a period of considerable activity with move and counter move. It soon became apparent that we were in the strong position and to cut a long and rather exciting story short we eventually achieved a merger on our terms and virtually took over Carbacid. We called the new company, Carbacid 61. Meanwhile we were negotiating the delivery of plant from Germany for the conversion of CO2 into solid dry ice. It is quite extraordinary, but the board began to regard me as the technical Director, because I was a scientist which none of the others were. Fortunately, we had engineers on the board and also we employed an engineering type as Managing Director. It would have been calamitous if I had been expected to advise on the engineering side. The time came for our home leave and the board asked me if I would look into commercial uses of dry ice. This I was happy to do. We were mostly interested in the application of dry ice in refrigerated transport that, of course, would be necessary if we were to make a market for our company in the vast areas of East Africa. In the UK I visited several companies that used refrigerated transport and I obtained much information that proved of value when I returned from leave. I found my investigation very interesting and rewarding. Carbacid 61 became a public company quoted on the Kenya stock exchange. We struggled for some years and we had problems with management and, not least, with the Chairman. However, the company began to show a small profit but this only became apparent at the time when I was preparing to leave Kenya. One of my colleagues on the board, Paul Wortley, an interesting, larger than life coffee farmer, was anxious to buy my shares and so I sold them to him. A few years later, I had to visit Kenya again in the course of my work in Edinburgh University. Carbacid heard about my projected visit and arranged a lunch in my honour in one of the Nairobi hotels. I was most flattered and all the more so when they presented me with a nice piece of Lalique glass as a mark of their appreciation of my help in the early days of the CO_2 project. I was gratified to hear that the company was going from strength to strength and was now paying a good dividend.

It was through my participation on the board of Carbacid 61 that I came to know Kitch Morson, and Kathy and I became friendly with Kitch and his wife, Millicent. They were both extraordinary people in their own ways. Kitch came from a family in Wales but was born in Kenya and was a very well known and highly respected businessman there. Millicent originated in South Africa. They had a large and thriving coffee estate at Limuru. They also grew very good peaches for the local market and for export to the UK. Kitch was a major shareholder in several companies in Kenya, among which was the biggest timber organisation in the country. This, no doubt, derived from his late father's timber mill on the edge of the Rift Valley. Kitch was also a keen sportsman, indulging himself in horse racing for which purpose he had a stable full of racehorses and even employed a professional jockey from England who had his own quarters on the farm. Among Kitch's other interests was deep-sea sporting fishing for which he owned a very powerful cruiser. He also owned a dhow that was kept at the coast manned by a skipper-cum-watchman who lived onboard the vessel. During our latter years in Kenya, the Morsons sold their farm in Limuru and bought a very nice house on the shore of Lake Naivasha. There they opened a furniture-making factory. The cruiser was transferred to the lake and our boys and I had the occasional thrash around the lake often much nearer to families of hippos than I thought comfortable.

Not long after we left Kenya, Kitch died very suddenly and very prematurely as he must have been only in his late sixties. Millicent was out doing some work in the garden on the lakeshore and decided to go into the house for some tea. Kitch had gone up to his bedroom for a rest after lunch, as was his wont. When the servants brought in the tea, Millicent called up the stairs to let Kitch know that it was ready. She got no reply and as Kitch's radio was going at full blast she assumed that he couldn't hear her and was probably still asleep. She went upstairs to rouse him but was shocked to find him lying on the bed, dead. While Millicent was a capable woman and took an active part in the Morson business, this came as a violent shock to her. Not only did the Morsons have interests in Kenya but they had a large piece of land in Wales, on the coast of Dyfed. It is still in the ownership of the Morsons and is a steep stretch running from the village of Marros down to the sea at the Pendine Sands. The house at the edge of the beach is a converted mill with the old millstream running past the side of the house. Millicent visits the property every few years and asks us to join her there. We have been twice and found it a charming and secluded place.

When we went to live in Kenya, my sister, Win and her husband, Laurie, had recently joined the East African Agriculture and Forestry Research Organisation which had just been established alongside the EAVRO. Laurie had been in the Indian Civil Service in the Forestry Service for about twenty-two years. After partition he and Win and their daughter Ann, left India and went to Zanzibar where Laurie was appointed to do an advisory job for the Sultan, in connection with the mangrove swamps. When that contract was completed, he was appointed to EAAFRO in charge of the forestry research. Ann, who had been working in Germany, took a job with Ethiopian Airways and was stationed in Nairobi. For a short time, she was able to find a place to sleep in our wooden house in Kabete. She had to do spells of night duty and we were a little apprehensive on those occasions when she had to go to the airport in the middle of the night, being picked up by an Airways driver and taken to the airport. Fortunately, for the short period when she had to follow this regime, all was well and nothing untoward occurred. She was later transferred to Mombasa and there she met and married John Rusby who had a rather hush hush job in security. My nephew, John, Ann's brother, had been at Bedford School and then joined the Fleet Air Arm. At this time he was flying sorties in various places having been posted as a Lt. Cdr. in aircraft carriers, flying, I believe, Gannets.

At Muguga, my sister, Win took a secretarial job in the labs. She enjoyed the work and social life, where she took an active part in the socials and entertainment associated with the two research organisations. She had the advantage of being a very accomplished pianist and so was very much in demand when musicals and pantomimes were being organised. I believe, when she was in South India, she played the Grieg Piano Concerto at a concert in Madras with the Governor's orchestra. However, Win had the misfortune to slip in the Muguga labs and broke her hip. There was no such thing in those days as modern hip replacement and she suffered badly. Laurie, who also had been suffering from ill health for some time, retired from Muguga and took Win home to be treated in one of the London Hospitals. The repair was not satisfactory and I believe she had to have a lot of sedation and drug treatment. When she was a little better, she and Laurie decided to have a holiday with Ann in Mombasa and so they flew out. I went to Embakazi Airport to see them briefly as they waited for the plane to Mombasa. When they arrived in Mombasa they were met by John Rusby who had just received the news that their son, John had been killed on a sortie in Ireland. The shock was too much for my sister and she died of heart failure a few days later on December 15th 1962. I went down to Mombasa for her funeral.

A person with whom we became very friendly in Kenya was Jani Schwartz, a Hungarian dentist who made a big impact on our lives in more ways than one. He, his wife and family were close friends of Henry Foy and Athena Kondi, whom I have already mentioned in connection with baboons. I happened to mention to Henry that I had a problem with my teeth and so we were invited to dinner with Henry and Athena to meet Jani and his wife. When I was a schoolboy I used to be irritated by small gaps between the lowers molars in my mouth. Small pieces of fibre in my food got trapped in these gaps and the gums became sore. I was in the middle of matriculation exams and the irritation became unbearable and so, one day, after morning school, I went out into the town and into the surgery of the nearest dentist. I asked him to extract two of the molars. This must sound incredible but it is true.

It happened that the dentist that I chose was a quack, it was before the law governing dentistry practice had been put on the statute book. Today, of course, a reputable dentist will do everything possible to avoid an extraction. Not so Mr Bumble or whatever his name was. He no doubt thought it odd for a schoolboy to demand the extraction of two perfectly sound healthy teeth. Nevertheless he did the extractions and pocketed the few shillings that constituted the fee and I went back into school. It was, of course, a very foolish thing to do and I have paid the price since. The lack of two molars in my mouth caused extra pressure to be exerted on my top incisors with the consequence of excessive wear on the backs of these incisors so that the teeth became very thin and, of course, very liable to be broken off. When we went on leave after transfer from Nigeria, I became very conscious of the vulnerability of my worn down incisors. So, I made a visit to a dentist in Whitby. He examined my teeth and said there was nothing to be done. I might just as well let them wear down or break off and then have them extracted and have a top denture. It was this story that I told to Henry Foy. He promptly said, "You must see Jani Schwartz. If anyone can do anything for your teeth he can." Thus I was introduced to Jani and Bruni Schwartz.

Jani was qualified as a medical doctor and had then qualified as a dentist and set up his practice in Nairobi. I made an appointment with him and that was the beginning of many hours in the dental chair in his office. He didn't believe in new fangled high speed drills but he did have a water cooled mechanical device that kept coming apart and spraying cold water down the patient's neck. He drove solid gold into the backs of my worn incisors and, over the years, into many other cavities. For the final insertion he used a sort of pile driver that was in the form of a heavy metal ring, which slid up and down on a stainless steel shaft. The assistant held the pointed end of the shaft against the gold insert while the ring was slammed down against a stop thus forcing the gold to become well and truly wedged into the drilled out cavity. My head ached for several hours after a session but Jani assured me that the inlays would probably stay in for ten years and so I was prepared to suffer. That was thirty-six years ago and the inlays in my incisors are still in place, while several other of my teeth, which received gold inlays, have in recent years had to be removed. By the time Jani had finished with me my mouth was a storehouse of gold which subsequent dentists in Britain have gazed at in amazement. The dentist I visited in Scotland gasped when he first looked in my mouth and pronounced, "Och! Gold must be cheap where you come from."

Jani and Bruni had a son who was also a dentist, a partner in his father's practice. He had qualified in Australia and had also changed his name from Schwartz to Short. He was very up to date and used high-speed drills. He was highly qualified and was the forensic dentist for the Kenya Police Department. I was one of Jani's special patients and therefore, could not be subjected to the modern methods applied by Chris Short. I spent many hours in the dentist's chair in long conversations with Jani on all subjects that happened to be of interest at the time. Jani had a little metal shelf that hung from a cord round his neck to rest on his capacious abdomen. This was used to collect the fine grains of gold that arose from the careful filing of my inlays into the correct shape to be hammered into my cavities. Jani decided that my jaw was not fixed firmly enough at the ramus which connects the two jawbones at the front. He insisted on fashioning a semi - circular prosthesis of gold. When finished, this was hooked onto the molars at each side and pressed into the backs of the lower incisors. It was a very fine artistic piece of sculpture in gold but it was extremely uncomfortable in my mouth. I persevered with wearing it for a few days and then carried it in my pocket so that if I met Jani, even in the street in Nairobi, I slipped it into my mouth as he was quite capable of peering into my mouth wherever we happened to be. He was very proud of this piece of sculpture. Some years ago I showed this prosethetic contraption to my present dentist, John Cooper, who was so amazed by it that he borrowed it to show to colleagues in the dental profession. Jani was a great friend and a very good dentist. Incidentally I never had a local anaesthetic for all the operations he performed on me except for one. This was for the destruction of the nerve in one of my lower teeth. He insisted that it was necessary for such a painful procedure. I'm sad to say that the anaesthetic didn't work.

I think that it was in 1963 that a group of ballet dancers from London came to perform a season of ballet in Nairobi. The Prima Ballerina was a beautiful Hungarian who had escaped from Hungary in the revolution and been taken on by the Royal Ballet in London. The lovely ballerina was made a welcome guest at the Schwartz home and a big party, to which we were invited, was held in the house and garden, hosted by Jani and Bruni. It was a great success with many distinguished guests. Amongst them of course, were Foy and Kondi. Henry was in his element and I saw him surrounded by a bevy of ladies explaining to them that he was a choreographer and had taught our guest of honour, whose name was Margitt Muller, all that she had learned about ballet. The outcome of the visit of the ballet for a season in Nairobi was that Chris Short and Margitt were married before the 'season' came to an end. Margitt gave me a signed photograph of her in one of her roles. I regret that this was lost, to my great distress, during one of our many moves of house since we left Kenya.

Henry was a great spoofer who could always keep a straight face and tell the most outrageous stories. One of Henry's stories concerned me. Foy and Kondi made a large number of trips abroad to international conferences and on one of these occasions, as a bit of fun, I asked Henry what time was their departure to be so that I could see them off at the airport and present them with a going away present. I explained that I had bought for them a particularly ornate brass pot containing a splendid Aspidistra. Some time later, Henry and Kondi had a visit from the eminent haematologist, Professor J.V.Dacie, who was on his way back to London after a visit to South Africa. Dacie was staying with Foy and Kondi and so the hosts organised a dinner party for the great man. Kathy and I were invited to the function to meet him. In the course of the evening I was sitting with Dr Dacie discussing various subjects and in the course of our conversation I asked him how his trip had gone and where he had stopped off *en route*. I enquired if he intended to fly directly to London when he left Kenya, which flight he would be taking and on what day. This, of course, was as a bit of polite conversation only. At this point his attitude showed a sudden change and he said that the actual flight had not yet been fixed. I was a little puzzled by his change of attitude. I mentioned this to Henry some time later and he said that he quite understood because before he introduced me to Dacie, he had told him that I was quite a nice chap but that I had a propensity for seeing people off at the airport, always presenting the travellers with a large Aspidistra in a big pot. He had told Dacie that he always gave Kondi the plants to dispose of and that she had told him that the ladies' loo at Nairobi airport was literally full of this vegetation.

Tragically, Jani and Bruni together with a grandson, produced by Margitt, were killed in a road accident on the way to Mombasa. It was a sad loss of good and stimulating friends and occurred about two or three years before we left Kenya.

In the late sixties the political situation was becoming less and less attractive. The country was now under the presidency of Jomo Kenyatta and was run by a one party government, the Kenya African National Union (KANU). New laws had been promulgated which militated against the employment of expatriates. Work permits were demanded of European employees and these were often refused and the replacement of such employees by Africans was enforced. For example, I would have to replace my secretary and bookkeeper and any European workers without professional qualifications, with African staff in a country, which had very few fully trained indigenous people. All the funds required by an organisation like mine came from London and, of course, were an asset to the country. I had kept a low profile politically, unlike some Europeans who formed relations with some government ministers and leading African politicians. So I seemed to be left in peace longer than some others were. However, this state of affairs couldn't be expected to last for long, and it didn't.

We began to get scruffy looking Kikuyus calling, armed

with literature on KANU headed paper, containing instructions such as 'Give this man a job'. Needless to say we did not employ such applicants. At that time there were many reports in the press of gangs breaking into European owned houses followed by assault on the occupants, robbery and gang raping of the woman of the house, often with the male members tied to chairs and made to watch the proceedings. There was a gang of thugs who escorted the frequent motorcades of Jomo and bashed up other road users, often damaging their cars and forcing the occupants off the road. These thugs were above the law and the regular police kept discreetly out of the way. Many expatriates were ordered out of the country with no more than forty-eight hours notice and no reason given. Should a Kikuyu have a grudge against an expatriate or a member of another tribe, he had only to lay a charge against the victim – usually an allegation that the person concerned had made a remark derogatory to the President – for that person to be ordered out of the country or to have his property confiscated. I could say much more about this deteriorating situation but the above is sufficient to indicate a change for the worse of a country that is so well endowed with attractive features. As I said above, I had kept a fairly low profile politically. In addition, Wilde and Wellcome had built up a very good friendly reputation among the local inhabitants and jobs at the WRL (EA) were much sought after.

In 1970 we left Kenya and at the time when I was getting everything straightened out for our departure, Kathy was convalescing from her hemi-colectomy. It was necessary to make sure that our financial affairs were in order as there was a limit on the amount of money that one was allowed to take out of the country. Income tax had to be dealt with which was an unpleasant process as the authorities were not at all helpful and seemed to delight in presenting obstacles. One had to reduce one's cash holding to a minimum and yet have enough to pay any dues they wished to demand at the airport without any left over otherwise the officials would be as unpleasant as possible about even an illicit 100 shilling note left in one's pocket.

Somehow or other we overcame the obstacles and flew away from Kenya at the end of March 1970, after many parties, presentations and sad 'goodbyes' from our many friends. Our sojourn in Kenya was thus a mixture of great interest, some success, many friendships, wonderful country and great appreciation of magnificent views, sunsets, mountains, beaches and brilliant blue and green seascapes. But there was also sadness; with the personal difficulties of Kathy's unhappy surgical problems, and our disappointment with the downward trend of what could be a happy and prosperous African country.

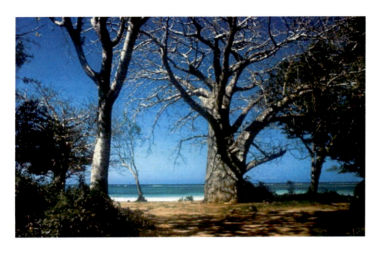

Baobab. Kenya coast

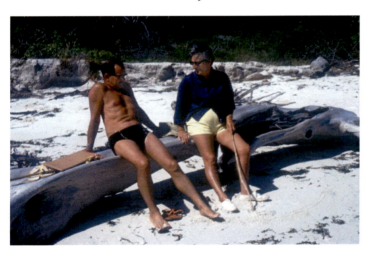

Jack and Kathy on holiday at the coast on Diani beach near
Mombasa.

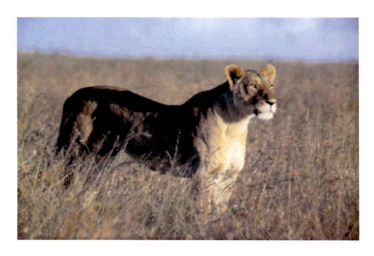

Lioness

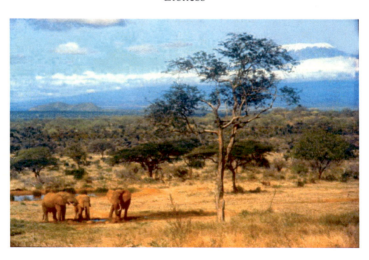

Tsavo Elephants – Kilimanjaro top right.

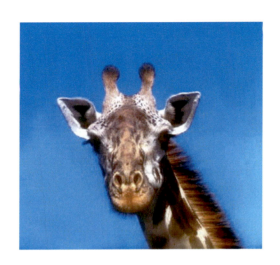

Beautiful eye lashes.

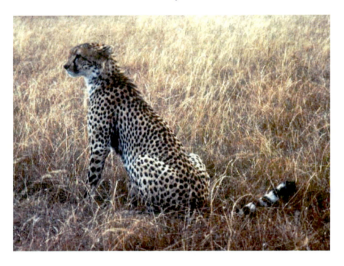

Cheetah

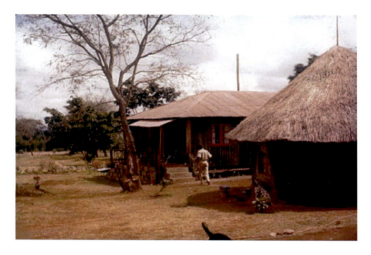

Early days in the development of Wellcome Research
Laboratories (EA)

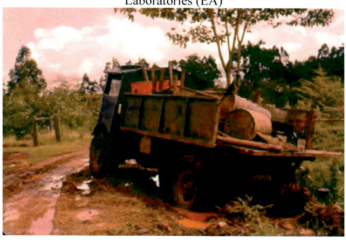

Building the wooden hut, drilling lorry in the mud, hoisting the
water tank

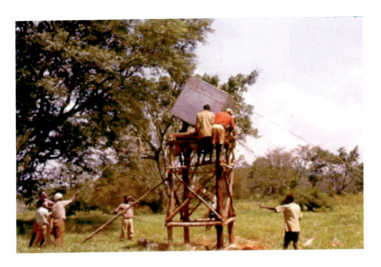

Temporary water tank

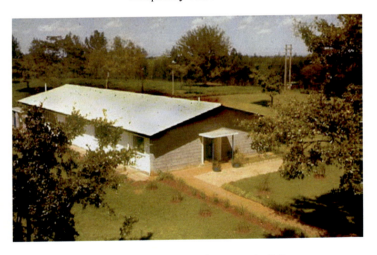

The newly built WRL laboratory building

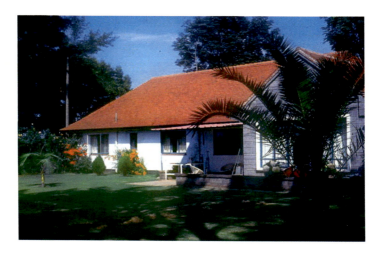

First house in Kabete ready

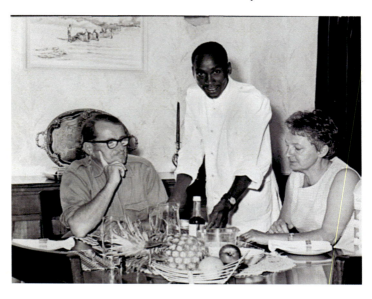

Jack and Kathy with George Gakubia

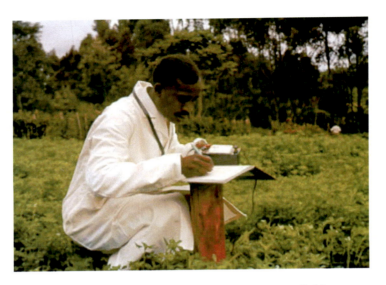

Benjamin taking soil readings in the lucerne field

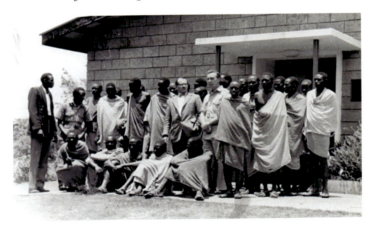

Public education – a group of Masai tribesmen visits the laboratory

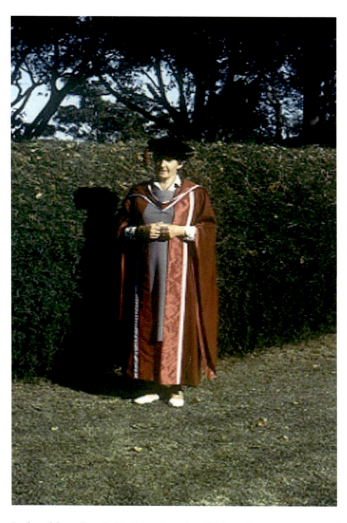

Jack achieved a ph.D. from London University as an external
student. Kathy tried out the academic robes!

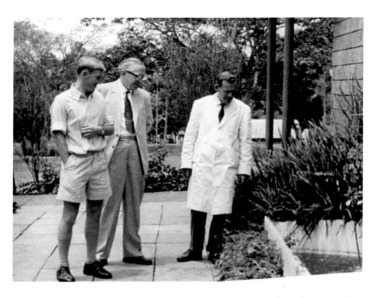

Duncan Brown (left) and Bill Macleod (right) showing round
Nick Falder, a Wellcome director.

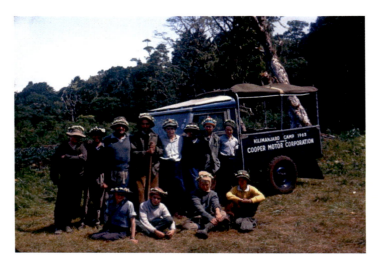

The school expedition to Kilimanjaro 1963. Group on the left shows Jack and James (third and fourth from left back row) and Peter (right front row).

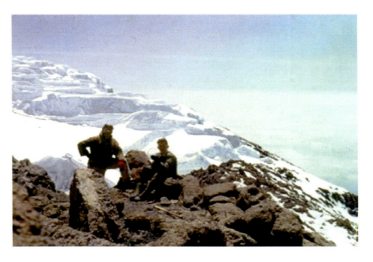

Jack with James at Gilman's Point, taken by Peter.

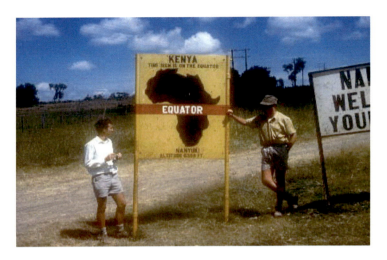

The boys on travels in Kenya. At the equator near Nanyuki.

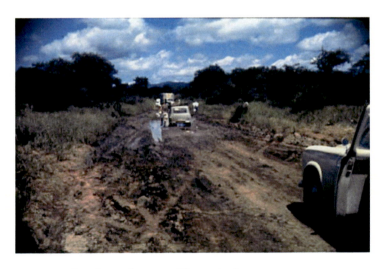

Road travels across Kenya in the wet season.

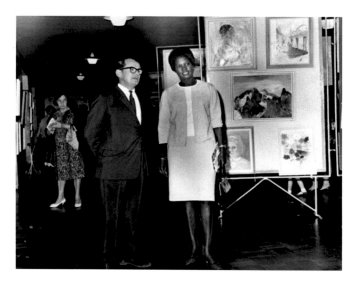

Jack with Ngina Kenyatta at a Nairobi art exhibition

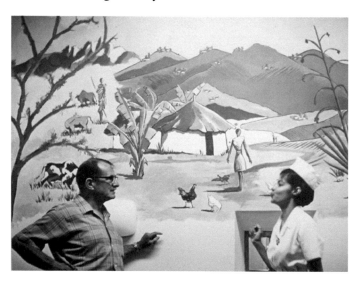

Part of the mural in the Cobalt bomb unit at Nairobi hospital.

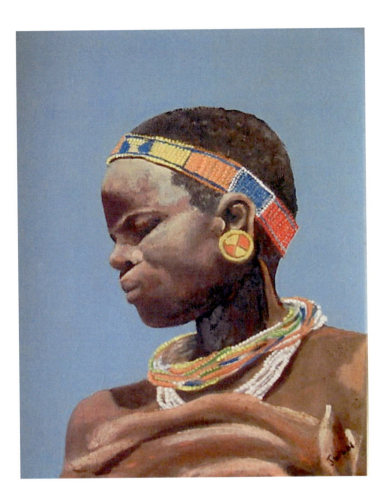

A young Gogo woman painted by Jack.

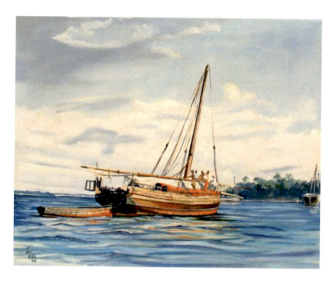

Arab dhow at anchor in Mombasa harbour by Jack

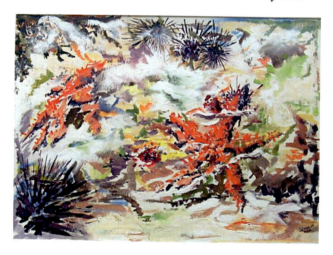

Underwater impressions of the coral reef by Jack

CHAPTER 7

Edinburgh

When we arrived in England we made straight for our house in Sleights, Whitby. Peter, who was a student in Liverpool, had come over to air the house for our arrival and so we could settle in at once. I had to go off almost immediately to Edinburgh to take up my new job. Through my old Company, I had purchased a new Triumph 2000, which was awaiting us at a garage near to the Wellcome Building in Euston Road, and so we were able to drive up to Yorkshire and then I was able to continue up to Edinburgh.

The Centre for Tropical Veterinary Medicine (CTVM) was a part of the Royal (Dick) School of Veterinary Studies, a faculty of the University of Edinburgh. It was housed in a modern, fairly new, custom-built block of laboratories and ancillary buildings attached to the Veterinary Field Station at Easter Bush, on the southern outskirts of Edinburgh. The fundamental work of the Centre was the postgraduate teaching of veterinary graduates from all parts of the world, who were involved in the treatment and control of animal disease. The department was divided into four main divisions, Protozoology, Bacteriology and Virology, Parasitology and Animal Production and Husbandry. I was appointed as Head of Protozoology and the other Heads were all people who had experience in tropical countries. The Director was Sir Alexander Robertson who had been an academic in the Royal (Dick) School for most of his professional life and paradoxically had never worked abroad. He had, of course, travelled widely and familiarised himself with all the tropical conditions and by his energy and tireless activity, brought about a strong body of support for research and teaching in the field of tropical diseases of animals. He was responsible for the establishment of a diploma in tropical veterinary medicine, the DTVM, which attracted students, from all over the world, mostly sent by their governments, to be trained for this prestigious qualification. It was through Robertson that the CTVM came into being and was funded and maintained by the Overseas Development Ministry of the Government. When the CTVM became established with its complement of tropically experienced staff, the University of Edinburgh authorised the award of the degree of MSc in Tropical Veterinary Medicine. The study course for this higher degree became a part of the teaching programme of the CTVM and we were responsible for the curriculum and examinations.

As in all science teaching institutions, the core of our work was research and in connection with this, we were able to take on students for the PhD degree of the university and a large part of my work was in providing lines of research for students who were either graduates of their own countries, or were graduates of British universities destined to work in tropical areas. During the almost ten years of my sojourn in Edinburgh, I took three foreign and two British research workers through to the successful attainment of this doctoral degree.

Having arrived in Edinburgh, I had to find somewhere to live and so all my spare time was spent in looking for a suitable house, in the right area, to make our home. It was not easy as I was a stranger to the city and its environs and so had no idea of what the various areas had to offer. I shall always be grateful to Gordon Scott, who had spent some time in Africa and who was the Head of Bacteriology in the CTVM. He gave me a large plan of Edinburgh and offered advice as to suitable neighbourhoods and I began to learn my way around the lovely city of Edinburgh and its surrounding countryside. One of our very good friends in Nairobi, Moira Dall, gave us an introduction to a solicitor (solicitors in Scotland are entitled Writers to the Signet) Douglas Graham. He welcomed us to his practice and became a very valued advisor and friend. In Scotland, in those days, house buying and selling was almost entirely in the hands of the lawyers and Douglas made it his duty to see that we got a fair deal in the business of buying a house. Estate Agents were few and far between and the purchase of a house was usually by means of the submission of a sealed tender which was handed in to the vendors' solicitor to be opened at a specified time and day in his office. He usually recommended the vendor to accept the highest bid at which price the purchaser was legally bound to seal the purchase and pay the sum, which he had offered on a day, laid down by the solicitor. This cut out all the hassle we have in England about exchanging contracts and withdrawing offers before the contracts have been exchanged or gazumping. In Scotland, if one makes a written tender for a house and this is accepted by the vendor, the sum agreed has to be paid by the due date and the deal is completed quickly and expeditiously.

The big snag about this method of house buying is that the choice of price to be offered demands a great deal of soul searching and, as it were, astute gambling. A purchase can be lost for a matter of a few pounds and in that case the search has to be taken up again. This can mean another survey with its costs and the chance that the sale might be lost again. It is quite exciting and in some cases it works in favour of the vendor, as the prospective purchaser, if he or she is very keen to get the property, will think of a number and then put on something extra.

For my first month or so in Edinburgh I had to drive back to Sleights for the weekends and then return on Monday, starting at about 5a.m. so that I arrived in time to present my first lecture at 9a.m. The journey was a rather tortuous one hundred and fifty miles in each direction. The weather in late winter and early spring was pretty awful and much of the journey was done in the dark and often in fog and snow. Of course, we were also involved in selling our bungalow in Sleights, which was an added complication.

After one of my weekend visits to Sleights I took Kathy back with me to Edinburgh and she stayed with me in digs that I had found near to Craigmillar in Edinburgh. We visited several prospective houses on the market but we had to return to Yorkshire without having found a suitable property. I was once more reduced to searching on my own. I saw a bungalow in Bonnyrigg, a suburb of Edinburgh near to Dalkeith, but after a look at it from the outside I moved on. However, I had second thoughts and went back and knocked on the door. The owner was a widow named Ella Hunter. She was a pleasant, white-haired woman, I suppose nearer seventy than eighty and she showed me round. The bungalow was of a very high quality as it had been built by a builder for himself and had been purchased by Mrs Hunter when the owner died. The front door was glazed with plate glass and opened through a porch into a hall completely panelled in oak. Above the panelling the coving was decorated with Scottish thistles in moulded plaster. The high quality was carried throughout the building and the master bedroom was large and panelled with large windows and capacious cupboards. There was quite a large garden almost surrounding the whole house and a reasonably sized utility room integral with the house but opening to the outside that housed the boiler for the central heating. The situation was on a corner, the front facing the main road and the side being on a lane bordering a golf course. Opposite the house, across the road, was a large field with a view across pleasant countryside to the distant Pathhead area. In Scotland, golf courses are sacrosanct and so I felt that the house was well protected on its north side. The field to the east was another matter and might well be open for development, but it is almost impossible to be secure against development unless streets and houses already surround your property. The price asked was, I thought, a bit high for the neighbourhood but the house was of a quality somewhat higher than most of the houses in the area. I rang Kathy and told her about my find. She agreed that it seemed to be satisfactory and left the decision to my discretion. I discussed the proposition with my solicitor friend. He suggested that I should take another look at the house and mentioned some things to be checked. The next day was a Friday and Bonnyrigg was on my way from the lab to the road for Yorkshire and so, after leaving the Centre, I stopped at the house and took another look. I discussed certain items with Mrs Hunter and decided that we should buy. I rang Douglas from the property and told him of my decision. He suggested that I should turn it over in my mind and if I had any doubts by the time I got to Jedburgh, I should ring him at his home number, otherwise he would commence negotiations and preparation of the necessary paperwork. I didn't change my mind and so that weekend we were committed to the purchase of Oakdene, Eskbank, Midlothian.

We didn't like the name and so we changed it to Suswa. This is the name of a mountain in the Rift Valley of Kenya and we felt that we would like an African name. We thought long and hard about African names and most of them would undoubtedly be mispronounced. Suswa we felt couldn't be mispronounced but we were wrong. It is amazing how such a simple foreign name can be complicated by British phonetics. Anyway, the die was cast and we moved into Suswa in the late spring and with not too long a delay, we sold our bungalow in Sleights, also called Suswa, in spite of our Whitby solicitor's insistence on calling it Soozwer.

We became very good friends with Mrs Hunter and before she left for her new home in Gloucestershire, she insisted on giving us several pieces of furniture and letting us have some more at knock down prices. One very large mirror has gone with us from house to house since and I still tap daily, the aneroid barometer, which came from her. The journey to my work through Lasswade and Loanhead was not onerous and we found shopping in Bonnyrigg and Dalkieth reasonably easy and, I think on the whole, somewhat cheaper than in the more up-market districts. At that time, academic salaries were poor in comparison with commercial and private practice incomes, but I was fortunate in that although my salary was lower than the one I had received from Wellcome, I now also received a pension from Wellcome and one from my Colonial Service. In addition, I was in the position of not having a mortgage, which was a drain on the income of my professional colleagues.

I soon settled into the work at the CTVM and became integrated into University life. Sir Alexander was not an easy man to deal with and most of my colleagues were rather frightened of him. I was not and could be frank with him and even argue with him, I never did this when anyone else was present but only when I bearded him in his den. I think that he was a little conscious of his lack of experience in the tropical field in which his subordinates were expert. He was, however, powerful and ruthless and could easily have destroyed anyone who crossed him. As head of a section in his Centre, I had to submit all papers for publication by members of my section to him before I could send them to the appropriate journal. I remember sending down to him a draft paper by Tony Luckins on a subject in the trypanosomiasis field. It was a very good paper and described some successful technical work. I always vetted these papers myself and made suggestions to the authors before I sent them for Alec's approval. The Director rang me and asked if I would go down to discuss Tony's paper. I went down and he started to pull it to pieces with quite undeserved criticisms. I said that this was a good piece of work and that far from criticising it he should be pleased that one of his young research workers was doing such advanced research and that far from being derogatory he should be sending an encouraging comment up to Luckins. He responded that he was only being devil's advocate and grudgingly accepted the paper. I then took him to task and said that he never gave praise to junior workers when a kind word from him could do much to encourage them. I said, "You know, Alec, I shall go and tell Luckins that you are pleased with his paper. I have to be a buffer between you and my staff."

He laughed and said, "You know, Jack, you're too kind. You should be more of a bastard like me and you might go far."

When I first arrived at the CTVM the new building had not been officially opened and we heard that the ceremony was to be performed by the Duke of Edinburgh and a date was announced. In the entrance hall there was, facing the main door, a large plain wall about six metres wide by about three metres high. Sir Alec thought it called for some sort of covering or decoration. After turning things over in his mind he came to me, knowing that I was something of an artist, and asked me if I could paint a mural on the space provided. I said that I could and I drew a cartoon design. Alec, who, I suspect was not very interested in art, thought it would be all right and so I decided on the use of acrylic pigments. I spent the evenings and weekends for two or three weeks working on the wall. The theme that I adopted was meant to show the connection between the research being done at the CTVM and the people, animals and diseases in the tropical field. It incorporated scenes from Africa with cattle and people down to the representation of viruses and bacteria in the lab with vignettes of workers in the lab. The mural was finished in good time for the official opening. When the Duke entered the building he didn't even glance at the mural as he was ushered into the lower corridor having to talk with some of us in the common room before he departed.

The protozoology section was mainly occupied with work on trypanosomiasis. I was keen to introduce work on East Coast fever and the other theilerial diseases but it had been firmly fixed in the minds of the university that these exotic parasites could not be brought into the British Isles. I discussed this with Alec Robertson and he felt that it would not be possible but if I were prepared to do all that was necessary, he would not stand in the way. I therefore commenced a long and testing process of trying to get authority to bring this little known exotic disease into the United Kingdom. I started on the Ministry of Agriculture and had many meetings with senior members of the Ministry Veterinary Service. I was amazed how little was known about the theilerial diseases in Britain and among British vets. I suppose it was only to be expected as most British veterinarians, if they had heard about East Coast fever at all, it would have been during their frantic last minute swatting before their final exams. Anything about it that they knew then would have been forgotten almost immediately after they had qualified. It was, therefore, my job to explain all the details about the epidemiology of the disease caused by the parasite *Theileria parva*. I explained how it was virtually impossible to transmit the disease from an infected animal to a susceptible animal except by means of a very small group of ticks, none of which were to be found in Britain. I went to great lengths to describe experiments in which masses of the parasites in the blood and spleens of infected cattle had been injected into susceptible animals by all possible methods without the slightest signs of the disease or the parasites in the recipient animals. Having convinced one senior Veterinary Inspector of this fact, it was then necessary to go over the whole argument with another. It took me several months to convince the Ministry of Agriculture.

I then had to start the whole process again on the medical profession and had long discussions with Medical Officers of

Health. They were even harder to convince. I had given them a long and detailed story of the history of East Coast fever, its epidemiology, its pathology, immunology, haematology and the tremendous effort that had been put into it's research, going back to the turn of the twentieth century. When I further convinced them that the disease was not transmissible to man, I finally won them over. Following this I had to consider the organisation of a suitable place in which we could experiment with the parasite and ensure that there was no possible chance of escape into the environment. I still had to deal with the engineering department of the Edinburgh City Council and the sanitary authorities and the final obstacle was the University itself. This was a hard nut to crack but I succeeded. I then had to find a place on University property, which could be adapted for our purpose. Finally I had to find the funds for the building modifications that would be necessary.

It took me three years to reach the point when we could start work on East Coast fever in Edinburgh. The building adapted for the work was an old property of the University, which had lapsed into disuse. It opened into a yard off the Cowgate, an area which was one of the haunts of the many 'winos' of the back streets of Edinburgh. In the work we now concentrated much of our effort on the problem of growing the parasite in tissue culture. I was pleased to be joined in the work by an old friend and colleague, Duncan Brown, who had done a large mass of research in the forefront of the East Coast fever work in a team led by Mat Cunningham at EAVRO in Muguga. This had led to a number of important publications from which arose great advances in our knowledge of the *Theileridae* and especially of East Coat fever. Duncan was able to continue this line of work in our Protozoology section and in collaboration with other workers, including some in the Wellcome laboratories at Beckenham, made it possible not only to treat the disease but also to immunise against it.

When I first arrived to head the Protozoology section at the CTVM, the section had been under the supervision of Dr Eric Wells whose responsibility it was to hand over to me. He had been doing this work for some time and was a very competent scientist. He naturally was somewhat resentful but he did not let this prevent him from helping me to settle into the job, for which I was very grateful to him and we became, and still are, on very friendly terms. Eric, however, was not on the best of terms with Sir Alec. He had expressed opinions of the way Alec organised affairs and had told him to his face that he was devious. His chances of promotion while Sir Alec was Director were not rosy and so when a job in one of the international organisations was offered, Eric took it. Soon after I joined the CTVM, Ross Gray was appointed to the Centre in my section. His was a very well known name in the field of trypanosomiasis and he had contributed very significantly in this field. He left the CTVM when he was appointed to be Director of ILRAD in Nairobi. Alec was a powerful man but I think he was always looking over his shoulder to see that no one was doing anything that might prejudice his authority and possibly have eyes on the Directorship. I was fortunate, however, in this climate as I was too old to be a candidate for the post when it became vacant. Indeed, Alec and I retired on the same day.

Much of my time was taken up with the supervision of students who were working for their PhD's. Most of our postgraduate students were from developing countries in the tropics, where the first language was not English. Occasionally we had a candidate who came to us with a scientific problem on which he wanted to work. This was a rare circumstance as most of them who were sponsored by their governments and were usually funded by the Overseas Department of our government just turned up and requested a subject on which they could apply for registration for a PhD of the University of Edinburgh. Depending on the country of their origin and the diseases of livestock from which it suffered, my duty, if they came to me, was to try to think up an appropriate field in which there was some work required and suggest that the applicant go to the library and look up some of the references on the subject. On some happy occasions the applicant may have come to me as he had heard that I was a nice man and very helpful, saying that he would like to work on some disease, which was not caused by protozoal parasites but was perhaps, a viral disease. Then I could say, with a sweet smile on my face, that this was a matter for Dr Scott's section and direct him to Gordon Scott's office.

In Bonnyrigg we were happily settled in our bungalow and did quite a lot of work, improving the amenities, redecorating and making modifications to the arrangements of bedrooms, dining and sitting rooms. I decided to hire an electric sander and improve the floor of the family room, which was at the front east corner of the building. I successfully sanded the floor, which was of parquet blocks, and sealed it with polyurethane. The instructions, on which I was basing my work, suggested that a first coat should be sanded lightly before the next two coats were applied. I assumed, wrongly, that this should be done very lightly using the machine and a very fine paper. I had just finished this part of the operation when a telephone message came from James to inform us that he was at Waverley Station and would like me to collect him and bring him home. This sort of thing often did happen with James, who was in the RAF and from time to time got a forty-eight hour leave and made for home as rapidly as possible. I left the scene of my activities, had a wash and got the car out of the garage. Darkness was now falling and before setting off for the station I went to take a look at the floor in the room where I was working. As I opened the door I was met by a blast of smoke caused by a smouldering dust bag on the sanding machine. I pulled the bag off the machine and stamped out the fire and made my way through the dense smoke to open the window. As I opened it, I was startled by the appearance of a policeman's face under the familiar police hat with its chequered band and the dour utterance, "D'ye know you're afire?" I explained that I had just discovered this for myself but not to worry as I had everything under control. What had happened was that spontaneous combustion had occurred in the polyurethane dust and that the bag of sawdust was not far from bursting into flames. Apart from a ruined bag on the sander and a scorched patch on the wood blocks of the floor, no harm had been done. This was a salutary lesson for me about the danger of compacted dust in a confined space. Since then I have always been careful to avoid leaving material such as sawdust or oily rags in a compacted or compressed state. The company who had hired out the sander was very understanding and didn't charge me for the ruined bag. It was very lucky that I had taken a look in the room before leaving for the station, otherwise I might have returned to a big conflagration.

I had bought a second hand Triumph "Spitfire" for Kathy's use for shopping or visiting when I was away at work. Peter was, at this time, at Oxford doing his medical course. He had purchased an old Morris 'Traveller' for his own mobility and he would come home for spells during vacations. On one of his visits he felt that his old banger was not satisfactory for such long journeys and so could he take his Mum's 'Spitfire' which he thought to be a much more appropriate vehicle for a student in his position. His mother agreed, as she didn't like the idea of his travelling from Scotland to Oxford in his old vehicle. We sold the Morris to a local mechanic who said he could put it into good order. If I remember correctly, he paid £50 for it and tacitly, the 'Spitfire' became Peter's although no one mentioned the transaction. The next time we saw the 'Spitfire' was when Peter brought his girlfriend Helen up to Bonnyrigg. Peter told us on the phone that they would be arriving well after midnight and that we should not wait up but leave the back door unlocked and we would see them at breakfast.

We met our future daughter-in-law at breakfast for the first time. Peter had let his hair grow long, as was the new idea at that time. Kathy and I had not been back in England for very long and the short miniskirt, long hair and cohabitation without marriage had come as a bit of a shock to us and I was critical of Peter's hair style and said so. At that, Helen just about jumped on me and said she could find nothing wrong with Peter's hairstyle, which suited her. Her brothers all had long hair and so I had no right to criticise. I was taken aback by what I regarded as a breach of the etiquette that should be observed between guest and host but I said nothing. It didn't help to enamour Peter's girlfriend with his parents. There was some coldness in our relationship for several years, but eventually Peter and Helen married and things became smoother between us.

One day, Kathy rang me at the lab to say that men with clipboards and dumpy levels were active in the field opposite our house. This was ominous; I don't like men with clipboards as they generally augur trouble. I made enquiries and learned that planning had been approved for the development of the field into a housing estate. We promptly set about looking for a new dwelling place. We had become customers of an outfitter who had a shop in Dalkieth and another in Bonnyrigg. He heard that we intended to leave and came to see us. This was most fortunate as not only was he interested in having a home half way between his two places of business but also he was delighted with the idea of there being a large estate with lots of prospective customers in his area. So a sale was agreed and while we had to bring our figure down a little we could start our search for something more to our liking with some confidence.

We looked at several properties in and around Edinburgh and saw nothing that attracted us. Winter came on and one day we saw a house advertised in a village called Broughton, lying between Peebles and Biggar. In my earlier searches I had been interested in a house in this same village, but on going to see it for a second time, the heavens opened and the road was flooded and so I gave up the idea. I was, perhaps, being a little illogical in this decision as the flood was a flash affair and was most unusual. We made an appointment to take a look at the house now on offer and started on our way. It was well after dark as I could only get home at about 5.30p.m. Furthermore, it had started to snow. Bill Macleod and Ivy had joined us as I had recommended Bill for a job as Chief Technician in the CTVM. They were living temporarily in a rented cottage that was in a village on our way to Broughton and they had said that they would like to go with us to see the house in Broughton and so I arranged to take them with us. It happened that my car began to play up on the way and so when we limped into the Macleods, Bill said we should go in their car and this we did. The snow became quite heavy *en route* and when we at last arrived in Broughton we had to find the house under difficult conditions, but find it we did. We drove up a steep drive to an area in front of the house and could see a faint light indicating the front door.

We staggered up the steps and applied the knocker. A grey haired, elderly man opened the door and we were ushered into the hall. There we made the acquaintance of Tom and Margaret Gibson, who had come to show us the house, which had obviously been unoccupied for some time. They were standing in the hall over one bar of an electric fire. It was a large house and as we were shown around, I was appalled by its size and its frigid coldness. I was all for getting out as soon as possible and returning to the warmth and comfort of our home. However, we completed the tour and had a verbal description of the outbuildings and attached land. Apparently the house had belonged to Margaret's mother and had not been occupied since her death some months before. Consequently, it had been neglected and needed a lot to be done to it. We made our farewells to Tom and Margaret and clambered into Bill's cold car. Before he had started the engine, Kathy said, "That's it. That's the place for us." I was dumbfounded, as were Ivy and Bill. At first we thought Kathy was joking but she assured us she was not and she listed what were to her overpowering factors in favour of our buying the place. The price for such a big property – it had six bedrooms – was cheap, the price of £12,000 reflecting the amount of refurbishment that would have to be done.

We rang Tom up and made an appointment to have a look at the house in daylight at the weekend. It was then that we really saw Drumsheugh in all its magnificence. It was an imposing Victorian mansion (to us) built in 1890. It stood in three acres including a paddock with stables and coach house, tack room and garage. There was a large kitchen, a small kitchen, scullery, washhouse and coalhouse. The sitting room, dining room and a third reception room were spacious and high ceilinged with ornamental coving and big panelled doors. The stairwell went up through the first floor to a glazed sort of cupola to give light to the centre of the house. There were six bedrooms and the master bedroom was large, airy and light with an attached dressing room. We were very much impressed by the fact that the name of the house, 'Drumsheugh' appeared on the ordnance survey map.

We bought the house and I searched around in what literature I could find, in an endeavour to discover the meaning or origin of the name, 'Drumsheuch'. The nearest that I could get to a meaning from a very limited access to local Lalance dialect was 'the ridge by the marsh'. This might well be quite the wrong interpretation but I stick to it until a better might turn up. Whatever the name means we had to get down to the work of modernising and renovating our new home. I was a little worried by the roof, which appeared to be made of a mat of black moss or lichen. We called in a roofing contractor from Biggar. He had just acquired a modern apparatus for steaming various parts of buildings which he had not yet used but decided that our house would provide him with the knowledge of how to use the apparatus and gain the skill, which was obviously necessary to operate this invention. Accordingly a mass of boilers, pipes, jets and electrical connections arrived in the front garden. I watched with some apprehension as the various parts were shuffled about until what seemed like the correct arrangement was achieved. Then male and female joints in the pipe work were assembled and disassembled until parts, which fitted, became apparent. A pipe from our water main had to be run out of the house and act as a water supply for the steam boiler. When steam and hot water jetted out of what was thought to be the right places, ladders were erected up to the roof and our expert roofer clambered gingerly up with a heavy pipe fitted with a jet tap. Things were pretty violent at first and I had visions of holes being blown in the roof but our fireman-cum-roof operative soon got the hang of things and, quite miraculously, slates began to appear as the thick coat of moss etc began to peel off. The roof proved to be in excellent shape and was of very sound Welsh slates. When it was completed, our heroic roofer was all for using the jet to clean up the quoins which were made of sandstone. This stone was very rapidly worn away into gullies and holes by the powerful jets and so I put a stop to experimentation in that direction.

We got a local plumber in to look at the water tanks and piping. In this department it became obvious that a lot had to be done. In the roof were two large, lead tanks, encased in heavy wooden panelling. Our plumber told us that they should be replaced by one large modern tank. The original tanks had obviously been installed before the roof had been completed and so we had to have them dismantled and removed piecemeal before a new one of a size that could be inserted through the available openings was installed. I was lucky enough to be put in touch with some members of the University maintenance staff who were prepared to work for us at weekends, in the evenings and during the summer, on the electricity, wiring and many joinery jobs. This was slower but cheaper and the chaps were experts and pleasant to have about the house. A senior technician in our animal houses at the CTVM, who was an excellent paperhanger, offered his services, and he and I started on the redecoration of the house. My helper was Jimmy Lowe. Unfortunately he was suffering some degree of painful lameness in his legs. This became worse until he had to give up his job at the CTVM and could no longer do the decoration work. Sadly he became bedridden and tragically died of what I later learned was cancer of the spine. He was a great loss and we missed his Scottish wit and fun and his ability to do the right thing. He was helping us for long enough for me to learn a lot of the tricks of the decorating trade and after he left, I went on to hang about 120 rolls of paper. I well remember the longest piece that I ever hung. It came down from the cupola in the roof and had to be cut into the balustrade of the upstairs landing and finished up at the foot of the stairs. It was eighteen feet long and, a very unusual thing, it went on in one go, exactly right. I was very proud of that.

We were, of course, involved in this work for several months but when we had finished, it had all been worthwhile. The result was that we had a beautiful house in a most delightful position with magnificent views all around us. Kathy's choice had proved to be the right one. True, even with our doing a lot of the work with the help of our specialist friends, we had to lay out something in excess of £20,000 pounds. This doesn't sound much in these days of so many multimillionaires but it was a lot in our position in those days.

A minor drawback to living in Broughton was that it was twenty-five miles from my work in the laboratories of the CTVM. I had to leave early in the morning to drive to Easter Bush and often I was quite late getting back home, especially on those occasions when I had to attend faculty meetings in the main part of the Royal (Dick) College in Edinburgh. It meant that Kathy had a long period each day on her own with no one to whom she could talk. We employed a woman out of the village to come to the house once or twice a week to help with the domestic work. She was Jean Carruthers, who became a good friend and was an amusing person. Her husband, Rob, was also a larger than life character who didn't seem to hold down any job for long and made a precarious living which was augmented by playing the double base in Jimmy Shand's well known band. It was said that Rob was the only person known to be able to continue on his feet playing his cumbersome instrument after having imbibed quite a lot of the hard stuff and even when he was asleep on the stage. His brother, George owned the garage in the village and was a very helpful man in this capacity. He was quite a clever engineer and could make parts when they were not readily available. He even invented and built a four-wheel vehicle, which could be driven off the road and up the steep hills of the farmland and over the roughest of tracks. I thought he should have been able to make a profitable business with this invention but he didn't manage to promote it. There must have been an inventive gene in the Carruthers family because there was another brother who lived in Biggar who was a lecturer in metallurgy in a college of higher education. He could fashion almost anything in iron and made a very nice fire poker for us and we have it still.

I was shunted into the job of being chairman of the local branch of the Conservative Party at the time when Ted Heath took us into Europe. I met him at that time and thought he was quite a genuine man but I have since changed my mind and realise that most politicians are activated by the need for self-aggrandisement. I was in office long enough to be involved in a general election in which we didn't have a chance as the majority of the electorate in our area was strongly liberal in persuasion and the sitting member was David Steele, whose father, incidentally, had been the Minister of the Presbyterian Church in Nairobi. He was the immediate predecessor of our friend, Robin Keltie.

We enjoyed our time in Broughton and made quite a lot of friends and had several of our old friends visiting us from time to time. I was persuaded into running an art class for the local authority, which was held in the school building once a week for the benefit of any village people who wished to join. There were usually about twenty present at the sessions. It was quite a success and we had a lot of fun, which the old ladies and gents of the village joined in with gusto. I ran this for two years and at the end of each summer we held an exhibition of the work of my pupils. They were thrilled with the success of these exhibitions especially as some of them actually sold pictures. The village policeman was particularly prolific and almost went into business as an artist. Kathy also played the piano for the keep fit class in the school and was quite chuffed to receive a minute stipend from the County Council.

Tom and Margaret Gibson, who had been instrumental in selling Drumseuch to us, were good friends and our weekly shopping visits to Biggar were invariably prolonged by a sojourn at their farm, Heavyside, to buy eggs. We were expected to spend at least an hour in the kitchen on Saturday mornings with Tom, Margaret and the family. Margaret was a wonderful provider and there was usually a great pan of vegetable soup bubbling away on the Esse stove while we chatted and exchanged views and news, some of which were often hilarious. Margaret made her own brew of sherry and didn't bother with such niceties as sterilisation of utensils and bottles. The finished article was always excellent and we were usually presented with a bottle. Margaret showed me how to make the brew and I was fairly successful but never achieved the excellence of her product.

We had to do something to keep the grass down in our paddock and so I bought a few sheep from Tom and he delivered them for us. In the late summer he came over again to shear the sheep. In the autumn he took them to his farm and brought them back in the spring after they had lambed. This made the keeping of a few sheep a very easy matter for me. Tom sold the lambs and fleeces and he kept the proceeds.

Some friends, Sheila and Andrew Innes and Sheila's mother, Dorothy McKechney, lived in an imposing house, Easter Calzeat (Pronounced Kalate) in the village. I knew Dorothy quite well as, for several years, I gave her a lift in the morning into Edinburgh where she worked as secretary to the Commandant of the Castle. Her late husband had been a senior officer in the army. The Inneses decided to mount a fete in their grounds and field for a charity and I was asked to help with the various arrangements. It was through their army connections that we managed to get the Red Devils Sky Diving team to do a drop into the fete, to land on a marked spot in the field. The whole thing was an outstanding success. The day was glorious and the sky was clear and blue so that the drop was perfect and a substantial sum was raised. The village people had an exciting and enjoyable day. Another pair of friends, the Gairns', lived in a house at the east end of the village. Jack Gairns was a solicitor practising in Biggar. He was a member of an old established family of solicitors and he and his wife, Bobbie, were well respected as being one of the old established local families. Near to the Gairns' but on the main road was the house of the Shearers. Tom was a horticulturist and every year in the spring, he made an entirely new layout of the garden with magnificent designs of lawn and brilliant bedding plants. The centrepiece was always spectacular, perhaps a large clock or coat of arms. I think the last one before we left featured the insignia of the Scottish National Party. Tom and Anne were strongly Scottish in political leanings. The road through the village was the A701, a main route from Edinburgh to Moffat, Carlisle and the south. In the season we had a lot of tourist traffic on this road and the Shearers was a point at which they all stopped in order to view the garden that was open and had a collecting box for charity. One day, when I was at work, Kathy saw that our sheep had come through the hedge, which separated the paddock from our front garden, and she was afraid that they would come through the garden and down the drive onto the road. She was wearing an overall and slipped her feet into a pair of wellies and taking a stick she ran down the garden and started to wave the stick and her arms to drive the sheep back into the paddock. At that moment one of the tourist coaches came on the scene and the driver pulled up and a mass of tourist heads turned to stare at this Scottish peasant driving her sheep into the field.

We had a rather smart pub in Broughton, called The Greenmantle, a name taken from the books of John Buchan who was a native of the next village along the main road to the south, Tweedsmuir, and from which place he adopted the name when he was elevated to the peerage as the First Baron Tweedsmuir. Local organisations held their annual celebrations in The Greenmantle. One of these clubs was that of the Broughton Curlers. Tom Gibson was the Chairman of this club for many of

259

the years when we were residents in the village. One Saturday in March when we made our weekly call on the Gibsons, Tom asked us what we would be doing on an evening a week or so ahead. We rather ingenuously said we were not doing anything particular on that evening. "Right," said Tom. "You must both come as my guests at the annual dinner of the curling club." We had no option but to accept this prestigious invitation. As foreigners and Sassanachs we were highly honoured but actually felt a little apprehensive. Scottish celebratory dinners were notoriously rather lavish in the flow of Scotland's prime export. Kathy and I, while being in no way teetotallers, have never been heavy drinkers and certainly were not imbibers of large quantities of the hard stuff. However, the evening arrived and Tom invited us to start the proceedings by having a drink at the house of our friends, Jack and Bobbie Gairns. It seemed rather strange that Tom should invite us to drinks at someone else's house. When we got there we found that some others had also been so invited. We expressed our apologies and our embarrassment to our friends *sotto voce*. They told us not to worry, it was just one of Tom's little idiosyncrasies. After the assembled group had imbibed liberally, we all repaired to the Greenmantle. When we got there, the pub seemed to have been taken over by a large crowd of merry young men who had already got into the spirit, in more ways than one, of the occasion. I was cordially invited to contribute to the 'Kitty' from which purchases could be made from the bar without having to dish out cash each time. As Kathy and I consumed two G&T's and a lemonade from the bar it was an expensive way of getting our drinks. The young man doing the collecting seemed somewhat taken aback by my liberal contribution. I suppose that he expected us to be making considerable inroads into the kitty. We managed to spin out our modest drinks until dinner was announced. We were to sit at the President's Table with Tom. There were about ten people at our table with Kathy next to Tom at one end and me at the other with Billy Marshall, our GP in Biggar. When the wine waiter came round, someone at Tom's end bought a bottle and Billy suggested that he and I should share the cost of a bottle for the people at our end. This we did. After the meal the fun and games began and it was obvious that the first thing was to use up the bar kitty and then collect for another session. Vigorous games of a violent nature were introduced with whoops and och ayes, interspersed with bouts of reels and other Scottish dances, performed with more enthusiasm than grace. The atmosphere was redolent with the fumes which had their origins in the stills of the Highlands. At midnight, Kathy and I thought it was time we now departed and left the more riotous part of the celebrations to the somewhat inebriated young but hefty curlers. We extricated Tom from an enthusiastic crowd of his sycophants and said we had better depart as Kathy was now rather tired. Tom was feeling no pain at this stage. "Well have ye enjoyed yoursels?"

"Yes, thank you very much" we dutifully replied.

"Good," said Tom. " Then that'll cost ye..." and he mentioned the cost of the dinner. I forget what it was but I had to go to the innkeeper to cash a cheque so that I could pay. We were rather taken aback but we had many a laugh about it subsequently with our friends who were well aware of Tom's tightfistedness with money.

During my tenure of office in the CTVM I was called upon to make eight visits abroad in the interests of furthering our work on protozoal diseases of livestock. These diseases were all arthropod borne and covered trypanosomiasis and the tickborne theilerial infections. In 1971 I visited Nigeria to consult with the staff of my old laboratory at Vom and paid a repeat visit in 1974, when I was accompanied by my colleague Gordon Scott. It was interesting to see how many of my old Nigerian staff had fared with their added responsibilities. I was particularly surprised to find my old Yoraba colleague, Jidi Shonekan, who had shown considerable aptitude as a very competent technician in my day, had left the service of the Vom Laboratory to take up the position of head of a small zoo and museum in Jos. It seemed to me to be a waste of valuable qualifications and experience of a senior Nigerian who would almost certainly have been able to offer considerable wisdom to the working of the laboratory which had established itself as the best known centre of veterinary research in West Africa.

The situation in Vom had been very adversely influenced by the bitter war which had erupted between the north and south of Nigeria. Fierce terrorist activities had occurred in Vom where there was great resentment of the southerners who held most of the more senior posts, in all the services, by the northerners in whose country the area was geographically situated. At that time, there was only one of the expatriate officers who were there in my time, who was head of the laboratory. This was Keith Nixon, who remained at the request of the Nigerians to act as a guide and adviser to the African officers who were now nominally in charge. Keith Nixon and his wife, Jean played a dangerous and brave part in protecting Nigerians who were targeted by the northern gangs. Keith put himself in very precarious positions to defend the senior southern Nigerians from torture and murder and to keep the work of the laboratory going for the benefit of the pastoral tribes of the country. Keith Nixon eventually left Nigeria and took up residence with Jean and his two daughters in Guernsey where he played an active part in the community of that island. Sadly, he died of cancer in 1999, a great loss to all his friends and associates among whom Kathy and I very much count ourselves.

On my last visit to Nigeria, I had to go to Lagos for a few days to discuss certain aspects of the country's veterinary problems and was appalled to see the state of the capital city. Crime and violence were rife and I was pleased to leave Nigeria with no desire to return. Incidentally, I contracted a bad cold during my last few days in Lagos and when we took to the air to return to the UK, for the first time in my life I felt acute pain in my inner ears. After arriving back in Scotland I experienced symptoms in my ears that I soon discovered were due to tinnitus. For some months I suffered symptoms resembling Menier's syndrome but these slowly diminished and I am left with the milder form of tinnitus that simulates the sound made by the passage of air through a punctured tyre. I am thankful that the condition has not developed to the maddening clattering and ringing that occurs in some unfortunate sufferers.

My first PhD student in Edinburgh was an Iranian vet, Parviz Hooshmand-Rad, from the Razi Institute in Teheran. He was a competent and pleasant person and the subject of *Theileria annulata*, a pathogen of considerable importance in the Middle East, provided the problems to be addressed in his research. His work was good but, as in all cases where a PhD thesis has to be presented in English by a worker whose first language is not English, the supervisor faces extra problems. Parviz's English was very good but the editing of a scientific research thesis demands a sound knowledge of the 'do's' and 'don'ts' of English serious writing. Much of what is written in scientific publications contains what the purist can only describe as jargon and many eminent writers fall into the trap of using it. I had learned a lot about this when I wrote my own doctoral thesis and on many occasions the editorial readers returned my early papers sent for publication with objections to certain forms of words. By the time I joined the CTVM I had gained considerable expertise in this field and my experience was of great use to me in supervising the writing of higher degree students and the papers of my colleagues submitting research reports for publication. I've no doubt that readers of these memoirs of mine, if indeed there will be such readers, will find many examples of slipshod descent into the use of jargon or journalese. However, it is now twenty-two years since I published anything serious or scientific and so I can hope for a little lenience on the part of the reader.

When he had successfully attained his doctorate, Parviz returned to Iran accompanied by his wife, Malak and young daughter, Roya. He was appointed to the post of Professor of Veterinary Pathology in the new faculty of Veterinary Science in the Pahlavi University in Shiraz. It must have been through his influence that I received an invitation to visit Iran to advise the faculty on the setting up of a research programme in tick-borne diseases with special reference to theileriasis. It was decided that I should accept this invitation and I flew to Shiraz via Teheran in April 1974. I had a rather worrying hour after landing at Shiraz airport, as there was no one to meet me. Parviz had assured me that he would be there to meet me but I could find no one who spoke or understood English and I had no knowledge of Parviz's address or the whereabouts of the faculty or, indeed, the university. After some efforts at making myself understood to anyone who looked like an official, without any success, I sat down on a seat in the concorse of the airport and awaited events. Not one official showed any signs of interest much less any concern for this obviously lost foreigner. After about half an hour, Parviz and his wife and daughter arrived and were astonished to see me already there. They had been given the time of arrival of my plane as one hour after the true scheduled time. However, I was warmly welcomed and taken to the Hooshmand-Rad home and, after a meal, on to my hotel. Next day, Parviz introduced me to the faculty and most of his colleagues. I gained the impression that the senior posts on the staff were allocated to the Iranian vets who returned from either the UK or the USA with brand new PhDs starting with the first to return who had been appointed Principal of the Veterinary School. Parviz was somewhere about the fifth or sixth and he was lucky to get the Pathology appointment. My stay was interesting and quite enjoyable although I was somewhat disappointed to find that the principle interest in the minds of these new professors and lecturers was just what were their chances of preferment for the higher posts in the veterinary world. These posts were, in their opinions, in Teheran, preferably in departments of government. A few of the more affluent of these new PhDs flew to Teheran each weekend in order to keep in touch with the influential heads of ministries in the capital. It was, of course, clear to me in retrospect, that there was a strong undercurrent of political feeling that not long afterwards, manifested itself in the overthrow of the Shah and the establishment of a very repressive regime.

My visit to Iran was busy and very interesting. I learned of some of the methods of farming, particularly of cattle, and the indoor feeding of cut grass. The poor and sparse distribution of pasture and the paucity of well informed veterinary advice were factors which made easy, productive farming virtually impossible. Indigent cattle owners had to rely on the veterinary advice of inadequately trained local people for help with animal health problems. These people received a modicum of training but my impression was that few, if any, qualified veterinarians and trained agronomists ventured very far off the tarmac. Among the mountains it was amazing to see tiny patches of soil retained in hollows between rocky outcrops utilised to their full capacity to raise grass and other crops.

Parviz was most helpful in organising our meetings and

safaris and he certainly smoothed out a lot of the difficulties that presented themselves. Through his efforts I was able to see the peasantry at work and to form opinions that helped me in advising on programmes of research and the practical application of existing knowledge, to the handling of tick borne problems. I was able to see some of the country in the south-west part of Iran. Parviz took me into the Zagross Mountains, which presented a truly stark and arid terrain. He also took me on a journey of some forty to fifty miles north west of Shiraz to the ancient ruins of Persepolis, a most interesting area.

I became quite friendly with some of Parviz's colleagues, joining them socially for meals and various discussions, but I was aware of an atmosphere of reticence, often when the discussions moved into the Farcy language and there descended on the group an air of secrecy and intrigue. Although I was very courteously received in Shiraz and my advice was readily accepted, I can now see how the minds of my Iranian friends were very much occupied by the political under current. When I returned to Edinburgh I maintained some correspondence with Parviz, but after the expulsion of the Shah, my letters were returned 'Not known at this address'. The last time I heard of Parviz he wrote to me from Sweden where he was apparently working in a research laboratory. His wife and daughter were with him. I was sorry to lose touch as he and his family were nice people and I am sure he was destined to make a mark in his profession.

During the winter of 1975/76, Alec Robertson, at one of our routine staff meetings, raised the idea of our organising an international conference on the subject of tick-borne diseases. We turned this over in our discussions and decided to have a go. As Head of the Protozoology Section the organisation of the event fell to me. It was no simple task and I had to get down to all the aspects involved in the setting up of such a complicated and far reaching event. The scope of the subjects involved the leading workers in these subjects, the invitations which would have to be sent out and the time scale involved in getting all these considerations satisfied before any details could be tackled, provided a daunting prospect. I anticipated that we might attract some hundred and fifty to two hundred delegates and their accommodation had to be arranged together with appropriate catering. The further I proceeded in this organisation the more complicated it became. All this, of course, had to be dealt with before any consideration of the real importance of the conference, namely, the actual contents of the papers to be presented and the choice of experts to be invited to present them, could be thought about. My colleagues were all helpful and supportive and the office staff came up trumps. Gordon Brown, the Chief Technician was a tower of strength as his knowledge of Edinburgh, its university and the people who mattered, was of great value. If anything showed signs of going wrong, Gordon would immediately get moving and things were miraculously put right. In this context, we managed to obtain accommodation for all the delegates who required it in the University Halls of Residence where the refectory would also be operated for us. I approached my former employers, the Wellcome Foundation to see if they would like to take part in the event. They sent Gilbert Macdonald, an old friend, to see me and the help they gave was phenomenal. Not only did they decide to set up a demonstration at the conference but also they provided an evening's dinner and entertainment in the Assembly Rooms in George Street and presented every lady guest with a tartan stole whilst the men received a half bottle of whisky. Indeed, the only material recompense that I received for my efforts was a roll of first quality Winsor and Newton artist's canvas, which Gilbert presented to me at the last function of the conference as an acknowledgement from the Wellcome Company. Among the functions, which were provided for the delegates, was an evening as the guests of the Lord Mayor of Edinburgh in Edinburgh Castle. This was a great success.

The planning of the conference meetings, choice of chairmen and speakers, the venues for the various sections, and all the apparatus necessary for lectures and demonstrations was an exercise of considerable complexity. In this, my professional colleagues played a vital part. The general support and help given to me by all members of the CTVM was excellent. It must be realised that this was the first time such a prodigious international conference had ever been mounted by the veterinary faculty of the University of Edinburgh and the occasion was unique. The Honourable the Lord Robertson, Chairman of the Advisory Board of the CTVM graciously agreed to open the conference.

When the conference was finished and was declared an outstanding success and the tumult and shouting died, I had the job of putting together all the scientific contributions and deliberations in a proceedings which had to be published. This was a mammoth exercise, which took up most of my waking hours, and, many of my hours normally devoted to sleeping. All the papers, and there were one hundred and two of them, I had to read and edit. It was necessary, from time to time, for me to consult colleagues and to contact participants at home and overseas regarding forms of words and factual items. Many of the delegates had not left me their scripts and so I had to contact them in order to obtain these. Some of them sent only abstracts and in many of the papers I had to interpret idiosyncrasies arising from quaint translations from the languages of scientists whose English was definitely a second language. The work was very exacting but eventually it was completed and then we had to find a publisher. We had limited funds for this part of the operation and of course, the natural publisher was The University of Edinburgh Press. I applied to them but things were not easy. They had plenty of work in hand and thanks to all the matter in the proceedings having illustrated papers with diagrams and complicated tables the press was not enthusiastic. This was where Gordon Brown's influence became vital. He was the friend of a crucial member of the University Press and after some prolonged discussions with a little give and take here and there, the Press agreed to publish the material and the work appeared in 1977 as 'Tick-borne Diseases and their Vectors' Editor J.K.H.Wilde CTVM, 1976 with a design by me on the cover and with 'Proceedings of an International Conference held in Edinburgh from the 27th September to the 1st October 1976 organised by the Centre for Tropical Veterinary Medicine', on the flyleaf.

When I look back on that piece of my professional life I shudder at the thought of what it entailed and I marvel at how I managed to carry out the duties, which fell to my lot. I am now so far from the science that was involved at that time that, when

I look at my copy of the book the contents are far above my head. Of course, I have been retired from veterinary work for more than twenty-three years. I knew that I couldn't possibly keep up with the work in which I had been engaged after I had quitted my place in the laboratory and I decided not to try to keep up with the great strides which were beginning to develop in the field of veterinary research. I think it was a wise decision. The work of those who were to follow me was already getting beyond me with all the developments in the new technology. Duncan Brown took my place when I left and his work has greatly added to knowledge and research in his chosen field. In 2001 Duncan retired and others are moving ahead. Many of my old friends and colleagues have tried to keep up with their subjects after retiring but I think it is a mistake. I have been lucky in that I have wide interests and also have my art to keep me on my toes.

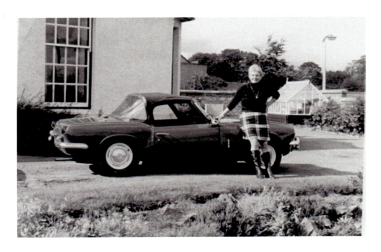

Kathy and the Spitfire at Bonnyrigg.

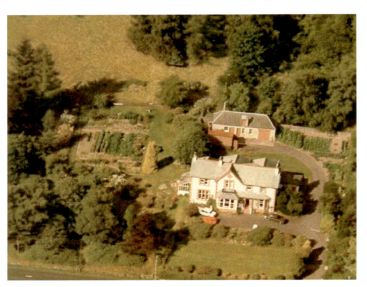

Drumsheugh from the air

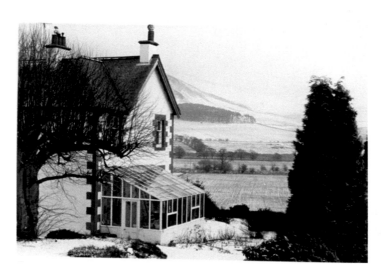

Winter view of Drumsheugh

CHAPTER 8

Colombia

In 1975, I was invited to a conference on tick-borne diseases, which was organised by Eric Wells to be held in Cali, Colombia. The hosting institution was the Centro International de Agricultura Tropical (CIAT), principally financed from sources within the USA. My old friend of Kenya days, David Brocklesby, was also invited and so we decided to travel together. We left Heathrow on the third of March and flew to Bogota via Antigua and Caracas. At Bogota, we had to change to a local flight to Cali. In Bogota we had very little time to make our connection and we were handicapped also by our lack of knowledge of the language. I rushed up to a desk and in my almost non-existent Spanish and a paucity of French gained an indication of the direction we should take to catch the Cali plane. We were carrying our luggage and I rushed ahead, David staggering along behind. He wasn't quite as good on his feet as I was. Fortunately, and with a lot of luck, my nose pointed in the right direction and I arrived at a lift that was crammed with a mass of Colombian businessmen and managed to ascertain that this was the way to go for the Cali plane. I indicated David who was puffing and blowing and the commuters, for this is what they were, held the door of the lift open until David arrived and we squeezed into the sardine-like packed space. It was very hot and we were perspiring freely. This we continued to do when we managed to get into the last two vacant seats in the last plane of the day to Cali. At Cali, we were welcomed by Eric and taken to our accommodation in the institute where the conference was to be held.

The members came from all over the world but principally from the USA, most of the South American countries and Australia. Eric took us to the condominium where he had an apartment. I noticed that the janitor at the entrance carried a handgun. Eric told us that this was the general practice in all the apartment blocks and warned us not to wear wristwatches or carry cameras if we walked in the town. I met several people whose names were familiar to me through the literature and the company was cordial and expert in the subjects on the agenda. From the technical point of view the meetings were very well worthwhile and the subjects were definitely brought up to date. Various trips were organised and some interesting places were visited. I remember being photographed by some of our American colleagues when one of the gauchos at an estancia, which we were visiting, persuaded me to wear his hat and get into the saddle of his horse. On a trip into the town, the strength of Eric's warning became fully apparent when some of our colleagues were mugged by thugs in the main square in broad daylight. They were South Americans themselves and only escaped further roughing up by managing to get into the nearby church and closing the doors against their attackers.

A rather hair raising two and a half hour flight across the formidable Cordilleras was organised to take the members of the conference to an agricultural research station at Carimagua. The plane was a very old DC3, in very dilapidated condition. I was seated in the rear part of the cabin next to the toilet, which had a door that didn't shut but swung freely to expose the only sanitary arrangement. This consisted of an old oil drum that had not been emptied after last used. The stink was strong. However, we took off and climbed laboriously to get over the massive, wild and craggy mountains. The weather was overcast with dark thunderclouds and from time to time we went through heavy rainstorms. I watched with bated breath as we approached one dark ridge after another and prayed that the engines would be up to the effort of climbing just high enough to get over them. We actually did succeed in flying over the Cordilleras and came into a valley to touch down on a grassy landing strip. I had noticed on the trip that at many points in the sides of the cabin and on the wings, there were patches of Elastoplast. As we were

270

disembarking, I asked the cabin steward what these were. He told me that on a recent trip to this same landing strip, the police had been alerted to the information that the plane was carrying a gang of dope smugglers and the aircraft was raked with rifle fire as it landed. The company had not had the time to repair the damage properly but had resorted to a sort of first aid by patching up the holes with plasters. Daylight was fading when the time came for us to return and I was, perhaps understandably, even more apprehensive about the pilot's ability to find his way and miss the most formidable of the horrendous looking peaks. I think that we all heaved a sigh of relief when we landed safely at Cali airport.

Some of the American delegation arranged a trip to a sugar plantation on one of our half days off and kindly invited me to accompany them. We travelled in a hired vehicle and with some difficulty found the buildings in the large area of the growing sugar cane. We were taken into the rather dilapidated, rough looking sheds where the cane was being crushed to produce sugar solution, which was channelled into large vats heated by wood burning fires. Each vat was in a different state of concentration of the liquor. The final product comprised large hunks of brown crystallised sugar. This rough sugar found a ready local market. The plantation that we visited was a family concern, its product, crude sugar, was used mostly by the surrounding peasantry. Larger commercial factories produced the refined sugar for export. The visit was very entertaining and instructive and we were made very welcome.

The conference was pronounced a great success and was a credit to the efforts of Eric Wells who was responsible for its organisation. The secretariat arranged our return flights. I decided to return a day earlier than David and was booked via Miami, Florida. I made enquiries at the secretariat to ensure that I did not need a visa to transit through the USA and was assured that this was true. Being a seasoned traveller through airports, I asked the secretariat to confirm that this was true by ringing the office of the carriers with whom I was booked to fly. This they did and told me that as I would not be leaving the airport at Miami no visa would be required. Accordingly I left Cali on the morning of Wednesday the 26th of March in an Avianca plane bound for Miami via Bogota. The Boeing 720 took off from Cali at 08.23 and touched down in Bogota at 08.49. As we had two hours to wait until our onward flight, most of us went into the city and had a quick look round and then, back in the airport we had a browse in the duty free shop where I bought a small sack of coffee beans. Our plane took off again at 10.23 and we had an interesting flight over the Caribbean, sighting Jamaica and Cuba and landing at Miami airport, Florida at 13.38 (14.38 local time).

Then the fun commenced. We were all herded into a large hall in which hundreds of people stood waiting to pass through immigration. After two hours standing and slowly shuffling forward, I arrived at the immigration kiosk. I was due to catch an onward flight to London via National Airlines scheduled to depart 4 hours after we had landed from Colombia, which was at 18.20 local time. Having arrived at the kiosk I immediately became a suspected illegal immigrant and was treated as such by the custom officials. This, of course, was because I had no visa. I explained that I was only in transit and had neither the intention nor the desire to enter the USA. My passport and flight ticket were taken from me and I was passed through the hands of a series of security officers and eventually put under the surveillance of a lady designated a security escort. Her duty was to accompany me through all the formalities and not let me have my passport or airline tickets until I was safely aboard the plane, which was to take me to London. This security escort was a Spanish lady, quite charming but with very little English as she had only recently emigrated to the USA from Spain. The first thing I wanted to do was to retrieve my baggage, which by now had been lying unclaimed for more than two hours. So we started towards the baggage hall where I was relieved to see my property in a corner near one of the carousels and took possession. I was surprised that the US authorities did not charge me demurrage. I then had to pass through the customs area where my escort and I joined another queue.

In this queue I was thrown into the proximity of a tall gangling American. He was surrounded by an assortment of impedimenta of all shapes and sizes, none of which had the appearance of normal baggage. He was in front of me and I had visions of suffering great delays while the officials sorted through this man's suspicious looking array of plastic bags with a large cardboard carton containing a black plastic disposal bag almost bursting with oddly shaped contents. This character immediately engaged me in conversation. He asked me about my life, where I came from, where I was now living, my antecedents and Scotland. When he heard that I had spent some time in Africa he switched onto the subject of bilhartzia. On this subject I was reluctantly forced into describing the disease, its symptoms and treatment. He then moved on to the horrors of other tropical diseases and their symptoms and effects on the local populace.

The rather tired old gentleman at the counter, at this moment, decided that life was too much for him. Chewing his gum with a sad expression on his battle scarred countenance; he gave up and departed. A black woman in an official uniform appeared to take over his duties. She asked my new acquaintance a few questions regarding his luggage and delved into his carton, which contained an odd assortment of personal belongings. He said that one of his many suitcases had disintegrated and so he had been obliged to improvise. The lady official seemed satisfied and stamped hieroglyphics on his card and he departed with a dark skinned Red Cap porter. The female official apparently decided that she had done enough for the time being or, perhaps, she had felt the urge for physiological functions as she stuck a notice on the counter stating 'CLOSED – join another line'. This evoked many irate outcries such as –'this is the great America! Etc'. I must admit that I joined in this show of annoyance and even my escort expressed her objections. However, we moved towards another line, then, just as promptly as the black lady official had disappeared she returned to remove the offending notice and I beat it back briskly to my rightful place. The lady was obviously tired because she passed me through without further delay.

I secured a porter and after some altercations between him and my escort, we eventually trundled off to the National Airlines check-in counter, which was a quarter of a mile away. There we joined another queue and waited. I decided to try to exchange an American Express cheque so that I could buy some duty free liquor and some perfume for Kathy. My security escort kindly looked after my baggage and, incidentally, my position in the queue while I went in search of a bank. I found one but it was closed. I then searched for and found a money-changing bureau and waited patiently behind a gentleman who was transacting a considerable amount of international finance. When he had finished, I asked the lady behind the grill if she could cash for me an American Express cheque. Not without my passport she confided. My passport was with my Security Escort who, on no account, could allow me to have it. However, when I returned and in my halting Spanish, acquired in the last two weeks in Colombia, I explained the situation, she kindly went off to the duty free shop and enquired if I could make a purchase with an American Express cheque. This, she assured me, could be done or at least that was my understanding.

After fifteen minutes or so, my ticket was checked and my seat allocated from the very few which remained unallocated. My escort and I moved off in the direction of the duty free shop. *En route* another escort who was in charge of an elderly foreign traveller in a similar plight to mine accosted us. This security lady was suffering from an urgent call of nature and asked my escort if she would act in her place for a few minutes. We duly performed this small service and then proceeded on the way to the duty free shop. When we arrived, the lady behind the counter was French and very friendly to another European. Once more, my life history was elicited and with a friendly 'Bon voyage, Doctor', I was sent on my way with my purchases, almost light-headed if not light-hearted. Eventually, after several tries, we found the right gate and stood in a queue once more to be passed into the enclosure that was to funnel me into the plane to whisk me away from the USA. My passport and tickets were handed over to an international official, who sealed them in an envelope and said I would receive them in the plane and once more become an honest individual. This official signed a form certifying my safe delivery and my escort made ready to depart. Meanwhile, I had learned much about her including that she had lived most of her life in Madrid, had five children, of whom the eldest was a lawyer in Madrid and that she had ten grandchildren. I bid her an affectionate *'Adios senora'* and sank into one of the few remaining hard plastic seats. It was almost four hours since I had disembarked from the Avianca plane and since I had last sat down. It was some five hours since I had last had a drink, which had been a coffee with lunch on the plane over the Caribbean. It was to be another fifty minutes before we moved towards the plane.

We had been flying for one and a quarter hours before I managed to get a drink and then I ordered two Budweiser's and began to make up for the dehydration losses. I was seated in the middle of one of the cross alleyways and this was the place where the large trolleys heaved about by the cabin staff, were parked. The staff seemed to have great fun in shunting them around the aircraft rather like schoolboys playing with electric train sets. The idea seemed to be to push the trolleys into the cross alleyway until they fetched up with a crash against my ankles. On making a vociferous complaint when this happened the so-called hostess said, "There just ain't enough room in these aircraft's," which is all I received by way of apology. People paraded about the craft all night, a favourite pastime being to play follow my leader up the aisles and across the space in front of my seat. Spice was added to this game when the trolleys were parked in front of us and indeed, at one point, I measured the space for my legs between the front of the seat and the trolley. It was just twelve inches. The only peace we had was when the movie was on and even then the stewardesses found the need to cross from one side of the aircraft to the other. Suffice it to say, I had not one wink of sleep the whole night. All in all, this flight proved the worst international flight I have had the misfortune to experience in more than forty years of flying around the world with a variety of airlines. The cabin crew was, I think, the most disorganised bunch I have ever known and I made up my mind never to have to suffer them again. Incidentally, I recovered my passport and ticket, after asking for them on several occasions, in the middle of the showing of the 'midnight movie'. It was a blessed relief to get home in one piece.

CHAPTER 9

Retirement

In 1978 I approached the time of my retirement as I attained the age of sixty-five in May of that year and I was to relinquish my post at the end of the academic year, September 18th. Alec Robertson and I retired on the same day and a party was held jointly for us both. During 1978, we in the CTVM, gave consideration to the lines upon which the Department should organise its future work. In the Protozoology section it was decided that work on the theileriases should proceed by expanding research into *Theileria annulata* which could well involve strains from countries in the Middle East and Asia. The Overseas Development Ministry, which was the supplier of our funds, was supportive of this policy and we had received encouraging noises on the subject from the FAO. We had also received requests from India for help in the research on the theilerial diseases of cattle suggesting that some of their workers might be given the facilities to gain training and experience in the CTVM. We appreciated that this was a very good idea for our future work. Professor S.B.Singh from the Punjab Agricultural University visited us on a sponsored visit to the UK. He had been very impressed by our international conference and spent much time in discussions with me. He made a suggestion, supported by the Indian National authorities, that I should go to India to advise those involved on the lines of research and control that should be followed. Much correspondence ensued and the suggestion that I should visit India began to take shape. The ODM was quite agreeable to my going after I had retired and to fulfil this function; the

Department would fund the assignment. I agreed, somewhat reluctantly, to accept this job.

At that time we had decided to sell our house in Broughton and find a place in the south west of England. We were very attached to our home in Drumsheugh but the upkeep of the large property and the three acres of land could become onerous as we grew older. Also, we did have doubts as to whether or not we could keep up the garden and property along with it having to withstand very late frosts in the spring and early summer and the very early frosts of the autumn. We were very sad at the thought of leaving the Borders and our many friends but accepted that we should make the move.

Peter had by now qualified in medicine at the Radcliffe Hospital in Oxford. He studied for and obtained his membership of the Royal College of Physicians, London and had decided to specialise in Radiology. I was rather surprised at this choice but events dispelled my doubts about such a decision. At the time when we were about to leave Scotland he was working in Bristol Royal Infirmary and so we naturally started our hunt for a house in the Somerset and Dorset areas. We made several journeys to the region, searching for a place that would suit our requirements. Over a period of about six months we must have visited and looked at sixty houses but had found nothing which interested us. We were apprehensive about the selling of Drumsheugh, which was a rather large property by ordinary standards, and our solicitor and friend, Douglas Graham, confirmed our feeling that we might have difficulty in selling. He thought we might be wise to 'test the water' by advertising the house to see if any interest might be attracted some months before I was due to retire. This we did and we were very surprised by the interest that was engendered. To cut a long story short we had a firm offer in a matter of a few weeks and Douglas advised us to take it, so Drumsheugh was sold and we were without a home. The couple who bought the house were pleasant people, a young man and his wife who were not in a position to make full use of the accommodation and they very kindly agreed to our stacking most of our furniture in the part of the house which had been my studio and which, furniture wise, they were not ready to develop. We had old friends from African days, Ian and Pearl Macadam, who had the lower half of a house, 'Oranmore' in North Berwick. Ian, a vet, had just accepted a post in the Far East and suggested that we should live in their property, Lower Oranmore, until I finally retired in about seven months time. We came to an arrangement and took up residence. I found driving into Easter Bush in the winter months a little trying but Kathy enjoyed being able to walk down to the seashore and to the shops when I was away at work. We settled in well and cleaned and organised the accommodation and got it to the standard that suited us. The fact that we kept the house in order and paid the rates and other expenses and kept the house warm in what was a very cold and bitter winter was reassuring to the Macadams.

Ian Macadam had qualified from the Royal Veterinary College in London in 1943 and came out to Tanganyika when I was in charge of the Mpwapwa laboratories. I liked him and helped him a lot during his career in the Colonial Service. Many of his colleagues found him strangely imbued with peculiar ideas and principles. He broke his service and went to the Glasgow Veterinary School and studied for a PhD in bacteriology. He joined me again in Nigeria as a bacteriologist and while on leave he met Pearlie, from Carradale in Kintyre, and married her. Pearlie came out to Nigeria straight from a Scottish fishing village. Kathy helped her a lot and we were good friends. In my later service I found myself defending Ian against all kinds of colleagues because he had strange ideas and seemed oblivious to the fact that very often he rubbed authority up in the wrong way. After I left the Nigerian Service he stayed on and then, later, took several appointments successively in remote parts of the world. He developed extraordinary ideas about sex and eugenics and he tended to frighten off potential employers. Pearlie was a most pleasant girl and we were very fond of her. I think that some of Ian's ideas rubbed off on her so that the pair of them developed a reputation for following an unusual lifestyle.

When we had settled in at Lower Oranmore, we were surprised to receive a telephone call from Edinburgh Airport late on a very cold wintry night, saying that Mrs Macadam had arrived on a plane from the Far East and was *en route* for North Berwick by taxi. Around about midnight Pearlie arrived. She

278

was attired in scanty tropical clothes and open-toed sandals and without stockings, just about frozen. We set about getting her warm and comfortable with an aired bed and some food. This arrival proved to be a prelude to the story that Ian had been sacked from his job and would be following her home. With his peculiar approach to his superiors, he had threatened to bring the Director, a local man of course, to court for alleged cruelty to a horse on the racecourse. In his usual forthright manner he had not considered the inevitable consequences of his ill-considered action.

The next few weeks were miserable for us. It soon became obvious that Pearl was drinking heavily, using all sorts of subterfuges to hide her addiction. We tactfully approached the subject with Ian who said that she had promised to stop drinking before Christmas and so we must be mistaken. We were very upset by the situation, as we had been very fond of Pearl for a long time. Ian tried to close his eyes to the state of affairs but eventually he could keep up the pretence no longer. Things became untenable for us. The management of the house was automatically taken over by Pearl and our living standards deteriorated. We tried to get Ian to see sense but he adopted the 'head in sand' attitude. He had brought home with him one of his many crackpot ideas. This one was based on the idea that society should be run by committees which would manage what seemed to be communes and the rights of members in the procreation of children should be governed by a points system determined by the committee. I tried to argue with him but he brought up what he regarded as support for his idea in the form of discussions with various people whom he had met in his last job and on his journey home. I remember him telling us about the enthusiasm of someone he had met in a station or on a dockside; I can't remember which. Meanwhile he was looking around for a job, as he now had no source of income. He went into Edinburgh and made enquiries of the Council and Social Services regarding his difficulties in getting a job. He decided to accept the offer to take a course in 'How to apply for a job and how to present himself to likely employers'. This was a man who was a veterinarian in his late fifties with a post graduate degree of PhD in bacteriology and many years of service in research in the overseas services, having held posts which demanded some considerable responsibility.

I explained to Ian that we would have to leave their home and find temporary accommodation elsewhere. He begged me to stay with them as they had no means of paying the rates etc., duties that we had been performing since their return to Scotland. We had purchased logs and had agreed to pay the bill for fuel oil. We also paid for food and other necessities, but when Ian managed to obtain a post as assistant in a veterinary practice in Hellensborough, we decided to leave. Pearl was still drinking heavily and we felt that we had to depart. We had no accommodation in sight but packed all our belongings in our trailer and the car and left for Edinburgh. We had no idea how to get somewhere to stay but found a motel in Dalkeith. Here we booked a room and, of course, had to leave our trailer and its contents outside the chalet with a tarpaulin tied over it to keep out the weather and, hopefully, human and other domestic predators. It was now snowing.

I had to leave Kathy in charge of our belongings while I was at work, and at work I made enquiries of my colleagues regarding possible properties to rent. One of my colleagues, Tony Smith, who was head of our Animal Husbandry Section, said that he had friends who owned a cottage in Peebles which they used in the summer for weekend holidays. He put me in touch with his friends and I rang them in their apartment in Edinburgh. They were a very pleasant couple; he was a lecturer in Edinburgh University. They agreed to our renting their cottage. When would we like to move in? "Today," I said. There was a horrified silence for a few seconds.

"But that will be impossible, we haven't been in the cottage since last summer and so it will be damp and quite uninhabitable." I explained our situation and assured him that we would take the place and get it into shape ourselves, otherwise we would be out in the snow. Thane Riney and his wife agreed to our taking over the cottage that was really an old lodge to a large house. Our home for the next few months was to be Kerfield West Lodge in Peebles.

When we found the lodge it was certainly rough. We lighted a fire in the open fireplace in the living room, connected some electric heaters up and started to straighten things out. Kathy soon had some bedclothes aired and got down to cleaning and smartening things up. How it happened, I do not know, but we got the kitchen working and in a few days we were reasonably comfortable. Kathy brought about a transformation and we became very attached to the old place and really enjoyed our sojourn in the Lodge. After a few days, Thane and his wife came to see us. They were charmed with the changes we had made. When the fine weather arrived they visited us several times and were so pleased with the lodge in its new colours that after we left in the September they sold their flat in Edinburgh and moved into the lodge where they stayed for some time until they sold up and left the country. I believe they went to Australia.

During our stay in Peebles we took every opportunity, when work allowed me, to have a few days off, to drive down to the West Country to look for somewhere to settle for our retirement. It was an arduous task and involved many miles of motoring and many laborious searches through all sorts of properties. By this time, Peter was living in a small village near Bath and spending all his free time refurbishing a small cottage that he and Helen had bought. He did some yeoman work altering the cottage structurally, doing demolitions of walls, which would have frightened me to death. He installed central heating and rewired the property. When we visited them the place was a mess, carpets under loads of rubble, cement and sand and very little of the comfort of a home. When the rebuilding and furnishing had almost been completed Peter and Helen suggested that we should go down to Bath, stay a night or two with them and then conduct our search from there. We duly arrived on a Bank Holiday weekend to find that there was no bed for us. Peter thought that we could construct one and so we made a plan that incorporated the function of being fixed to a wall by means of hinges so that when not in use it could be folded up. The foot of the bed was also hinged so that when the bed was secured to the wall the footboard dropped down so conserving space. Peter said that he knew of a good place for us to purchase a spring mattress at rock bottom price and so off we went into the environs of Bath. The furniture warehouse was closed. So we made for Bristol and managed to buy in John Lewis's, a suitable mattress that we had to carry down to the street through the goods entrance and then tie onto the roof of the car with string and tape kindly supplied by the store. We had to keep the car windows open in order to pass the string under the roof and over the mattress. Helen was driving and we set off at great speed. I think Helen was operating on the assumption that the faster we went the less time there would be for the mattress to be blown off. As it was, Peter and I had to put our arms out of the window, one at each side, and try to hold the mattress down. The mattress had a mind of its own and bounced and lashed about most alarmingly. The front part flew upwards and bent over tending to pull the strings to the rear. However, we got back to their home, Dolphin Cottage, with the mattress still hanging on precariously. We then had to find a local joiner's yard where we purchased the necessary timbers, screws and hinges and got down to the actual construction. Amazingly, this was reasonably successful. We had a very strenuous and fraught job getting the bed up the cottage stairs but we won. Remarkably, the bed was quite comfortable and the engineering worked. This bed became a feature of Dolphin Cottage and I believe it helped to sell the property when Peter and Helen moved to Bristol.

While we were at Dolphin Cottage, Kathy developed a painful back. Peter looked at it and said, "You've got shingles, Mum, and there's not much we can do about it." And that was that. We started our search for houses and moved west into Dorset and Somerset. Our efforts were pretty fruitless. We had various provisos that were germane to our choice of residence. We were not tied to any particular area or any requirements such as schools for children. We wanted somewhere quiet in a pleasant rural situation with, preferably, some seclusion. We had to have a place that had at least two rooms large enough to accommodate our large Persian carpets, with three bedrooms and at least two loos.

Our search over about four visits of length varying from four days to two weeks covered a range from Winchester in the southeast to the north end of the Quantocks and to Wellington in the west. In the east we were guided by James's wife, Sue whose parents lived near to Winchester. James, on the insistence of

Sue, had left the forces and had moved from Germany, where he had been stationed, to the area of the Wallops where he had found a job. It was during our visit that originated with our bed-fabricating episode, that we were exploring the region near Stogumber in North Somerset. Kathy's shingles were developing painfully and at one point we stopped near a little piece of bushy, rough pasture for the usual necessary physiological reasons. Kathy squatted behind a bush on a weedy slope. She had the misfortune to overbalance backwards into a bed of nettles. It was not a happy day.

We must, by now, have visited and actually investigated some sixty properties without any success. We did find an attractive thatched cottage on the road from Taunton to Williton, near to Lydeard St Lawrence. When we visited we found a very pleasant and spacious house which was being personally refurbished by a retired army officer who had made a profitable hobby of buying decrepit property and renovating it with very convincing results. When we arrived, the major was already showing some people around and so we had a look at the interior and found it most attractive. It was pristine, with an inglenook fireplace and an open staircase to the bedrooms above. The party of prospective buyers that preceded us moved off and the major turned his attention to us. We were very interested and extracted all the details from him. We thought the house was rather expensive especially as there was not a single fitting, not even a cooker or electric installation included in the deal. We said that we liked the property and would like time to consider it. He said that the previous people who had just left were also interested and that they would be giving him a firm offer on the following day. We decided to return to Scotland and giving the major our address we departed. A few weeks afterwards the major phoned us to say that the deal had fallen through owing to the failure of his prospective customers to sell their current house. This news came to us in the week before Easter and so we said we would go down to see the cottage again at the weekend. The major said he would not be able to meet us at the property as he had to go to Bisley for the shooting competitions but that he would leave the keys at the pub some hundred yards down the main road. So, once more, we made the long journey down to Somerset. We booked into a hotel in Taunton and on the Saturday before Easter Day we proceeded to Lydeard St Lawrence. By this time, the newly refurbished house had been named 'Yeomans' and we pulled into the pub car park which was on the left side of the road about a hundred yards beyond the house as we drove northwards. We contacted the publican's wife who handed over the keys. Then the problem became apparent. Yeomans was on the other side of the road from the pub and the business of crossing the road became frightening. Huge queues of traffic obstructed our crossing. We had to wait minutes before we dared to run across the road in a brief gap in the line of vehicles. Having achieved a foothold on the other side of the road we decided to take the risk of struggling up to Yeomans in single file. We went into the house and still found it attractive but the noise of the traffic was intense as the garden between the house and the road was just a narrow strip of rough grass. We returned to the pub, suffering the same hazards that had impeded us on the outward journey. We both agreed that if this was the traffic position at the beginning of the Easter break, how impossible it could prove in the height of the summer holidays when the better weather might incline us to the taking of tea in our garden on a sunny day. Sadly, we returned to Scotland.

In the summer, I had accumulated quite a lot of leave and so we made another trip to the West Country. We decided to devote a couple of weeks to house hunting and made contact with estate agents in several areas and visited several properties. We eventually pitched up in Dorchester and, after looking at some properties in and around this Dorset county town, could find nothing that attracted us at all. We decided to book in for the night at the Kings Arms and the following day, take a look at the Glastonbury area. Peter had done a little reconnoitring for us and had told us about an estate agent in Glastonbury who had impressed him as a sound type of chap and so we decided to try him. We spent the next morning visiting two houses which proved to be entirely unsatisfactory and then moved on towards Glastonbury. We arrived in the main street at about five o'clock and booked a room in the George and Pilgrim. I expected the estate agent to be closed by this time but, after locating our room in the hotel, we walked up the street and found the agent mentioned by Peter, who was still open. His was a one-man business and we were pleased to meet the proprietor, Dick Rhind. We found him to be a straightforward, likeable chap and we later became very good friends. He told us that he remembered Peter visiting him and knew what we were looking for. He added that he had nothing on his books that would suit us. "In fact." he said. "I can think of no properties in this area which would fit into the specifications which your son explained to me. Most of the houses on the market now are small and none on my books has the size of rooms which you require." We told Dick Rhind that we were booked in at The George and Pilgrim and he suggested that we call on him in the morning before we left Glastonbury. We had decided that if our visit to him failed to turn up something worth looking at we would leave the area and take a look at properties in the Lake District, on our way back to Scotland. At the hotel, a rather ancient hostelry, the bedrooms were named after members of monasteries such as 'the Abbot's Chamber', 'the Prior's Room' and so on. I can't remember which monastic member had given his name to our bedroom, but it must have been some one of undoubted eminence as the chamber was richly draped, if somewhat gloomy, and the double four-poster bed was situated on a high dais. Climbing into bed was an exercise of some difficulty and no little hazard. I said to Kathy that it was fortunate that we were used to heights.

The next morning after breakfast, we went back to Dick Rhind's office. The boss was not in but had left a message with a young man who was helping in the office. It was to the effect that details of a new property had come from an estate agent in Bruton who sometimes collaborated with Dick. It was this estate agent's son who was helping Dick and he explained to us that the property was under offer but that the vendor had expressed a disinclination to accept the offer made. Perhaps she would be interested to let us see the place. The young man rang up the owner to ask if she would be prepared to let some prospective buyers, us, see over the house. The lady asked when. Our young man said "Now." She seemed to be taken aback and said that it would not be convenient at the moment but that we would be welcome after another half-hour. I immediately had visions of hurried preparations being made to hide the more obvious defects so that the property could be seen in the best of condition. Dick's young assistant gave us directions as to how to find the house and we started off for the village of Barton St David and a search for the lanes that would bring us to the cottage, which was on the edge of the village. We arrived a few minutes under the half-hour and knocked on the door of 'Haygrass', which stood in about an acre of garden and orchard, surrounded by farmland and with a nearby farmstead.

The door was opened by a rather grumpy looking old lady who dispelled our first misgivings by saying that the house was not hers but her daughter's and that her daughter was not at the moment available, but the gloom was dispersed by a clattering down the stairs of a very pretty young woman, who excused herself for not being ready to meet us as we arrived because when she received the telephone call she had been just about to step into the bath. Her name was Anne Morris and her husband was an accountant with his office in Castle Cary. He was called Gerry. Anne showed us round and we liked what we saw. The property had originally been two cottages for farm workers which had been quite attractively converted into two storeys with an open stairway leading up from the quite large living room to three bedrooms and bathroom with a loft running the whole length of the house. There was a fireplace in the living room with a chimney serving also a fireplace in the adjoining dining room, the doorway of which opened into a spacious kitchen. The back door opened into the orchard. There was a large barn near the front gate which had double doors at each end and alongside it was a garage.

Whether we were influenced by a sort of desperation or were really pleased by the property, I do not know, but we decided to make an offer. Anne Morris was delighted. She said she had received another offer but was not attracted by the person offering and was perfectly ready to turn the other offer down in favour of ours. She rang her husband, Gerry, at his office and it was arranged that we should all go to the George Inn in Castle Carey for lunch and to sort things out. We duly had lunch together and we were mutually favourably impressed and clinched the deal. I rang Dick Rhind and asked his advice about a suitable solicitor to draw up the agreement. He recommended a firm of solicitors called Gould and Swayne of Glastonbury. We phoned them and made an immediate appointment with their Mr Alec Wyllie and went to see him to start up all the necessary procedures. At about 5p.m. we left Glastonbury and made for Scotland arriving in Peebles late that night. It had been a long and eventful day.

When I retired from the CTVM, we moved to our house in Barton St David. We changed the name of the house from 'Haygrass' which we thought was not very attractive, to 'Bramleys'. The orchard behind the house contained several old Bramley apple trees that proved to be very prolific fruit providers so that the name was truly appropriate. A lot had to be done to get the house into good order. The conservatory running along the west side of the house had been damaged by the exceptionally hard winter of the previous year and much of the supports and the glass had to be replaced. Fortunately, there was a good general builder in the village and he proved to be very useful in many ways. We purchased and had installed new equipment such as a washing machine, dishwasher and cooker and by the time winter weather set in we were snug and comfortable. We discovered the local supermarkets and did most of our shopping in Street and Glastonbury with occasional visits to Yeovil for more exotic items. I set up material and equipment for framing my pictures and the necessary impedimenta for dealing with our rather large garden, in which, incidentally, there was a very good well that was expertly lined with red brick.

When we were fairly comfortably settled in Bramleys and had got over our first Christmas in retirement, negotiations for our trip to India were commenced and in February we started our journey to the subcontinent. We planned to take the train from the nearest station, that was Castle Cary, about four miles away from our village. The weather was very cold and wintry but in the interests of keeping down our luggage weight we took very little warm clothing and that which we did include, was not the normally heavy winter clothing that we would have worn during a winter at home. Anyway, we argued, we should only be exposed to outside winter weather at the station and during the changeover to the bus at Woking and then when transferring from the bus to the concourse at Heathrow. Of course, Sod's Law had to come into effect. When we got into the cold, unheated station at Castle Cary, we were informed that there was a delay due to problems on the line near to Exeter. However, this would soon be put right. A later announcement informed us that the delay had been further extended. The pattern was repeated several times and when the train actually arrived we had been standing shivering in the miserable unheated waiting room for more than two hours. Of course, we missed the bus connection at Woking and had to spend another half-hour in that station which was nearly as cold and uncomfortable as the one at Castle Cary. Eventually we flew to New Delhi with a stop at Qatar. Our main contact in New Delhi was Alan Jackson of the British Council Division of the British High Commission in New Delhi. He was most helpful to us throughout our visit and, indeed, was most diligent in seeing that all the arrangements for our travel and accommodation were as satisfactory as possible. We must have caused him some headaches, as affairs can be somewhat fraught in India.

CHAPTER 10

Indian Assignment

My invitation to visit India was for the purpose of advising on schemes for the furtherance of research into the very important disease of cattle, caused by the tick-borne protozoal parasite *Theileria annulata*. In discussions with various authorities, including Indian veterinary research workers, it became apparent to me that I would have to concentrate my time and effort at a small number of sites where work on the subject was already being carried out. I was fortunate to have, working in my department at the CTVM, a veterinary research worker from the Veterinary Research Institute at Izatnagar in Uttar Pradesh in India, Dr M.N.Malhotra. He was able to give me much valuable information on the situation in India. After a considerable amount of discussion by mail and in person with him and Indian colleagues, it appeared to me that the institutes on which I should concentrate were three in number. They were the College of Veterinary Science, Punjab Agricultural University, Ludhiana; the College of Veterinary Science, Haryana Agricultural University and the Veterinary Research Institute at Izatnagar (UP). These centres were selected as the places in which serious work on theileriasis was included in research programmes, and where workers in this field had established their names with publications in the international literature.

After our arrival in New Delhi the British Council Officer, Alan Jackson, who was responsible for all the arrangements for our visit, took me to meet senior officers of Government to discuss the programme. Dr J. M. Lal, Joint Commissioner of Animal Health and the Ministry of Agriculture suggested that I include in my itinerary, a visit to the Veterinary College of Muthura where some work was being done on the chemotherapy of the theileriases. He said that as Muthura was near to Agra, we should take a look at the Taj Mahal. Dr Lal also invited me to make recommendations regarding schemes of work on theileriasis requiring financial support from the Indian Council of Agricultural Research (ICAR).

We travelled to Muthura by rail on the Taj Express and disembarked at the small station where I expected to be met with transport from the Veterinary College. The station was small but we were soon surrounded by a noisy crowd of rikshaw men who, without any understandable English, were obviously anxious to take us anywhere we wanted to go. I said "Veterinary College," and they all indicated vociferously that they knew exactly where it was and pointed in several different directions, it was quite apparent that they hadn't the slightest idea of what I was talking about but they were eager to take us there. I was beginning to get worried. The station-master came out of his office and he was as deficient in communication as all the others were. I had to become a little forceful and indicate quite firmly that we were not going to let any of them take us anywhere. Half an hour must have elapsed and we were beginning to have visions of sitting on the station until the next day when we presumed that another Taj Express would be coming through. However, a cloud of dust appeared on the road to the station and a dilapidated old Ambassador car pulled up and an equally dilapidated driver slowly climbed out. I was relieved to see, under a thick coating of dust on the car door the words 'Veterinary College'. The crowd of clamorous rickshaw men, when they realised that our transport had arrived, melted away. I seem to remember that the college was some three or four miles from the station so where we would have got to if we had accepted the offers of one of the crowd, goodness only knows.

When we arrived at the college we were accommodated in a bungalow and lunch was provided. Two of the Senior Lecturers visited us to see if everything was in order and then announced that the whole college was to be assembled in the main lecture room ready for my lecture at 2p.m. This came as a bit of a shock as no one had invited me to give a lecture and I had assumed that I would just be expected to have discussions with those research workers involved in the work on chemotherapy. However, needs must when the devil drives and so at 2p.m. I walked into the theatre and after being introduced by the Dean to the assembled college, gave a lecture on the latest research in which I had been involved in Kenya and the CTVM. The staff seemed to be highly satisfied and we had tea and retired to our bungalow. The accommodation was spartan but we survived the night and in the morning were taken by road to Agra and checked into one of the prestigious hotels in the town, which is a very popular venue for tourists from all over the world. We recognised in the foyer, one of the passengers who sat near to us in the Taj Express the day before. We had exchanged a few courteous words on the train when he and his wife advised us on our choice of breakfast from the menu. Now he greeted us as long lost friends. He was the owner of the hotel and so we were well looked after during our sojourn there. We had already noticed a characteristic of India in the matter of wealth and poverty. There are some obviously wealthy people living in big houses with resplendent walled gardens. On one side of the wall, ostentatious plenty, and on the other side, abject poverty. It all seems to be taken as a matter of course. As we looked out of our hotel room window and over the high wall which surrounded the building we could see a drainage ditch in which peasant women were washing themselves and their family's clothing. Not far away, buffaloes were drinking and defecating in the same ditch. We had already seen from the train, villagers attending to their morning ablutions and also their other physiological functions.

Of course, we visited the great tourist attraction, the Taj Mahal. The Taj itself is a brilliant structure with its white marble and encrusting jewels and we were very pleased to have seen it. The approach to it, of borders and ornamental pools was, when we were there, a little shabby and neglected and the imposing archway entrance was beset by scores of vendors of photographs, souvenirs and knickknacks of all kinds.

From Agra we travelled by British Council car to Hissar and the Haryana Agricultural University. Here, we were quartered in the College Hostel, which was reasonable but somewhat reduced to the bare essentials. Dr O.P.Gautam,

Professor and Head of the Department of Veterinary Medicine was our host and we were made very welcome. The hostel was under the direction of a retired Indian Army officer known to all and sundry as 'The Captain'. The Captain's response to any request from us was invariably "Why not?" and then at length the required service or item was forthcoming. One of the commodities, which seemed to be in short supply in all the academic institutions, which we visited, was paper. This applied to toilet rolls, which were not much used among the indigenous population, and when they were produced, the rolls were very skimpy with a much larger inner cardboard roll than is usual in the West with a corresponding paucity of tissue. Occupying the next room to us in the hostel was an American scientist on a similar mission in his own field, as mine was in animal disease. We noted how much more lavishly he was treated by the American Embassy than we were by our High Commission. The latter organisation was housed fairly luxuriously in a compound of its own in New Delhi, where the many amenities such as swimming pools and sports facilities were jealously guarded against intrusion such as might be threatened by such visiting specialists as me and, I was given to understand, even against members of the British Council who appeared to be regarded as second class British. One of the great privileges that they enjoyed was the provision of duty free imported items.

Our next visit was to the Indian Veterinary Research Institute, IVRI, at Izatnagar in Uttar Pradesh. Here our hosts were Dr Subramanion and Dr Malhotra whom I have mentioned above and who spent some time with me in the CTVM in Edinburgh. They were doing splendid work in difficult conditions. The Institute has a close relationship with the Mukteswar Veterinary Research Institute, which was set up in the nineteenth century by the British and became one of the most prestigious veterinary research organisations in the tropical and sub-tropical world. The names of the directors and research workers in the Mukteswar Institute comprise an outstanding list of brilliance. When I was working in Africa the research publications coming out of the Institute were of top class quality and Africa had much for which to thank these eminent scientists. They did work on which much of our success was based. I expressed my interest in this institute to my colleagues at the IVRI and the Director, Dr C.M.Singh, kindly made arrangements for me and Kathy to be transported to Mukteswar and to stay there for a weekend.

We were taken by car from Izatnagar along a road that climbed into the foothills of the Himalayas. We were fascinated by the beauty of the masses of rhododendrons and the spectacular terracing of the steeply sloped mountainsides. The farmers, in cultivating their crops, must have had to descend and climb hundreds of metres every day. In the earlier part of this journey we passed through several villages. At one of these we stopped and explored the small dukas in one of which we bought some handkerchiefs that were very cheap. I have used these handkerchiefs ever since and some of them are still giving good service. In this village was a small railway station and so Kathy and I thought it would be a good opportunity for us to relieve our bladders. Our driver sought out the station-master who opened the station and unlocked the ladies toilet. I asked where the male facilities were. Whether there were any male facilities or not, I do not know but the station-master told me that I should use those provided for the ladies and so I did just that. The drive up the mountain road was not for the faint-hearted. There were numerous hairpin bends. The road was rough and narrow and I dreaded meeting a vehicle coming in the opposite direction. At some points the offside wheels were perilously near to a sheer drop of hundreds of feet. It was, to say the least, exciting. Our driver, however, took it all in his stride and eventually we arrived safely at Mukteswar which was a small settlement near the top of a mountain called Naini Tal, one of the foothills of the Himalayas, some 3,000 to 4,000 metres high.

As we arrived in the early evening it was very cold. There was a large fireplace in our bedroom but no fire. I asked the servant allocated to us if we could have some firewood. He went away and returned with an armful of large logs. Again we experienced the lack of adequate supplies of paper and so I spent some time whittling some of the smaller logs to produce a small pile of kindling and by dint of searching through our pockets and luggage obtained a few pieces of paper, including a few old bus tickets and receipts and attempted to light the fire. Our efforts were not very successful and so we went to the dining room where we were given a meal The next morning we were rewarded by the wonderful view from our bungalow of the great mountain range, of which the highest peak, Everest, had been conquered for the first time, by my second cousin, Sir Edmond Hillary, and Sherpa Tensing. Although our view did not include Everest, the view fulfilled for me, a lifelong dream.

I found the Institute most interesting. The library walls were adorned with large framed photographs of the directors, all British, who had established this laboratory which had contributed to so many branches of tropical veterinary medicine. It was pleasing for me to see that those now responsible for the work of this centre were proud of their predecessors and acknowledged freely the debt that they owed to them. The fact that I knew the work that had been done at Mukteswar and had actually met some of those whose photographs were on the walls established us as welcome visitors. This generous attitude we found also in other places we visited and in which I worked in India. In the Punjab, for example, those with whom we made contact, would point out railways, water schemes and other engineering developments, which they proudly informed us, were left for their benefit by the British at the time of the close down of the Raj. To me, having lived and worked in Africa before and after the change over from the colonial administration and independence, it was particularly gratifying when I thought back to the new African rulers who did their best to obliterate as much as possible of the signs of our colonial rule.

Our return to Izatnagar was, if anything, more frightening than the outward journey, but it was without untoward incident and we arrived back at the laboratory and our resthouse safely. We finalised our discussions and were booked on a night sleeper to New Delhi. Several of our friends and their wives from the Institute came to the station to see us off, even though the train was scheduled to leave at midnight. In the event, the train's arrival at Bareilly was delayed for about an hour as further back up the line it had been ordered to wait for the arrival of one of the government ministers who was having a send off party, presumably with his constituents. We felt concerned about keeping our hosts up so late at night but they insisted on seeing us safely settled onto the train. We found that we were assigned to a four-berth sleeper which already had two of the berths occupied. As morning dawned it transpired that our fellow passengers were two Delhi lawyers. Kathy found this a bit disconcerting but as we approached Delhi and ablutions had been performed, they proved to be very pleasant and sociable gentlemen who were most helpful in organising our disembarkation at the station.

In Delhi we had meetings with several government officials and discussions with Alan Jackson and others concerning our next visit that was to be to the Punjab Agricultural University, where I was to help in the setting up of specific experiments in Dr B.S.Gill's department. We were informed that for the duration of our stay in Ludiana a guest bungalow would be provided for our sole use. There would be full service but we would be wise to take our supplies of food from Delhi as the bungalow was on the college campus and most provisions available would not include many European foods. We had, therefore, to start on a shopping spree. Alan suggested that we make a list and he would try to buy the items from the shop in the British High Commission. He warned that he might not be successful, as while he had certain privileges in the high commission shop, they might not agree to sell if they knew that the goods were for us and not for him. I thought this an extraordinary state of affairs. Here was I, a so-called expert, sent to India by the British Government on a mission for the benefit of and at the request of, the Indian authorities and not entitled to purchase necessary food at the High Commission shop. It confirmed in me a feeling that I had acquired from other experiences in territories in which British interests were in the hands of a High Commission as opposed to an embassy. I have already commented on the marked difference in treatment of American nationals by their representatives abroad. Alan risked disapproval of the High Commission, he purchased our foodstuffs for us and we were packed off to Ludhiana.

When we arrived on the campus we were informed that the bungalow in which we were to stay was being repaired and redecorated and so was not available. We had, therefore, to share a bungalow with another member of the college staff. A delightful elderly couple, Musti and his wife, looked after us. They were very kind and did their best to see that we were as comfortable as possible. In the Veterinary department I was allocated a small laboratory and an assistant, a young Sikh vet, Mr Harsharanjit Gill Singh. This young graduate was very bright and always anxious to do anything he could to make things go well. He came to see us regularly in our bungalow and Kathy became very fond of him.

I spent approximately a month in the laboratory at this centre working on the plans for extending the current work in progress. I was instrumental in drawing up a detailed model for a future scheme which was based on a project submitted to ICAR by Dr B.S. Gill entitled 'Establishment of a Centre of Excellence for the study of the Haematozoon Diseases of Livestock and their Vectors'. This scheme was under consideration by ICAR but it was unlikely that funding would be available for a further sixteen months. I, therefore, had to advise on the work to be carried out in preparation for the final approval of the scheme.

I do not intend to elaborate on this work here as the details of all my investigations and advice are contained in a forty-three page report to the British Council, and through them to The Overseas Development Ministry of the United Kingdom. This report covers observations and advice on all the research institutes visited and includes recommendations on staff, equipment, research methods and objectives and ancillary activities.

Some aspects of my visit and experiences and my reactions to the conditions we encountered are, perhaps, of general interest and I will touch on these and will then include a record of impressions written by Kathy who, perforce, was left to her own devices when I was at work. I was struck by the difficulties that faced the local professional workers and the stoicism and ingenuity with which they overcame them. They were obviously grateful to the British Government for the help given and to me personally and to Kathy for being so friendly to them when they felt that she would have been more comfortable at home in England. When we were on the institute campuses they were most anxious to make us feel at home and welcomed us into their own homes to meet their families. They were most solicitous as to our health and wellbeing, adjuring us to be careful what we ate and drank. In this respect we were very lucky until very shortly before we were due to come home when, knowing that I was interested in art, Harsharenjit was anxious for me to visit a friend who was an artist in Ludhiana, who had a studio in the main street behind his father's shop. His forte was in copying pictures by the great masters such as Rembrandt, Titian, Leonardo da Vinci and the Impressionists. The pictures were brilliantly executed and I particularly remember a copy of the Mona Lisa. I don't know where he found a market for his work. However, before we left, the artist's father asked if we would have some refreshment. I politely declined but he pressed me to have something to drink and suggested a Coca-Cola. I thought that, as it was bottled it should be safe and so I accepted. The old man went out into the street and came back with bottles for all four of us and flicked off the crown tops with an opener and we drank out of the bottles. As we left, I noticed outside the door was a case of Coke bottles, presumably the source of the ones which we had consumed. Along the sidewalk at the edge of the baked earth roadway ran the open town sewer. I was apprehensive and my apprehensions were confirmed in the middle of the night when I had violent bowel pains with diarrhoea and vomiting. I was very ill and spent two days in bed. Musti brought for me supplies of curd, which he assured me, was a specific for my condition. My colleagues from the lab, organised into watches, ensured that at least one of them was constantly at my bedside. I had to get out of bed and stagger to the bathroom at frequent intervals. I think that on the first day this operation was repeated some twenty times but my solicitous friends sat stolidly on. Of course, I recovered and made my rather frail stagger to the lab on the third day. So concerned was Dr Gill that he detailed one of my assistants to accompany me to the loo attached to the lab which was of the Asiatic squat stance style, whenever I felt the urge to go.

I was very interested to visit the large animal clinic run by the veterinary faculty, which was a hive of activity from morning to night every day. Here the students, supervised by their lecturers, treated animals belonging to the local populace, suffering from many infections or other conditions, very commonly lameness or accidental wounds, digestive disorders or even malnutrition and parasitic infestation. The owners, some of whom had walked for miles with their cattle or water buffaloes, gathered in the compound outside the clinic and patiently sat around on the ground and even rolled themselves in a blanket and slept overnight with their animals. In some cases, where surgical operations were necessary, the owner and animal might spend some days in the compounds but, as far as I could determine, there were no complaints.

Part of the College campus was like a small village with a row of small shops, which supplied the basic requirements of the inhabitants such as flour, sugar, chapattis and other household requirements. My observations in this area showed, once more, the phenomenon of the countrywide shortage of paper goods. Commodities such as rice, maize and wheat flour were dispensed in bags rolled into a pointed shape, such as was common in England, when I was a boy and went to buy sweeties. On the campus, however, the paper used was examination papers from the university examinations, covered by the laborious script of anxious students sitting their degrees. I got hold of a few of these bags and tried to decipher the answers written, no doubt under great stress.

The roads in India can provide nightmare conditions for anyone wealthy enough to own a car. They are usually packed with carts and other vehicles drawn by oxen, buffaloes, camels, sweating human beings and motor scooters. There are some cars, mostly Ambassadors and mammy wagons, which are old lorries converted to act as buses. Little attention seems to be paid to any rules of the road if, indeed, there are any. I went one day with Dr Gill to Amritsar, the important Sihk centre with its spectacular golden temple, to discuss some matters relevant to my terms of reference. It was one of the rare occasions when he was granted the use of the College Ambassador car. I was welcomed and very graciously treated by the Government officials with whom we had meetings and we were invited to the home of one of them for a meal. The journey there and back was in my estimation about two hundred miles. It was a long, hot and tiring day, but it was most interesting. On this trip we stopped at various places and B.S.Gill pointed out many features characteristic of the Punjab, which is sometimes described as the main agricultural provider for the subcontinent. One of these was the means of irrigating wide areas using canals and pumping systems, which had been installed by British engineers.

Kathy and I would take a walk round the campus and village in the early evening before dark. Sometimes, Harsharanjit would accompany us. He would tell us of his family and home in the country, giving us an insight into the difficulties of rural life in the Punjab. I remember him telling us how his parents utilised the dung heap to generate methane gas, which was piped to their house and used for cooking and heating. One day we walked through the park that had obviously been laid out with pools and waterfalls but had fallen into an unkempt state. The channels were cracked and certainly could not hold water and while there were lamp standards for electrical lighting of the area, few, if any, were functional. At the bases of these standards were cover plates, presumably to give access to the wiring. Many of these were broken off so exposing the wiring and the connections. I pointed out to Harsharanjit this rather dangerous state of affairs and expressed my alarm that they could cause electrocution, especially of children. He replied laconically, "Life is cheap in India." There were a few beds containing some hardy rose bushes bravely lending colour to the rather drab scene. This gave the answer to a question that we had asked ourselves about the bunches of roses that Harsharanjit brought to Kathy on occasion and which helped to brighten up our quarters.

When I was away at the lab in the daytime, there was little that Kathy could do to pass away the hot and stuffy hours in our lodging. The garden had no shady trees or other means of protection from the scorching sun and reading in our dull rooms soon palled. Kathy, after organising some of the local labourers into the job of emptying the furniture and carpets from our rooms and giving them all a spring clean, probably the first such disruption they had suffered since the house was built, decided to write an account of our Indian experience. So she purchased an exercise book from one of the dukas in the village and started to write. I'm very glad she did because it made me aware how our visit affected her. I am, therefore, going to include her account in this story, verbatim.

This does, of course, mean that there will be a certain amount of duplication but it does express Kathy's impressions.

Here, therefore, is much of our visit seen through Kathy's eyes.

It took me a long time to decide to go to India. I didn't want to go but on the other hand I didn't want to stay on my own for five months. Neither did I want to spend time going around to stay with relations, tho' I could have stayed the whole time with my sister, Nancy. Jack wanted me to go as it would be his last professional assignment abroad and it would be much nicer for us to go together to see India and we would be able to speak of our experiences together in our later days. Having returned to the UK I'm pleased that I went, as we were company for each other, and would have shared experiences to reminisce about. I think that we felt a certain amount of isolation, I more than Jack who was busy most days. We had to go through the usual injection routine and all the business of banks, insurance and clothing and the complications of leaving the house into which we were barely settled. We had not been to India, but as long as I can remember, people had told me what a fabulous country it is and I really thought I should not miss this chance to see for myself. Well, now I have seen it! There is a saying 'See Naples and die'. If you see India, you are damned lucky if you don't die. After living most of our married life in Africa, we did not expect it all to be easy going. Travel never is, and we were quite clued up about living in tropical conditions. We were quite prepared to accept discomforts, heat, food, hard travel and a bit of sickness perhaps, but the isolation and lack of hygiene were most unpleasant. The living standards of very many people were so low and for millions of people there are no standards at all. Let me make it quite clear from the start that the people with whom we came into contact fell over backwards to make us as comfortable as possible. The sad thing is they just did not know what we expect to be normal; jugs without handles, dirty tumblers and crockery seem to be the norm. I often visited the kitchen to get boiled water (I watched it boil) and at the same time while waiting for the kettle to boil I had a good look around. The crocks were washed up in an old chipped sink, no dishcloth (maybe as well), no soap and a horrible old drying up cloth which I think made things more contaminated than they were to start with. Tablecloths and napkins were always on the dining table but they were old, badly washed and of a medium grey colour. I bought two napkins for our own use, but enough about that. I don't think I can describe what I've seen this last ten days. There is nothing pleasant, beautiful or nice. The trees are not yet in leaf or flower, apart from a bit of hibiscus and bauhinia, and they are too dusty to touch. Even the birds look as though they need to be brushed. Speaking of birds, one place where we stayed was swarming with green parrots. They roosted in some gum trees close to the guesthouse in which we were staying. Each morning at dawn they screeched off to the wheat fields and returned at sunset. This was in the Punjab State where the wheat and other grain crops were magnificent, much better crops than we see in this country. The ugly old vultures seem to sit for hours in the trees, just waiting, what for I never found out and I didn't see anything worth waiting for.

We visited the great Taj Mahal in Agra; fantastic but like everywhere else, the approach was thick with vendors plying the usual trash with people rushing up and offering their services as guides (unofficial of course). We were told, "Ah, but you should see it in the moonlight," I'm sure that must be better because you wouldn't be able to see the muck. Before going in to see the tomb we had to put some rather dirty cloth overshoes over our shoes. They were made in stripes, checks and even tartan. No reverence was displayed about the great Taj, it seemed to be treated as a rather vulgar money making tourist business. I'm sure the Mumtaz would have turned in her gem-encrusted tomb if she could have seen all the activity.

Our journey from Delhi (via Muthura) was by train and we had to start very early in the morning so that we could not have breakfast in the hotel. Delhi station is a story in itself. The platforms are covered by what look like large bundles of rags but underneath we could see people sleeping. One had to step over and around them. They were awaiting trains and of course could not afford to spend a night in a hostel. They just had to get down on any old mat or, if they were lucky, a bedroll and sleep the night on the spot. There is nothing illegal about this squatting and nobody tries to move them on. Where could they go? There were hundreds of them. There were little stalls where tea was brewed for sale and some guys had little fires and were cooking chapattis and other spicy snacks for the waiting masses. People were urinating at any available place. A porter, who seemed to know which train went from which platform, appointed himself to our service, grabbed our bags and heaved them onto his head and made off into the crowd. Fortunately, we could see our luggage above the masses and we followed as best we could. The atmosphere was very unpleasant but we got to the train and felt, as we boarded it, that we had got over another hurdle. Little did we know what a lot more hurdles lay ahead of us for the next few months.

Our seats had been reserved for us and so all seemed well but we were thirsty and hungry. Soon after the train had started we heard an Indian servant taking orders for breakfast. Across the gangway a pleasant couple ordered omelettes and coffee. These passengers, presumably a Hindi and his wife, seemed very confident and at home with this breakfast routine and so we ordered the same meal. The meal eventually arrived on a rather nasty looking battered aluminium tray. As the waiter could not get the complete order on the tray, he had the omelettes in the other hand. I'm not trying to make this sound any worse than it looked. There was a plate on his hand with one of those tin covers intended to keep the food hot. There seemed to be a frill hanging over the edge of the plate onto his hand and as he approached our table I saw that it was part of my omelette. My breakfast comprised a very indifferent cup of coffee and a piece of dry toast. I couldn't bear to look at my plate and turned away to look through the window only to see, squatting at the side of the rail track, men and children performing their morning defecation. This was the time of day when nature seemed to call. As these people of the plains have only poor dwellings of very insubstantial construction they have no running water or regular sanitation and make do with the village pond, which they share with the water buffaloes. I lit a cigarette only to be told, "I wish you would stop smoking, dear." It seemed to be the only sterile thing for miles.

We had to break our journey at a place called Muthura,

where we were to pay a short visit to the College of Veterinary Science and Animal Husbandry. Plans had been made for us to be met by someone from the college and taken the next ten to fifteen miles by car. There was no sign of anyone, who might be expecting us, only bicycle rickshaws. No one spoke any English, the train had gone and we didn't know where the college was. We had a harassing half-hour fighting off the rickshaw men. Then a scruffy driver turned up and we saw he was from the college by the lettering on the vehicle. And so off we went, feeling hot, hungry and more than a little doubtful about our prospects in India. We were given some food and told that the college was waiting for this certain Dr Wilde to give a lecture. I'm ashamed to say that I dozed through most of it. About a kilometre away, there was a most interesting museum full of exhibits, some of which dated back to 200 BC. We were given a guided tour of this museum before we left Muthura by road for Agra.

By this time I had developed a very heavy cold and my first day in Agra was spent in bed. Incidentally, my cold lasted three weeks but I had to keep going as every day we had our itinerary to follow and any change or delay could mess things up badly. Back to Delhi again. Everything, at that time, seemed to involve visits to Delhi.

Our next move was to visit and stay on a university campus where Jack was to be working. This place was Haryana in Hissar. The people were very kindly and helpful and anxious to please but again fell short on essentials. Our journey to Haryana was by car over a bad road with lots of traffic. We weaved about and in places missed oncoming lorries by the odd four or five inches. Transport varied from pony and trap, buffalo cart, camel cart, bicycles, rickshaws and dozens of motor scooters. I think motor scooters must be in a ratio of thirty to one with cars. It is a common sight to see several members of a family on one scooter. Father drives, possibly with two small children sitting on the tank; two small children sit behind father and mother in a flowing sari sits side-saddle behind them all. All the ladies sit side-saddle and appear to be calm and comfortable but I don't think they would be so placid on the roads in Britain dressed in their flowing robes. The food in Haryana was grim. The menu was about the same every day. The chap in charge was an ex army officer and was known as 'the Captain'. He had once been to the UK and stayed in Birmingham. 'Wonderful place and wonderful people'. He would exclaim. He never offered us anything but if we requested something he usually obliged, saying, "Why not?" The man who was in charge of the department in which Jack was involved reminded me of Dick Emery when he wore the prominent false teeth. He was a very pleasant and kind man but had the awful habit, which I have observed in Asians in East Africa, of hawking up phlegm from the back of the throat. This he did about every seventeen seconds. Very off putting! He told us that his wife had died about five years before. She must have been a wreck, poor thing, probably could stick it no longer. In this campus house very little cleaning was ever done and as in all places where we stayed, I washed all things down with Dettol or Savlon and used articles of clothing such as disposable pants, socks and pyjama bottoms as cleaning cloths. Action started at about 6.30 in the morning when a boy brought tea. We drank it while we were still half asleep and so didn't notice the weakness of the tea or the quality of the cups and saucers. About ten minutes later a chap scratched at the door and shouted 'Cloths' meaning, 'Have you any washing?' Another ten minutes and a scruffy old sweeper man came in to clean the loo and shower cubicle. These servants always referred to this area as the bathroom. It comprised a grey cement floor with a drain in one corner. The sweeper used to throw a pail of water over the floor and at the loo and then roughly wiped round with a dirty old cloth which was used for the loo, wash basin, the floor and the table in the bedroom. The process took about five minutes flat and that was the cleaning for the day. I always made our own beds and went round with Dettol and disposable underpants. They proved most useful and I would recommend anyone who was to visit India in the same way as we did to take a supply of old, unwanted cloths and worn out underwear. There was no shortage of mosquitoes and there were no nets. The mosquitoes were so big they seemed to me like flying prawns. We were suffering a spell of cold weather; some kind soul brought us a one bar electric fire but the power failed so often that from time to time we had to get into our beds with our dressing gowns on. Snow and hail fell on the plains while we were in Haryana and this was unheard of. Some local people expressed the view that the end of the world must be at hand. Next door to us was an American scientist. I was telling him how our loo leaked onto the floor. He said we were lucky as his didn't work at all. All the loos where we stayed were European pedestal style; they didn't all work but then, as the locals were wont to say, 'This is India'. What a sad reflection.

Between assignments we went to New Delhi for a short break and the comfort of a first class hotel. This was bliss but the stays were usually of short duration, as we had to be off again to the next campus. The 12th March 1979 is a day that I shall never forget. We had to leave Claridges Hotel where we had a pleasant room, a hot delightful bath in a marble bathroom with all mod cons and where the cuisine was of a high standard. Unfortunately our departure had to be in the early hours of the morning as we were booked on the Bareilly Express scheduled to leave New Delhi station at 6.30a.m. First class accommodation had been booked on this train for us. A car from the British Council collected us from the hotel well before sunrise and took us to the station. Here our nightmare started. Fortunately, the driver of the car who was a very pleasant fellow, accompanied us into the station and found out which was our train. Here we had to make the usual progress over and around the mass of sleeping bodies with inadequate lighting on the platforms. Our driver assured us that the completely dark and unilluminated line of coaches was our train. When I saw what we were going to travel in, I was sure that someone had made a big mistake. I was terrified. Our driver, whose name we now knew was Gupta, made enquiries and with his help we found our coach and the compartment with our name on the door. There were no lights in the train but as a smoker, I had a box of matches and was able to shed a faint flickering light on our surroundings. What we could see was depressing. The place was filthy. Gupta was obviously embarrassed by the state of the compartment. However, we managed to get our luggage aboard and the driver tried to dust the seats with his handkerchief but he made no impression. We were repeatedly assured that this was the Bareilly Express. After about ten minutes we felt a movement of the train and realised that we were being coupled up to a steam engine. Then the lights came on. Gupta politely asked if he might take his leave and then we were on our own. Thinking that if this really was an express train and, as we had been told, the journey from Delhi to Bareilly was only 157 miles, we could resign ourselves to four or five hours in this mess. We perched on the edge of the seat and awaited the arrival of daylight. When it came we could see the full horrible state of affairs. What we hadn't seen in the dark was there all around us and we could do nothing about it. From ceiling to floor was filth. There were four old fans in the ceiling, which had long since ceased to function. The bunks were covered in old leather, the original colour being quite indistinguishable. There were two upper and two lower bunks that were more like benches with no padding. The window had iron bars fitted and the glass was covered with mud and dirt no doubt thrown at them by children. The inside of the window was well covered by squashed flies and dirt. The floor was thick with dirt and there were wet patches, which were due either to spilling or people relieving themselves or both. The train had filled with local people and our coach, supposedly first class, was packed. From time to time people pushed against our door in an effort to enter but Jack had managed to lock it. We eventually began to move and the Bareilly Express proceeded at a snail's pace and literally stopped at every village on the route and often at places which didn't even sport a single dwelling. When we were moving we opened the window a little to let in some air as it was now insufferably hot. As soon as we approached a village the flies swarmed in and we had to close the window and swat the flies. Fortunately we had a newspaper and so could use that, rolled up as a fly swatter. We now could see why the windows were almost obliterated with swatted flies.

The time came when we felt the need to relieve our bladders and so Jack opened the door and went in search of the loo. He virtually had to force his way down the corridor that was packed with bodies on the floor and even filling the luggage racks at the end of the coach and also the space between the coaches and around and in the loos. When he managed to get back he said it was no good my trying to go to the loo. The time came when I just had to do something about it. Fortunately, I had handy in our luggage, a plastic shower cap and so we brought this into use. Jack held it at the back and I held it at the front and then we emptied it through the window and let the shower cap follow on. Jack made a joking remark about who would be wearing it next. By this time we were getting very grimy. The heat was such that we had to open the window for short periods between stops and then the effluent from the steam engine blew into the compartment carrying with it the odds and ends that blow out of steam engines. At one point a splash of hot water blew in through the window over me. It was the only water we experienced on the whole journey. Towards the end of this nightmare I just could not believe it could be true. I wondered if I was really dead and this was hell. I felt that God had forsaken us.

At about 3.30 that afternoon we felt the train coming to a stop for about the twenty-fifth time and there on a board, printed in large letters was the information 'Bareilly Junction'. This was our destination and I calculated that our average speed on the journey had been a little short of eighteen mph. We were met by two research officers from Izatnagar who had been waiting for us at Bareilly for three hours. They were horrified when they knew that we had been booked on this train, which had a notorious reputation. One of the two was Dr Malhotra who had been a student at the CTVM under the guidance of Jack. They told us that they had actually written to the British Council on the occasion when another visitor had been booked on this train by the Council telling them about the deficiencies of the Bareilly Express and suggesting a much more efficient train which was not only faster but also left Delhi at a more civilised hour. Jack brought this fact to the attention of the British Council at a later date. Malhotra and his colleague, Dr Subramanion, were very concerned for us. Fully aware of what we must have endured on our journey. I must say that they were two of the kindest people one could wish to meet. They drove us to the guesthouse on the Izatnagar campus where a very welcome pot of tea appeared and it was then that I took a Valium as I could not stop trembling. We dropped off our clothes in a heap and got under a shower and began to feel human again. These two men and their wives could not have done more for us. They were wonderful. We went early to bed and had a restful night.

When moving about in a new country, it's amazing how each new experience seems to make the last one less important. Here we were in a place Izatnagar, where we awoke to find that our first day there was a public holiday or as the inhabitants called it, 'Holi day'. This particular day was the one where every one goes slightly mad throwing coloured dyes at each other. Everyone wears, on this day, old clothes, which become multicoloured by the end of the celebrations. Needless to say, with our limited wardrobe, we kept a low profile, which gave us the opportunity to unwind and rest. However, we did see some oddly coloured, people, cars, scooters and even cows. There seem to be so many religions in India and they all have their own gods and goddesses and it seems that every few weeks or so, it is some one's special day. Religion seems to play a big part in the lives of the people. To us it seemed a little artificial and not very attractive, especially when some temples start belting out prayers at very early hours of the morning by means of high-powered loud speakers.

It was from Izatnagar that our hosts took us on a mountain trip to see the Himalayas. Our transport was a Dodge van belonging to the Institute. We went round more hairpin bends than most people have seen. Up and up until we were at 7,000 feet. It was quite cold and although we had a wood burning fireplace in our room it didn't do much towards warming us as the wood was not very plentiful and what we had was in such large lumps that we found it difficult to make a good fire. You might be thinking, "Why didn't you cut it?" but you can't make much headway with a penknife. Anyway, the mountains were out of this world; in fact I had the feeling that it probably was another world. The mountains are so huge and so high even when seen from so far away as we were.

The food at this place was too bad to describe but we were invited out for some of the meals for the short time we were there. The breakfasts, however, we had to suffer. The hills and valleys all around us were terraced and cultivated and it made us wonder how on earth the farmers worked the land. It was a great place for apple orchards and I'm sure that at the right season the blossom must have been a sight to see.

We had to return to Izatnagar and we were told that it was worse going down than coming up. Our informants did not exaggerate. At some of the bends in the road there was a drop of 1000 feet or more and the wheels of the van were inches from the edge. Again I took Valium and didn't feel nervous. Jack was shattered by the time we got to the bottom as we had an extra passenger on our return and he, Jack, was pressed against the left door and so had a birds-eye view of the sheer drops a few inches away.

Back at Izatnagar, we had a bath, the first for three days and a meal and then went to bed for an hour or two. We were booked on a sleeper to return to Delhi after midnight. Our hosts and their wives came to collect us at midnight to take us to Bareilly Junction. The train was one hour late. Some Government Minister was responsible for the delay but our hosts stayed with us and saw us on the train before returning to their homes. We were shown into our compartment, which was four berthed, two berths being occupied. As it was the middle of the night, we didn't put on much light in case we might disturb the two sleeping passengers, but kicked off our shoes and got onto our bunks. I slept quite a while but imagine my surprise when I awakened in the morning and found two Indian gents opposite me! We all had our bed tea, rubbed our eyes and weighed each other up. The gentlemen then went, one by one, to the toilet and dressed and really we found them very nice, but even so, I couldn't help feeling as a female, the odd one out. A car from the British Council met us and took us to Claridges Hotel.

On our first stay in New Delhi we were booked into the Janpath Hotel, which we did not like and so after that we were accommodated in Claridges Hotel that was superior and we were made very comfortable there. Our room was spacious and the *en suite* bathroom was resplendent in white marble. The hotel was air-conditioned and we could have meals brought to our room at no extra cost. The dining room was pleasant with a live orchestra at lunch and dinner. I thought that I recognised one of the instrumentalists and so I asked him if he had ever played on ships. He said that at one time he had played in the Uganda. So that was where we had seen him before which is quite amazing as the lapse of time between when we were travelling in the Uganda and when we were in India must have been about ten years. How we enjoyed the luxury although it was only for a few days, clean bath towels each day, clean bed linen every night, lashings of hot water and a large thermos of iced water to drink. There was a radio and also a TV in our room but they were not of much interest to us. Our short stay gave us the chance to do a little shopping and as our next stay was to be in Ludhiana where we were to be for at least a month we bought such items as water sterilising tablets, soap and some tins of food as special treats. Some of the foodstuffs we managed to get from the British High Commission shop, which is only for the service of the 'crème de la crème', the officials of the BHC and their families. This transaction had to be carried out with some secrecy by our friend, Alan Jackson in the British Council. This was a little nauseating to Jack who, as a British expert, sent out by the British Government to India was, apparently a second rate citizen in terms of the High Commission hierarchy. It was degrading to have to go through this back door arrangement to obtain a few piffling items through the BHC shop.

The time had now come for us to depart once more for the real India. And we were taken by British Council car from the metropolis to Ludhiana, a journey of about six hours. Our driver was smart and pleasant and pointed out to us the features, which he thought might interest us. He had been born in Burma and certainly resembled his countrymen. At the far end of this journey we had to keep asking local people the whereabouts of the Punjab Agricultural University. No one seemed to have heard of it. Ludhiana is an industrial town and on the outskirts were scores of small factories. We were told that they could make anything from screws to tractors. I think, perhaps, they were right. Some of these workshops were at the roadside and the conditions in which the men were working seemed to be grim. Young boys of ten to twelve years old were wielding heavy hammers and we were told that they did this for 8 hours a day.

We had travelled miles over the plains and we saw better fields of grain than any I had seen before. The Punjabis had built canals so that there was no shortage of water for the crops as

310

they have a pretty good idea what the weather is going to be like. There is no wind or rain during the growing season; consequently you can see all the crops standing like ramrods. The farmers know to the day when the crops are ready to be harvested.

There are all sorts of slogans on placards at the roadside but no one seems to bother about safety in driving. One slogan said, 'Drive like HELL and you are sure to get there'. Our driver was very good and got us to our desired destination safely. We had been told that there was a guesthouse for our sole use with servants and transport for the duration of our stay at PAU. Everything would be to our satisfaction. Of course the intention was there but the actuality, as in many other things we have found in our travels overseas, was not quite up to the intention. We soon realised that there was quite a lot of sorting out to be done. We were greeted by the old man in charge, 'Masih'. He was white haired and seemed tired in the heat of the day. In the sitting room of the guesthouse was a group of doctors and the Acting Dean, waiting to welcome us. We could see that the atmosphere was somewhat apologetic; something was wrong. We were informed that there was another occupant of the guesthouse and all we were offered was a room with adjacent bathroom, which we would have to share with some unknown person. I turned it down flat. A third, bigger room with another bathroom was then offered to us and, on the understanding that we would not have to share the bathroom, we accepted. It appears that there was another guesthouse being built for visiting academicals but this would not be ready for another month or two. They did offer to take us to see two other empty houses, which were in a rather poor state, but they could get them white-washed for us. We decided against that and settled for the room in the guesthouse.

My first activity was to send out for scouring powder, disinfectant, paraffin and dusters and I cleaned the place thoroughly paying special attention to the loo in the bathroom, which was of the European style. The bath itself had to be seen to be believed. I can't describe its condition. I demanded that it should be scoured out completely and immediately a student arrived accompanied by a cleaner with a bottle of acetic acid

311

with which he was instructed to scrub out the bath. The job was done and made little, if any, difference to the appearance of the bath but at least we knew that it was chemically clean. Then we had trouble with the hot water, electric geyser. It was leaking over the floor and the wiring was exposed. It appeared to us to be messy and a potential danger. A workman came and took his life in his hands and he managed to achieve a little improvement but the drip, while being reduced a little, continued to wet the floor but we just had to live with it. We met a certain degree of fatalism among the ordinary people. At one place we saw a man trying to weld the tank of his motor scooter with the tank half full of petrol. We moved away rather smartly. The attitude as expressed by one of our Asian friends to us was that life is cheap in India. On the first evening the power failed. There was an old oil lamp in the room but it had no paraffin in it. Fortunately, I remembered the bottle brought in for the cleaning and there was some paraffin still left in the bottle. We filled the lamp and then the power came on again. I left the oil lamp in the bedroom and then when the power failed once, twice and sometimes three times in an evening we could, at least have a little illumination.

Masih produced a reasonable meal and as we were very hungry, we tucked in. We went to bed that night feeling a bit fed up with India but slept quite well, not a bad bed, but double. Next day was some other god's holy day and as most people were having a day off, I spent a lot of time cleaning furniture. I made a great cleaning cloth by cutting open a pair of nylon socks and then stitching them together down the side. This may sound trivial to anyone reading this; but believe me that was a very valued possession. With this old cloth I washed the headboard of the bed, the chair arms the table and all the doorknobs and handles. There was a carpet on the floor and a sweeper came in with a home made broom. All he seemed to be doing was raising a lot of dust and spreading it about to settle on the bed and everywhere. I felt it wasn't for me to tell servants what to do and I didn't want to hurt his feelings by making too many obvious changes myself. After two days I found that this chap had no feelings at all. I think that if I'd kicked his backside he would have said, 'Thank you, Memsahib', and smiled. I decided to take a new line. I called up the dhobi and told him and the sweeper to lift up the carpet and take it out and beat the hell out of it. They were flabbergasted! They didn't know how to start this project and so I took on the job of charge-hand. It was very hot and although I was dripping with perspiration I got them going like cats on a hot tin roof. The dhobi was a very slight thin man and I felt a bit sorry for him. Then I mixed a good strong solution of Dettol and hot water and made them scrub the whole floor of our room before bringing the carpet back. By the time they had got everything back in place, I had these chaps laughing and they seemed to think I was a great memsahib and thanked me for driving them. Sad, isn't it? Lots of flowers were blooming in the garden and I picked two big pots full and the room took on a different appearance. Even our Mr Mustih came and admired the room and in his broken English said, "Ah it is very beautiful, the cleanest room in the house." I spent a lot of my time in it as it was too hot to sit outside and the flies were tiresome.

By this time I had got to know two chaps from the lab who were outstanding for their kindness and patience. One was a Hindu called Dr Bhattacharyulu but I called him Charlie. The other was a young Sikh, twenty-two years old and his name was Harsharnjit Gill Singh but as it was also difficult for me to remember I called him Harchi. I have never met two such nice people. Charlie was the senior and was doing work in which Jack was interested. Jack said that his lab was dirty and he went to town about it and about the importance of cleanliness in the laboratory. How could they expect any reliable results to come out of a set-up like this? Poor Charlie listened attentively to every word of the criticism and accepted it all in good part. He seemed to be so pleased that someone was helping him and trying to advance his work. He was from southern India and although he knew English very well and even gave his lectures in English, he spoke very quickly and hardly opened his mouth when speaking. I found him most difficult to understand and even after seeing him every day for nearly a month, I still couldn't distinguish his words. He had a nice wife and three small sons and was finding it hard to pay for them to get a good education. Charlie and his wife were most anxious for us to have tea with them and to see their house. We went but said that we would like to have a cup of tea with them but would rather not have anything to eat. The house was on the outskirts of the town, very small, one living room, one bedroom and a kitchen. It was very hot and seemed to be hemmed in by many other buildings. However, one could go up some steps outside which led onto a flat roof overlooking the park, and what a park. All was quite clean but Charlie's wife had gone to the expense of buying a lot of sticky buns for tea. Where she procured them I hate to think. We politely declined to eat but no doubt the children would have a treat after we had left. They were so delighted that we had come to take tea with them that as we left they insisted on presenting us with some mementoes. Sadly they were not particularly of use to us and were things which might well make our luggage overweight, and so we eventually gave them to an Asian chambermaid in Claridges Hotel.

Now about Harchi, he was my favourite. Maybe, his age and attitude reminded me of my own sons. He was my brown-eyed boy. He was married and his wife, Geeta was studying home science. She had spent eight years and been to school in the UK and had just that bit more about her than the other women I met. Harchi spoke better English than his colleague and I found that if I wanted to purchase anything his advice was invaluable and he would make sure that what I bought was right and at the right price. He soon became my right-hand man and he or Geeta would bring me a large bunch of roses nearly every day. His parents were farmers and lived quite a long way off near the Pakistan border. We often pulled his leg when he made mistakes in his English but he took it in good part and was only too pleased to be corrected. We are hoping that he will be able to come to Britain to further his education. Geeta is coming very soon, as her father is a British citizen. I hope we shall be able to help them as they have helped us. Each time I thanked him for the flowers his answer was always, "No problem, it is my duty." After being at this place for a week we had got on very well with Masih who turned out to be a very good cook. I think he must have thought that we were the right type as he had been a servant to British people in the days of the Raj. Someone had told us that he had a wife and in the visitors' book most guests had referred to Mr and Mrs Masih.

It was at this point that he told us about his troubles. He had two sons who lived in Lucknow and one of them was in hospital having kidney stones removed. His wife was in Lucknow with the son but was to return soon. She arrived one morning at 7.30 after an overnight journey on the train. From the minute she arrived she seemed to have brought new life to the place. Her first job was to get her husband tidied up. She sent him for a bath and got him dressed in clean clothes and he seemed so happy to have her back. She was a treasure and her cooking was delicious. The two of them worked together so well although it was only Mr who was officially employed but all the work she did, and that was at least fifty per cent, was in order to enable her husband to retain the job. They were marvellous and we became very fond of them. Her name was Shanti.

It was about this time when we heard that another guest was expected to arrive the next day. This, of course, caused us a good deal of worry. Three bedrooms and two bathrooms to be shared between three reservations! The guest was a male so surely the obvious thing was for him to share the Sikh's bathroom but not a bit of it. The Sikh just locked his door and refused to share his bathroom with anyone. The new guest arrived, Professor Watkin Williams, from Reading University, a man of fifty-seven years or so. As soon as he came the situation was explained to him and he was very upset. However, we could not dream of him having to have an argument with the Sikh and agreed to his sharing with us. It was a case of calling 'All clear' each time we had used it. We became very friendly with the new guest, as can be imagined, when we were all thrown together in this situation. There was some embarrassment at first but we got over it and the incident was put into the back of our minds but we did feel that the sooner Jack could finish his job the better and we began to think in terms of going home. During this period, our Asian friends were in and out of our quarters many times a day to see if they could do anything else to help. Then we both had upset bowels and that didn't help things. We had with us a bottle of whisky and one of gin. They were litre bottles and so permitted a drink most evenings. The Prof. also had some whisky, a bottle of brandy and some nice chocolates which he had bought at Heathrow. He was only with us for less than a week and we had some pleasant social evenings. I still say that the Asians with whom we were associated were very patient, very helpful and very kind. They were so anxious to please, but they were unable to get things done. Jack learned that there was a good deal of personal rivalry between the senior members of the various faculties in the university and influence was brought to bear on the Dean and the administration by various devious means. He thought that this had been at the bottom of the trouble about our accommodation. B.S. Gill, apparently, was having a lot of trouble with those responsible for the allocation of funds and some so called colleagues had ganged up to thwart his ambitions to transform his faculty into a centre of excellence in animal disease research. Jack told me that he felt that this unfortunate chicanery existed at all levels and he felt depressed about getting his views accepted in the higher levels of the Indian Government, because of the methods of influencing the higher echelons in the administration.

The weather was heating up. Once or twice we had thunder and every time a black cloud appeared the power went off. I was hoping for a good shower of rain, firstly to cool things and secondly to wash the trees and the ground but we didn't have much rain. During one night we had a few hail storms and our Mr Masih thought that would cool us (even he felt the heat) but the next day was just as hot as ever. The Indian summer was almost here, the trees and shrubs were coming into bloom and the mango trees were fairly groaning with the weight of their blossom. Our stay was well into the last half and we were beginning to think about the UK. Up to this point we hadn't thought much about home, it would have made me homesick. We had very few letters from home and were getting anxious for just a bit of news. Someone lent us a radio but reception was bad and when we did get world news it contained little about Britain.

Prof Williams had to move on. He was going to Hissar where we had already spent a week. We could let him know what to expect. We missed him a lot as he was the only person we had met from our own country outside New Delhi. We gave him a present which he put in his bag and we assured him that he wouldn't see many of them in India. It was a precious toilet roll.

We now had a definite date for our departure. The British Council was sending a car to return us to Delhi. When members of the department to which we were attached heard of the date all hell was let loose. All our associates insisted on giving us a party and wanted to hold it in one of the halls of residence on the campus. We were a little bit worried because we knew that they would go to a lot of trouble to gather together the appropriate eatables which would be an expense to them and be of unknown origin. Jack told the organisers that he didn't want another bout of bowel upset and was being very careful what he ate and where he ate it. Nothing would put them off and it was decided to have the party in the guest house where it would be prepared by Mashi and his wife. Preparations started at 7.30a.m., Mr and Mrs Masthi were going at it all day. We gave each of them a wee dram later in the day as they were exhausted, but the whole thing was out of our hands. They said that they were very happy to be doing this for us. Shanti was crushing and grinding spices between two stones for two solid hours. A huge curry was being prepared as well as sweetmeats. The table that evening was loaded with food and confusion reigned and at 6.30p.m. I was ready for bed. People started to arrive and, of course, there were several whom I had not met but no one seemed to bother about introductions. It was unrehearsed pandemonium. The rooms filled up quickly and the heat became more intense and the noise would have shot the decibel scale very high if there had been a meter. At one point I found myself in a room with women only, apparently the usual practice. Only about three out of the thirty odd present spoke any English but they all seemed to get the gist of the conversation because when I asked if any of them would care to come to my bedroom or use the loo there was a swish of saris and a stampede. They seemed to be interested in my bottles of various lotions, which I had accumulated. They consisted of Jeyes Fluid, Dettol; insect repellent to things like, Johnson's Baby Lotion and Madame Rochas perfume and other toiletries.

The gathered throng was called to order for a presentation ceremony. A photographer was flashing his camera and I saw out of the corner of my eye a large brass ornament, which was obviously going to be presented to us. My heart sank, as I could see I was going to have to accept it graciously, but how could we pack it and how much would it weigh? I thanked them and said that it was just what I wanted. We were in our beds by midnight and I felt very happy knowing that in the morning, quite early, I would be in an air-conditioned car on the way to New Delhi.

Having sorted out our belongings, we passed quite a lot of things to Mr and Mrs Mastih. They were delighted, like children after Santa Claus had visited. We had to explain what some of the items were to be used for and we had a good laugh together. There were tubes of embrocation and we warned Mastih that he should wash his hands well after using the stuff as if he went to deal with any other part of his anatomy it might be unpleasant for him. The next thing I knew was parrots screeching and prayers being chanted through the loud hailers on the top of the nearby mosque; a feature of the area to which we had almost become accustomed. It was now early morning. Our old caretaker and his wife were up and about but they looked quite sad as they prepared breakfast. We had grown very fond of them and they seemed to regard us with respect and affection. With sad farewells we drove away, probably never to see them again. It was a very touching few minutes, as we knew that they would not be appreciated by their own folk in the way they deserved. Two people we shall always remember very kindly.

Our drive to Delhi was very pleasant, thanks largely to the air-conditioning in the car and the fact that we had started very early in the morning. Even so, the roads were busy with the usual buffalo, camel and many other forms of transport. The large brass pot, which had been presented to us on the previous evening, was on the seat beside me and I kept wondering in which bag we would have to pack it. Arriving in New Delhi was becoming a familiar experience by now. We had come and gone so many times but this time was something special as it was to be our last. Back in Claridges Hotel we made straight for the bathroom. No words can express the luxury of clean hot water, a new tablet of toilet soap and a large clean towel. We were to stay here for our last three days in India and so we did our final shopping and visited the Red Fort and other tourist attractions, all of which were swarming with people. We had to fight off the usual mass of vendors of cheapjack trinkets and souvenirs. I saw a few Europeans about and they seemed to be buying peacock feathers, some of which had been made into fans. I didn't feel like flapping these dusty things into my face. The tourists clutched them in their sweaty hands as though they were carrying the Crown Jewels. We were invited by Alan Jackson of the British Council and his wife to have dinner with them in their home after which we would be driven directly to the airport for our flight home. The day before, I started having pains in my inside and was confined to our room. This really was bad luck as I had managed to stave off the enteritis bug but it got me in the end. Thank goodness we had our own bathroom and loo! Our last night in India was very disturbed and it was a very hot night. As I made my frequent journeys across the bedroom at night I glanced through the window and the trees never showed a flutter, the air was completely still. I began to worry, would I be able to get onto the plane, then out of our magic medicine box which we had carried about with us, I found and took a dose of something guaranteed to stop this distressing condition. I got back into my bed and slept the rest of the night.

Well this is the day, I played it very carefully; I had no choice really because I just hadn't any strength left. I stayed on my bed until the evening when we had to go out to dinner. A car came for us and it was wonderful to be in a home where the decor and customs were familiar to us. The food looked so tempting I had a little but lack of air and the heat got me again. I felt I was on the way to leaving this world and I must have fainted because I found myself on our hostess's bed in an air-conditioned room. I was given glucose. It was about half an hour before I felt able to take any interest. I heard someone say, "She can't possibly fly tonight," there was no way they could have prevented me going. It's amazing how one can force oneself to cope. The very thought of being so close to getting on a plane and flying away from the heat, the poverty and from the poor state of hygiene was the only thing in my mind. The urge to get away became stronger and stronger when we were being pushed by human masses through Delhi Airport. The crowd was so massive in the concourse that we couldn't even see which were the checkout desks. There was only one thought in my mind and that was to get through this human bedlam and onto the aircraft. An Asian porter suddenly appeared at our side, grabbed our bags and presumably took them to be weighed and checked. He disappeared instantly and I don't know how, but we found

319

ourselves being checked-in by a big fat, Sikh gentleman in uniform and as we thanked him in his own language he smiled and shook us both by the hand. Then the porter turned up and asked for a very large tip. I suppose we had to thank him for getting us through the melee to the checkout and no doubt we overpaid him.

I still don't know how we finally boarded the plane, but we did and it was nine tenths filled with Indians, mostly with large families. It was a long haul back to London and I salute the cabin crew who did their best to feed us and attend to our needs. By the time we got to Heathrow we were sitting in the dirtiest aircraft that we have ever been in. The floor was covered with food, some of which had been trodden into the carpets. Paper napkins, earphones, string, clothing, paper cups and bags of sweetmeats were scattered everywhere. It was almost impossible to get to or into the loos as unruly Asian children, who took all the toiletries and paper from the loos and blocked up the drains with toilet rolls and paper towels, continuously occupied these. The parents didn't seem to think anything was wrong in this activity and exercised no discipline whatever. The cabin staff told us that this was the norm on this particular service and they could do nothing about it. They all hated being on duty on this run from India. As we left the aircraft we could see Asian children carrying little bags of soap which they had pinched from the loos. If ever I hear anyone grumbling about British airports I shall feel like telling them to go to India and then see if their ideas change.

This brings me to the end of Kathy's notebook on her impressions of our trip to India. When I read it I realised quite a lot about our Indian experience. I was working and so I was meeting people who were in my profession and I was busy assessing the difficulties that faced them in their efforts to overcome the obstacles to their progress. I was, therefore, fully engaged in learning the difficulties and in trying to devise means of overcoming them. Kathy was in a very different position, more or less tied to the quarters in which we were housed and dependent on servants and casual visitors for any conversation. Of course, out of working hours we went about together and I was made fully aware of all the things she observed. I think the nadir of our time in India was most certainly the train journey on the so-called 'Bareilly Express'. My sister, Win and her husband Laurie, lived in India for more than twenty years and that was in the days before partition, when members of the Indian Civil Service were, perhaps a little pampered. They travelled and lived in a manner suited to their position in the Raj. When we were in New Delhi we saw a reflection of this way of life in the High Commission and other European officials. Perhaps much of the splendour had gone, but I think that European representatives of the Western Countries still lived somewhat apart from the ordinary teeming millions. My brother-in-law might have had some experience of the poorer areas but I don't think my sister could have envisaged what we experienced on the Bareilly Express.

CHAPTER 11

A Brief Stay in Somerset

Peter and Helen, when they knew the date of our return from India, came down to Bramleys for a few days in order to see that all was well with our house and to get the beds aired and have some food ready. It was a kind thought on their part and in exploring the larder they went to open the deep freeze cabinet, which was in the garage. They landed themselves with a dirty job as, when they opened the freezer, they were appalled by the stench. Apparently, there had been a big thunderstorm soon after we left for India and the switch of the freezer had tripped and, of course, the power had been off for most of the time we were away. We had arranged for a lady who cleaned for us to check the house weekly but none of us had thought of including the freezer in the checking programme. The entire contents from plums and apples to fish and meat had been converted to a stinking black fluid mess. Peter and Helen very bravely tackled the job of dispensing with it and it must have been an awful job. We were most grateful to them. They dug a deep hole in the orchard and laboriously emptied the cabinet using plastic buckets and disposing of the stinking fluid in the hole, subsequently filling it in. We were fortunate to come back to a clean, if empty, deep freezer.

We soon settled back into our Somerset home and started getting it into the sort of shape and condition that we wanted. We registered ourselves in the Glastonbury Health Centre and with a dentist, John Cooper, also in Glastonbury. I became a member of an art club associated with a business in the High Street called the 'Glastonbury Experience'. There were some very competent artists in the club, one of whom, Les Jeffries, became a good friend and fellow artist. During our time in Somerset, I held a one-man show of paintings that was more successful than I had expected. Les and his wife, Dorothy were employees of the well-known footwear manufacturers, Clarks of Street, a town near to Glastonbury where we did most of our routine shopping.

Our village, Barton St David, was a rather scattered farming area and our house was on the edge of the village. Our next-door neighbours on both sides were farmers. The farmhouse of one was very near to our property. In fact, our house had been constructed from two farm workers' cottages and our garden had formerly been part of a field. The farmer was, in my opinion, a poor farmer who did little more farming than buying in young stock and trying to make a profit by grazing them and selling them later. He was too parsimonious to pipe water into his fields and so had the job of moving them daily to a trough where they could water. This movement, of course, reduced the grazing time of the beasts and also detracted from the object of the business, which was to put meat on them. The buildings were allowed to deteriorate, as were fences, gates and hedges. The farmer and his sons were not very pleasant. The nicest member of the family was his wife but we saw very little of her. The farmer's real interest lay in keeping a few, far from new coaches, with which he made a living, using them mostly as school buses.

Two real characters owned the farm on the other side, the cider apple orchard of which was contiguous with our garden and orchard. They were brothers of dyed-in-the-wool Somerset stock. We didn't see anything of them at first as they were described as somewhat reclusive. We eventually ventured onto their farm and asked if we could buy eggs from them. Amazingly, they welcomed us and asked us in and plied us with eggs and from that day until many years after we had moved to Dorset, we bought our eggs from them almost exclusively. We became very close friends and we could walk into their house at any time. The door was always open for us and a huge teapot, filled to the brim was there to be dispensed for us. Charlie and Bill Hart had never married and had lived in the large, three-storey house, Lower Farm, since their father had built it when they were small boys. They were a few years older than we were, Charlie being the elder. He was about 5ft 2ins tall with a bent back and powerful strong arms. He really was the boss and drove the tractor but couldn't drive the car. That was Bill's job. He was a little taller than Charlie but that was possibly because he wasn't bent. Soon after we got to know the two brothers they sold all their stock and implements, keeping only the chickens, which were really Bill's hobby.

The keep of the fields was sold off on the farm by a local auctioneer and was the main source of their income. The day of the auction was something of an annual get together. All the local graziers came and there was food aplenty and the whisky bottles were opened to be emptied. We were always interested in the way the knock down prices for the keep on the fields varied from year to year. Money didn't seem to be much of a consideration to Charlie and Bill. They lived a frugal sort of life starting each day with a breakfast of rice pudding with a couple of raw eggs stirred into it. Long after we left Barton and came to live in Leigh in Dorset, eighteen miles to the south, we made the journey to Low Farm, Barton, ostensibly to buy eggs but really to have a bit of crack and a good laugh with 'the boys'. If Bill was away with the chickens when we arrived Charlie would go to the door and roar out at the top of his voice, "Bill! Bill! The children are here!" A handful of tea would be put in the pot and the pot was filled to the brim with boiling water. The cupboard was always stocked with every kind of biscuit. If Bill saw a type of biscuit in a shop that he hadn't seen before, he would buy it and it was added to the stock in the cupboard.

It would take a large book to tell the full story of these two loveable and delightful characters. I wish I could have the time and energy to write the story of Charlie and Bill with their quaint customs and anecdotes and their use of Somerset words and sayings. Sadly they are now gone but their memory will stay with Kathy and me until we follow them. I cannot leave this subject without telling how Charlie's great passion was auctions. The two brothers would travel miles to an auction, Bill driving the old car with its home made trailer behind and then he would sit in the car while Charlie went to bid. He was well known to all the auctioneers for miles around. He wouldn't bid until the boxes of rubbish, which couldn't attract a bid, were put up and then the auctioneer would turn to Charlie and say, "What about you, Mr X?"

"I'll give you a couple of bob."

"Come on, Charlie, that's a poor bid."

"And that's a poor lot of rubbish."

"Knocked down to, Mr Hart." And then he would proceed to the next lot. Meanwhile, Bill would be sitting in the car reading the paper, but if the sale was in or adjacent to a garden he would wander round it snipping off the odd cutting that might take his fancy. His great delight was his garden around the house at Low Farm. The house itself was a veritable museum of all sorts of items, some of them of little but others of great interest and possibly of value. Every space, from the living room to the spaces under the eaves, was crammed with books, pictures, bric-a-brac, sheets, bedspreads, towels and other textiles which had come from auctions in Somerset and Dorset. These had been sorted by Charlie and had been washed and cleaned if their condition so required. In the dining room were innumerable cases and shelves full of books, ivories, porcelain and antiques that could have supplied the material for several years of antique road shows. In the middle of the dining room was a full sized snooker table with a polished mahogany cover over the baize playing area which itself was completely obscured by piles of antiques of many kinds. Indeed, in the years over which we visited Lower Farm, we never saw the mahogany tabletop, let alone the baize and snooker pockets. Every wall in the house was hung lavishly with paintings, photographs and other wall adornments, some of little merit but some of undoubted value. Built-in cupboards were crammed with books, magazines and, in addition to biscuits, preserves of various kinds, mostly made by Bill from the fruits of the orchard and gardens.

The workshop next to the now unused dairy was literally filled with tools, anvils old furniture, carefully dismantled by Charlie and carefully stored in their component parts. For example, there were veritable fascicles of rail back chair spindles, chair seats, bed ends and literally dozens of tins, boxes, buckets and barrels of screws and nails of all kinds, sorted by Charlie according to size and type. If I was short of nails or screws, Charlie would just squeeze into the workshop and give me generous handfuls wrapped up in an old cloth or put into a suitable tin or box. I once wanted a couple of large 'G' clamps for my frame making. I had searched for the type I wanted in various hardware shops and found them to be very expensive. Kathy suggested that we should see if Charlie had any of the right kind. Accordingly we went down the lane to the farm and I explained what I wanted. "Oh I've got plenty of they," said Charlie and led the way to an old barn across the yard. There, clamped to the wooden streamer of an ancient hay cart were more than thirty clamps of all shapes and sizes. "Which ones do you want?" enquired Charlie. I chose two, which were suitable, and asked Charlie how much he wanted for them. "You just borrow them," he said.

"Don't be silly, Charlie," I said.

"I don't want to sell them," he answered. I pointed out that he wouldn't be able to use all of them if he lived to be a hundred and ten. I eventually persuaded him to sell me the two that I had chosen and so he said, "Would fifty pence hurt?" Anyway, I acquired the clamps and I have used them ever since for all sorts of jobs.

On one occasion a lady from the village came down to Low Farm to see if Charlie could supply a small white blanket for her grand daughter's cot. The lady and her daughter arrived with the baby in a pram. There was a little consternation, as it became very obvious that a nappy change was required. The young mother blushed when her mother asked Charlie if he had something that could be used to put the matter right. "Oh, you want a clean nappy?" Charlie asked, "I've got plenty of they." And he darted off upstairs, returning with a handful of spotless white Turkish towelling nappies. He said that he'd picked them up in a job lot at an auction and he insisted that the young mother should 'taken on' which was Charlie's way of saying have them as a gift.

Barton St David has a rather fine church, which is almost unique, in that its tower is an octagonal structure. When we lived in the village it also had a unique vicar. He was a rather reclusive man who lived in a large vicarage, which was almost completely hidden from view by an overgrowth of trees and weed. He was responsible for three parishes and having no car he walked from one to another to conduct the Sunday services. In our church he took the services, read the lessons and played the organ. There was not a lot of enthusiasm among the congregation, varying in number from about three or four to about fourteen on a good day. Having pronounced the blessing at the end of the service, he was usually the first off the premises, armed with his umbrella and raincoat striding out to his service in the next parish. From time to time he would walk round the village distributing notices. The first time we saw him on this perambulation we were in the garden and asked him in for a sherry. He accepted the invitation with alacrity and apparently enjoyed his stay in our sitting room and the sherry we provided. We became a regular stop on his notice distribution days.

One day when he called on Charlie and Bill, which he did very often although neither of them attended services, he sat down and accepted a whisky. Bill, not being a drinker himself, had little idea of the volume of a normal tot and erred on the lavish side. The good vicar was tired and in need of a rest and so accepted a second and then a third. When he decided that it was time for his departure he rose to his feet rather unsteadily and promptly fell back into his chair. "You'm all right, Vicar?" enquired Charlie. The vicar replied rather indistinctly that he was but it became obvious that he wasn't all right and so Charlie and Bill had to stagger him out to the car and with Charlie supporting him in the back seat, Bill drove the rather somnolent vicar back to the vicarage. They rang him later to ensure that he was reasonably *compos mentis*.

Bramleys was a pleasant house and we did quite a lot to make ourselves comfortable in it. The upstairs windows provided us with good views. We could see the Mendip mast and from the north bedroom we could see Wells Cathedral. There were three bedrooms and a bathroom upstairs, kitchen with loo near the back door, very useful when working in the garden, dining room and sitting room from which an open stairway ascended to the upper floor. On the west side a conservatory ran the full length of the building. In the garden we had several Bramley apple trees, two very prolific fruiting walnut trees and a black plum that was weighed down with fruit at harvest time.

A snag about our garden was that it had been made from a farm field and was infested with harvest mites to which Kathy was very susceptible. It was, however, our neighbour with his old buses and the fact that we were somewhat isolated that made us decide to look for a new place in which to live. We started looking around, once more hitting the house-hunting trail.

House-hunting is a tedious and tiring occupation but as we were looking for a place in the West Country it was easier than when we had to travel from Scotland. We tended to concentrate on the area from south Somerset to the northern part of Dorset. We had a little knowledge of this region and so could discriminate when studying the adverts in the local press. Much of the property available we could discount and restrict our search to areas, which we found promising. Nancy, Kathy's elder sister, came to spend some time with us and so she enjoyed being driven around on our property searches. At 4 p.m. on a fine day we were attracted to a house in Stoke Sub Hamdon. A village in south Somerset. The house stood at the top of a steeply sloping drive and commanded a beautiful view over south Somerset with vistas over a full semi-circle of countryside. We looked round the property, which had been, until recently, a mess for three senior officers in the Fleet Air Arm. It had been redecorated and was almost like a newly built house. We fell for it and so we drove as fast as we could to catch the agents in Yeovil before they closed their office for the day. I wasn't very familiar with Yeovil at that time and had difficulty in finding a car park and then in finding the appropriate office. However, we made it just as the staff of the estate agents was about to leave and the boss returned to his desk and we sat down to talk. The asking price was, in our terms at that time, somewhat higher than we felt like offering. I did some rapid mental arithmetic and finding that the property had been on the market for some months I made an offer that was £3,000 lower than the price asked. The agent adopted a rather unencouraging expression and said he would get in touch with the vendor who was a titled lady whose name I have now forgotten. We left our telephone number and made for home. The following morning, the telephone rang and the agent came on the line to say that his client had accepted our figure and we could go ahead with the negotiations.

I immediately rang our good friend and estate agent, Dick Rhind and asked him to put Bramleys on the market. He sprang into action immediately and within twenty-four hours our house was advertised in the local press and in some other more prestigious journals. The next day while I was out, the telephone rang again and it was the agent from Yeovil who explained to Kathy that we could not have the house. He apologised earnestly and said that his agency was not the main one for the property, but that the prior agent was Jackson Stopps and Staff and they had already accepted an offer on the same day as mine had been made and that the offer had been for the full asking price and, furthermore, the offer had been made by someone who was selling his present house by auction a month or so ahead so that the purchase price would be available on that date. This was a sad blow and we had to start afresh our search for a new home and had to withdraw Bramleys from the market.

Some four or five months later, and curiously, Nancy was visiting us again and so was accompanying us on our perambulations, when we went to look at a house in a village in West Dorset named Leigh (which we were informed is pronounced 'Lie'). The house was called 'Brookside Cottage'. When we found it, we were put off by the fact that it was directly on the side of the village street and the window frames were painted light blue. "We are not going to buy that," said Kathy emphatically.

"We must go to have a look inside." I said. "We have an appointment to view."

Kathy agreed grudgingly and turning to Nancy she said, as I parked the car near a farm gate opposite, "Don't bother to get out, Nancy, we'll be back in a few minutes."

We were admitted by a lady who proved to be a neighbour from next door, called Sally Dearling. She took us through the house to the garden behind where the owner, Mrs Dorrie Brownsell and her elderly mother were having tea with some friends. Mrs Brownsell was crippled by advanced osteoporosis and Sally seemed to do a lot to help her. I think it was Sally who started to show us round the house and we were agreeably impressed by many of its features. It appeared that it had been the village store until it was purchased by Mr and Mrs Brownsell some six years previously and converted into quite a pleasant and spacious dwelling house. Mr Brownsell had died soon after they had moved in. Sally told us that the house had been on the market for some months and there had not been a lot of interest shown in it. Mrs Brownsell was unable to climb the stairs and desperately wanted to buy a bungalow nearby. We could see that our large carpets would fit into the rooms and we were so impressed that I was sent out to the car to bring Nancy in to see it. Amazing to relate, we made a tentative offer for the property, which was promptly accepted. We went to the local pub, The Carpenter's Arms, for sandwiches and a drink and had a chat about the village with some of the regulars of whom the apparently most regular was a man called Goldsack.

The upshot was that we bought the house and changed its name to 'Lamu'. Before we exchanged contracts we received particulars of the house in Stoke Sub Hamden for which we had offered. These came from the agents who had stepped in to prevent our clinching the deal. The price was £5,000 less than the original asking price, £2,000 less than we had offered. Presumably the person who was going to be able to buy the house on a certain defined date had let them down. Had they accepted our offer they would have sold the house for £2,000 more than they were now asking and several months earlier. I wouldn't let Mrs Brownsell down at this stage but I felt some satisfaction in telling these agents that they had had their chance and so we took possession of a house which was entirely different from the one we had determined to find.

Bramleys was sold to a couple, Eric and Margaret Hayward. Margaret was the Head Teacher of a big comprehensive school in Bridgewater and Eric had been something fairly high up in airways, but had taken to life as an entrepreneur and was avoiding as well as possible, his first wife who was doing her best to squeeze more money out of him over and above the original divorce settlement sum. She had a nasty habit of having writs served on Eric which caused him much hassle as these demanded his presence at courts in odd and far away places at awkward times and so, naturally, Eric did his best to keep his whereabouts secret from prying eyes. We liked this

330

friendly couple and our property, Bramleys, suited them very well as Eric was keen on sailing and had a large sailing boat for which our outbuilding made an excellent boathouse. Margaret invited me to be the guest of honour at her school speech day and to present the prizes. I remember that in my speech I stressed the importance of reading and I was presented with a nice turned piece of wood that had been made in the school woodwork room. The Haywards have moved on and now live on the coast but we still exchange Christmas cards.

As I write these memoirs in our house, Lamu, we have lived here for twenty-two years, longer than either of us had spent in any other house including those in which we spent our youthful days. It is a funny old place but we have added to it and made alterations so that it has served as a comfortable family home.

CHAPTER 12

Life in the Village of Leigh

In my professional career, many of my colleagues who reached retiring age, have found it difficult to step down and leave the ambience of their duties. I can understand their feelings and I experienced the same reluctance to let go of the reins and relinquish such influence and authority as had been accorded to me in the exercise of my profession. I determined that I would not try to continue to contribute to work that would be carried forward by my younger colleagues. I decided to make the cut final after I had completed the Indian assignment. Our research was in very good hands and I knew that it would be carried forward by Duncan Brown who was in my team and took over my post and in later years expanded and developed its objectives and successes with excellent results. And so the break was made.

I had many interests and, indeed, I was rather a 'Jack of all trades', with the well known remainder of that quotation. I had hoped to be able to spend much more time painting and I made a start when we were living in Barton St David, by joining the art group associated with the 'Glastonbury Experience'. I soon discovered that retirement was not the relaxed period of rest and enjoyment that is anticipated by most workers when they approach the end of their working life. As I now look back over the period of twenty-three years that have elapsed since I left my last professional post in Edinburgh, I realise that I have virtually had a second career filled with interest and human contacts and many aspects of life resulting from settling in a Dorset village. There is no doubt in my mind that we made the right choice when we made this delightful county our home. Of course, a number of the people around us who have become our good friends are also 'incomers' from other parts of the British Isles but we have, I venture to suggest, made a lot of friends among the real Dorset people. Indeed, I feel that we have been accepted into the community. I have been very active in the church, St Andrew's, Leigh, in spite of my having abandoned my quest for faith and acceptance that I am atheistic. I have made this quite clear to members of the church who know that Kathy and I try to base our lives on the Christian ethic. I attend evensong and matins and am a member but I ceased to take Holy Communion many years ago. I have helped in fundraising and when I was a member of the Parochial Church Council, I suggested and organised a sponsored cycle ride that raised over £400 for the fabric fund. Some time after this, the Dorset Historic Churches Fund initiated an annual sponsored cycle ride for the benefit of all Christian churches in the county and I serve as the parish organiser for St Andrew's Leigh.

When we lived in Barton St David, we signed up for our central heating oil with a supplier called Kellands. They had a grandiose scheme whereby they would keep us supplied with oil without our having to watch our tank level and order when we were getting low. In addition they would attend to the servicing of our boiler and replace, as necessary, any worn parts. It was not quite as simple as all that but we paid up promptly and without question. When we moved to Leigh, some twenty odd miles away across the Somerset/Dorset border, Kellands were only too pleased to continue supplying us with oil. A local friend one day happened to ask me what we paid for our oil and when I told him he was astonished and pointed out that any one of the local suppliers would provide us with oil at a much cheaper rate. He mentioned one supplier whose price he knew and it appeared that I was paying at least £50 more for a six hundred gallon tank full than was necessary. In my sublime ignorance I had assumed that the price of oil would be reasonably standard irrespective of which company was the supplier. I hadn't realised that to acquire a new customer the method seemed to be adopted by the tanker companies of offering a lower price for the first order and then, sufficiently lured into acceptance the customer would not bother to check on current prices for his or her next fill up but would happily carry on ordering from the same supplier. This led to a few of us ringing around to find the cheapest source of oil. Monica Jackson and I started to cast around to see if we could find a supplier who would supply us at discount rates if we would group together and order so that the tanker could supply several of us on one visit. Monica and I rang several oil companies in an area within a radius of about twenty miles from Leigh enquiring if they would be prepared to supply at a cheaper rate if we organised this sort of bulk buying. None of them would countenance such a deal and some of them were almost rude in turning down the idea.

We therefore cast our net wider and I found a young supplier in Bridgewater who had recently set up in business and was keen to accept custom in our area. I took on the duty of organising the purchases. When we started we comprised four tanks. After a few years, the business had increased to thirty tanks on my list. The owner, Craig Lamont, called his company Western Counties Fuels but later, when he had expanded to three tankers he moved his office and changed the name to "Western Fuels". It was an onerous job for me, with no remuneration, and at times it caused me quite a lot of hassle as people would not follow my suggestion that they should let me know when their tank level fell below half so that I could organise supplies to make the tanker journeys worth while. If someone was desperate I would rush or telephone around to see if any more members of the group could take a top-up. Craig was very straight in his dealing and would even send a tanker over if only one member required oil and they still got the supply at the discounted price. The driver making the delivery would call on us and check the tanks needing oil and after a cup of tea would make his way round the village. I have a feeling that some of our members took it for granted that I was a paid agent. This was certainly not the case. With all my telephone calls and driving or walking round the village, I think that the oil cost me more than it cost the other members of the group. At one time Craig said that he would knock £5 off my bill but after a few such recompenses this activity slid into disuse. I didn't mind as he was struggling in a very competitive market in which the big suppliers could command lower prices at the port. I did receive a bottle of sherry and a diary at Christmas and a supply of calendars that, of course, I had to distribute. In 2000, I 'retired' and it was agreed that all members of my group would get the bulk price provided they gave Craig a week's notice of order. I was involved in many things and had two cataract operations that prevented me from driving, Kathy's health was deteriorating and my time was limited. I had done the job for about thirteen years.

In 1995 the architects employed by the Church Commissioners declared the bell frame in our church tower to be unsafe and the ringing of the bells had to stop. There followed a lot of discussion on the subject of the new frame as to whether the new one should be of oak like the existing structure or to be of steel that would last for a very long time. A steel frame would be much more expensive and, of course, money was a matter of great importance in a country village the size of Leigh. A new oak frame would cost about £17,000, a steel one would be in the region of £20,000. Most of us felt that £17,000 would be miles out of our reach but the argument for the steel frame won and the project of fund raising was the big problem. The figure was obviously beyond our reach but the effort was launched. Alan Woodward, a semi-retired accountant, was chosen to lead the appeal. He did an unbelievable job, chasing up all the current inhabitants and seeking out many more who had resided in the village in past years, some as far away as Australia. Local projects of all kinds were set up and amazingly the required sum was raised in six months. One of the projects was the mounting of an art exhibition which, I think, was suggested by me and it was strongly supported by Alan who joined me to organise the project. It was quite successful and raised a small but significant sum of money.

I took a great deal of interest in the activities involved in the replacement of the old frame with the new one and the restoration of the retuned bells in their new steel frame. I spent much of my spare time in the tower and helping with the work of removing the old frame and the lowering of the bells to ground level and their transport to the factory of Nicholsons Engineers of Bridport. Much of the work was done by members of the church and village community under the guidance of Percy Read, the Bell-Captain, ably assisted by Dennis Fudge. There was a lot of work associated with the removal of the four hundred year old oak frame and the measuring up for the fashioning of the new steel frame. I did my best to get a photographic record of the whole process and also helped with the winching up and down of all the items which were involved. I found it most fascinating and instructive and marvelled at the way our local people mastered the problems that arose at every stage. The largest of our six bells is the tenor, weighing more than ten hundred weight having first been installed in 1681. It was recast in 1888. The smallest and latest addition to our ring was hung in 1897 and carries an inscription, which reads, 'Added to the Peal by subscription as a Memorial of Queen Victoria's Diamond Jubilee Reign'. When the bells had been retuned and the new frame was ready, a party of us who had been closely involved in the work went to the factory to see the new frame, assembled with the bells in the big workshop. It was a most interesting and memorable occasion.

The bells were installed in time to be rung at Christmas 1996, nine months after the beginning of Alan Woodward's campaign to raise the funds. This was really a remarkable achievement. Apart from this episode in our life in Leigh, I had become very familiar with the church bell tower. For several years I had been responsible for the raising of the appropriate flag on the mast at the top of the tower for the various occasions. This had to be done irrespective of the weather and many was the time when I had to reach over the castellations when stormy winds blew the end of the flag rope far over the church yard which seemed very far below. Now the old worn steps of the spiral stairs inside the bell-tower have been replaced by more level steps. In 1993, Elizabeth Linehan, Secretary of the Parochial Church Council, very diffidently on the instructions of the council, came to tell me that I should not perform my flag raising duties any more as I had attained the great age of eighty and anything could happen to me, I might have been found dead or disabled at the foot of the tower.

Leigh is a very pleasant Dorset village with a large number of kindly people who are very helpful and ready to make life pleasant for their friends and neighbours. Some of those born and bred here have most amusing anecdotes to relate. I wish I had the time to write some of them down and also to include stories and incidents resulting from the activities of some of the incomers who have happily found Leigh as a place for their declining years. We have in our village bounds, an ancient maze and we also have a unique wild tulip which grows in a spot which is kept as a secret by those who know, as in the past people have pulled up the bulbs to take away and only a few remain. We have a most flourishing bakery that has established itself so successfully that Fudges products are sent to many places in the country and even to Harrods the well-known London store. The village can boast several most competent artisans. We even have a gunsmith who shows a remarkable skill and ability in fashioning parts of such prestigious weapons as those bearing the name Purdey or Holland and Holland.

We are remarkable in this village in having, every year, a candle auction. This is an old custom that, I understand, used to be a common feature of many country areas. The use of a burning candle in making important sales goes back several centuries. Allusion to it is even to be found as early as the seventeenth century. Samuel Pepys refers to it in connection with the sale of ships. Reference to it in France is to be found in the literature which indicates that this method of selling by auction was widespread and covered deals in many and varied sales of merchandise. It is believed that the well known saying 'Not worth the candle' had its origin in the practice. In recent times this method has slipped into desuetude, the last uses having been in connection with the disbursement of charitable funds.

The candle auction in Leigh is the method of allocation of grazing rights or use of the aftermath, over two plots of land from the 1st of August to the 14th of February. The auction in Leigh is presided over by the Chairman of the Parish Charity Commissioners, who, ever since I first attended, has been Alan Hill. Every year, two parcels of land, Bere Mill Mead and Alton Mead, are presented for auction by the candle. Anyone wishing to obtain the use of these pieces of land for the approaching season must attend the candle auction. The chairman brings to the meeting two short pieces of candle and at the appropriate moment he calls the meeting to order and announces the auction

337

of the first parcel of land. He explains the details of the land and the period of time for which it will be available and then lights the first candle. At the start, there is silence until someone makes an opening bid. Silence falls again, occasionally broken by witty remarks or amusing repartee. As the candle burns down and begins to flicker, another bid will be made and then, depending on the state of the flame and the size and shape of the remaining wax, more bids follow and the observation by the assembled audience becomes more and more intense and the interested parties tend to lean forward in their seats. I have seen the flame at this stage, suddenly go out. At others, the flame flickers, reddens and may suddenly grow larger, possibly to resume its steady burn or without warning to become extinguished. This is the point at which the bidding and counterbidding become exciting and the interested parties watch with concentrated attention, each trying to judge the critical moment. The last bidder before final extinction then goes forward to write a cheque to a burst of applause. The second piece of land, Alton Mead, is then auctioned in the same way.

There is a group in the village, organised by Stanley Waterfall, with special interests in conservation and which had the bright idea of obtaining the use of Bere Mill Mead as a conservation area. I was a member of this group and we were successful in obtaining the aftermath control of the area. Enthusiastic members worked on the Mead, which had been rather neglected and had become a rough scrubby, sometimes flooded piece of woodland. Selective cutting out of scrub and brambles and the clearing of pleasant paths produced an attractive site for observation of birds and other wild life. Nest boxes were installed, one of these being aimed at attracting owls. Of course, we had to bid for the land at each annual candle auction. One year, I think it was our second, Stanley was away and I had to bid. I think that I bid shrewdly and won the auction for £15. Since then, the bidding has become more competitive and the cost higher so that now, in order to hold onto the land we have to arrange fund raising events in order to retain the group's control of the Bere Mill Mead as a conservation area.

Kathy's health had deteriorated sadly for several years and she had to be taken by ambulance, at night, to hospital in emergencies on four occasions. The first of these was a heart attack when she was admitted into the Coronary Care Unit in which she had a cardiac arrest followed by resuscitation, which left her with a broken rib. The other episodes comprised a dissecting aneurism of the aorta, an attack of what appeared to be a stroke and a double seizure. Each time I suffered agonies and waited for news of what seemed to be the inevitable end. Amazingly, she recovered each time thanks to her terrific resilience. We had to take great care over her diet and medication but later episodes caused deterioration in her condition. She was diagnosed as diabetic and I had to control this by careful attention to her diet and had to monitor her blood glucose level using a Soft Test apparatus. I felt awful about this as she so hated the prick that was necessary for the blood test. Over the last three years of her life, while she was reasonably mobile, I had to take Kathy at regular intervals to a haematology clinic in the Yeovil Hospital, where she had to undergo venesection for the removal of four hundred mls of blood. This became more unpleasant as it became progressively difficult to find a vein that would accommodate the comparatively large hypodermic needle. Poor Kathy became so weak and lost much of her mobility so that it was necessary for someone to be with her full time. I, of course, assumed this responsibility. Our doctor was John Tuke with whom we had established a very good relationship. He was a caring and very competent practitioner and a good friend. Furthermore, he was a resident, with his wife, Judy in our village. When he retired, his place in the group practice was taken by Charlie Middle. Again we were lucky. Charlie was also assiduous in looking after Kathy and he was a frequent visitor to Lamu. In spite of all our efforts, Kathy's condition continued to deteriorate and it was made clear to me by Charlie, our son Peter and all our friends that I should have to get some help with the constant caring and close attention for Kathy. We took advantage of the fact that there is, in our village, a very good residential care home, run by a friend, Annie Sinnot. I had two separate weeks of respite while Kathy was in the home, The Old Vicarage, very well cared for by Annie and her helpers, so that I was able to catch up a little on such matters as correspondence and housework.

This was manifestly, not enough and I set about trying to find some competent help in looking after Kathy and keeping the house habitable. I was, unexpectedly lucky in this quest. I found Dot Page who had been a nursing auxiliary for many years. She proved to be a gem and she got on so well with Kathy and all our friends and neighbours that I was given a well-needed breathing space. Things were easier for me and I was able to have three hours off on Tuesdays and Thursdays to play short mat bowls that I had taken up some three years before. Also I could manage to do the household shopping without having to rely on the kindness of friends to do it for me.

Sadly, four months after Dot started coming to help, Kathy died, on the 5th January 2002. I had promised her that as far as it was in my power she would not be sent to hospital again. She died in her own home, in her own bed with me there with her. I have been overwhelmed by the friendship and love that has been demonstrated by so many neighbours and friends from near and far. St Andrew's Church, Leigh, was packed for the funeral and cards and letters were received from between a hundred and hundred and twenty people who knew Kathy. She wouldn't have believed that she could attract so much kindly thought.

I decided to close my memoirs at this point although there were so many things that I had hoped to include about our current friends and village affairs. They will remain in my memory for as long as I can avoid the final lapse into senility of one form or another. I close with two items. The first is a contribution to our village magazine 'The Wriggle Valley Magazine' written by our good friend Stephen Neal upon the event of Kathy's death. The second is a transcript of a letter that was received from our Medical Group in Sherborne. Instead of flowers at the funeral, there was a retiring collection to be handed over to the Bute House Medical Equipment Fund as a mark of appreciation for the devoted manner in which the Medical Group treated Kathy in her great need.

A Yorkshire Lass

In late 1945, a young woman from Robin Hood's Bay who had never seen the world much beyond the Yorkshire borders, set sail from England to join her young husband whom she had married that September in Sheffield. The trip she embarked upon, unaccompanied, aboard a rather rusty and primitively equipped troopship, was to East Africa where Jack was a colonial veterinary officer. The young woman was our Kathy Wilde and the journey she was taking was to last over fifty-six years and destined to end at Leigh.

To say that Kathy's early experiences in Africa must have come as a culture shock would be an understatement in the extreme. However, her good staunch North Country upbringing and huge strength of character, allowed her to meet life there head on, undaunted and undimmed. She steadfastly supported Jack in his research career both in East and West Africa, organising and socialising with uncanny ease, sometimes in the most difficult circumstances, and meanwhile raising two fine sons.

Eventually, after twenty-five years Kathy returned to Britain with Jack and settled in Scotland where he had taken a lecturing post. On his retirement, they came south to Barton St David in Somerset before finally settling in Leigh some twenty-two years ago.

It was here that so many of us came to know, respect and love her. Although Kathy's formal education had been fairly elementary, no honours or degrees, her natural wisdom and talents shone through, for instance her self taught ability at the keyboard. She had an astonishing memory, especially for names and small details – although the punch line to that joke often evaded her – and sometimes we wished that it had. Her honesty and directness, her humour and wit, were always genuine, often refreshing, sometimes notorious. A spade was never anything but a spade.

Kathy was a remarkable individual, a 'one –off', and knowing her was a rare privilege and one to be savoured.

Doctors D.W.Townsend, I.A.Bartlett. R.A.Childs and C.E.Middle.

Dear Jack,

My partners and I at Bute House Surgery were delighted to receive the donation to our Equipment Fund in memory of Kathy.

The generosity of that donation was a reflection of the affection in which she was held by so many people.

As you know, I personally grew very fond of Kathy and it was always a pleasure to look after her. We all share in your loss and our thoughts continue to be with you at this difficult time.

Kind regards.

Yours sincerely,

Charlie.

Dr C.E.Middle.
26 February 2002

343

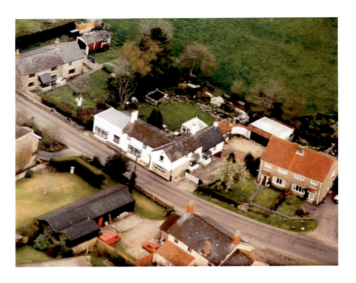

Lamu, our house, from the air.

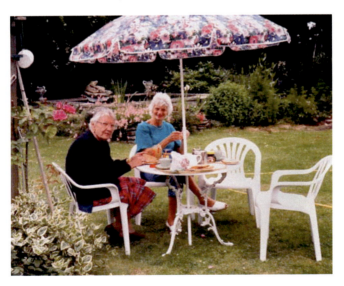

Kathy and Judith taking tea at Lamu.

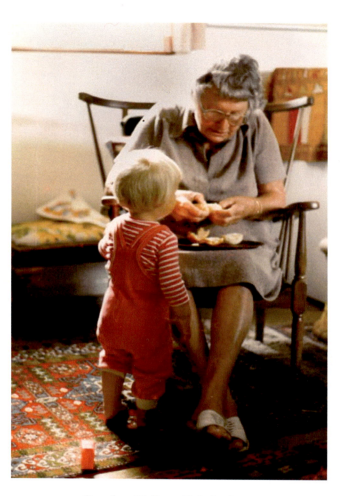

Grandma Kathy with baby Jane.

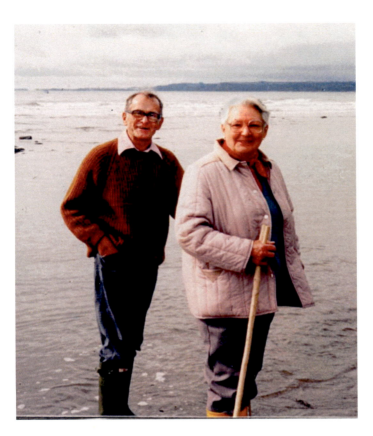

Jack and Kathy in Wales.